Art /
Fashion
in the
21st
Century

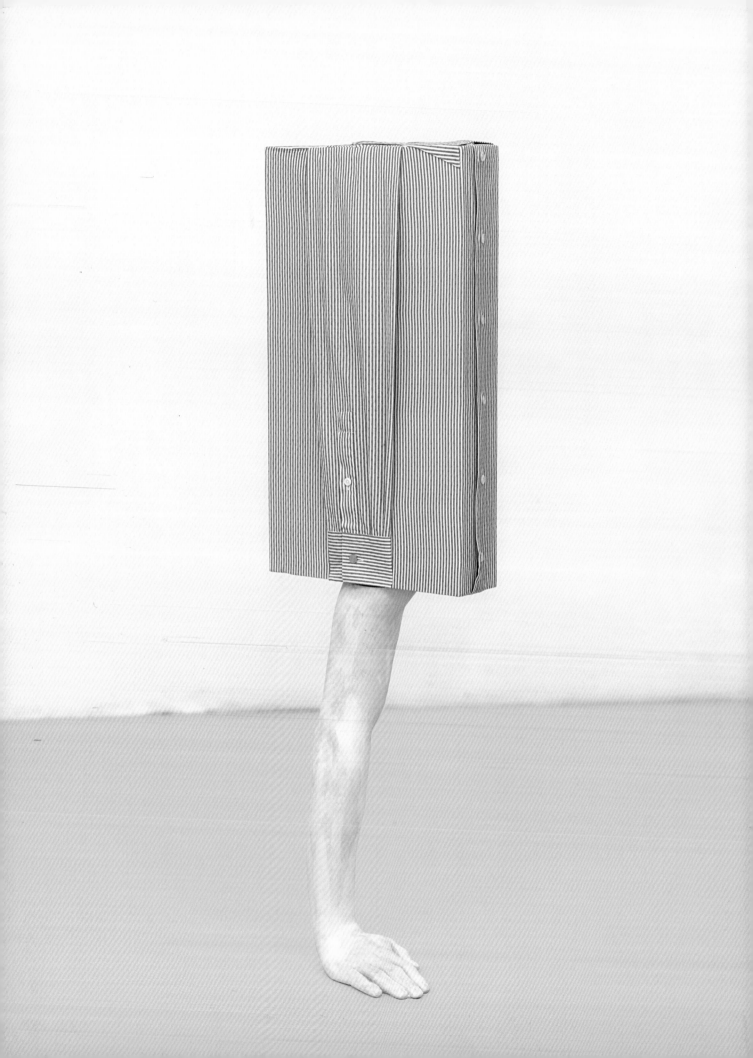

Art /
Fashion
in the
21st
Century

Mitchell Oakley Smith
Alison Kubler

With a foreword by
Daphne Guinness

238 color illustrations

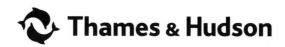

Thames & Hudson

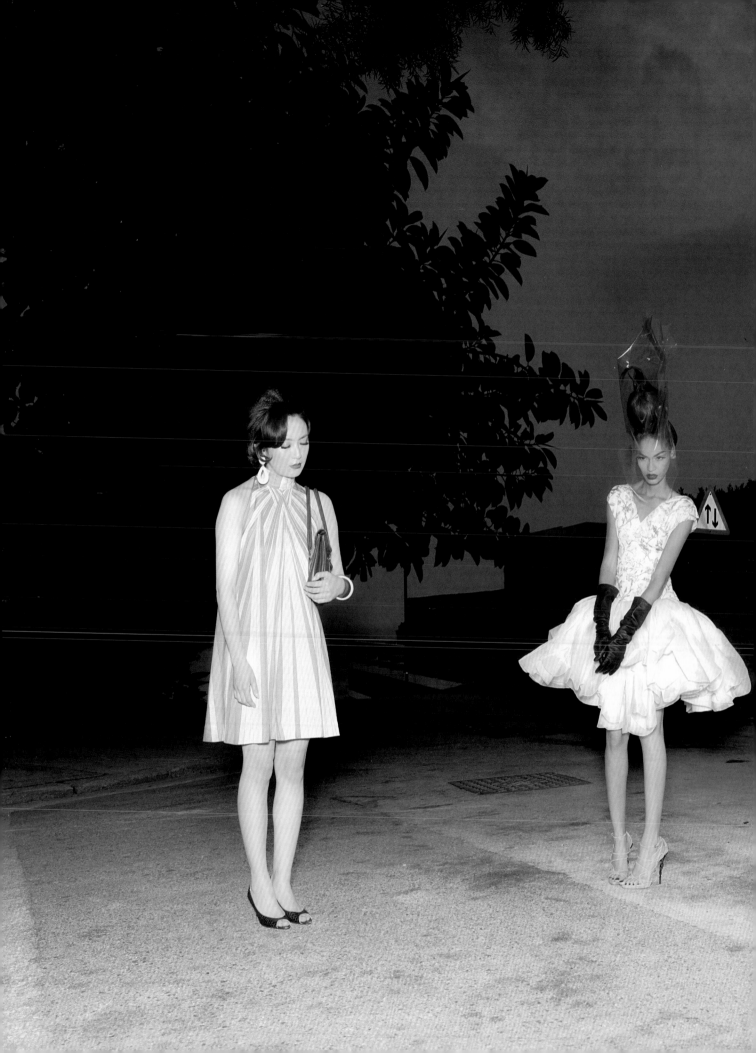

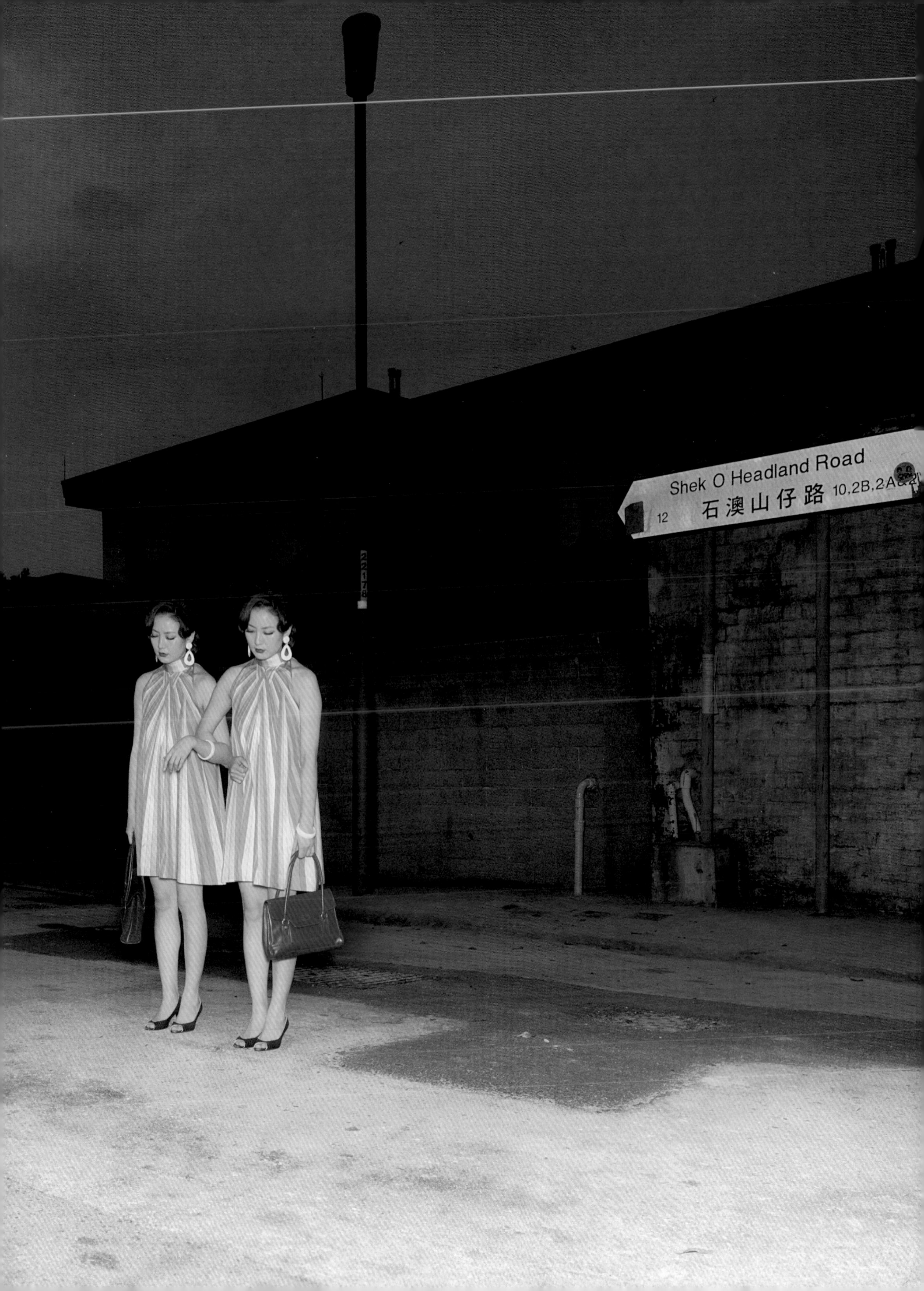
Shek O Headland Road
12
石澳山仔路
10,2B,2A

Contents

More than clothes: Fashion as art
24

Art meets fashion: Collaboration
94

Eye candy and ideas: Fashion as exhibition
152

Beyond the photoshoot:
New fashion media
202

From boutique to gallery:
Fashion, art and architecture
246

Page 2: Erwin Wurm, sculpture from his *Untitled* series
created for Hermès, 2008.

Pages 4–5: Quentin Shih, *No. 02*, from his *Hong Kong Moment*
photographic series created for Christian Dior, 2010.

Foreword:
Daphne Guinness

The links between art and fashion are more apparent now than they have ever been. To my mind, the best of our designers are indisputably artists; it just so happens that they have chosen fabric as their medium instead of paint or clay. Whether or not they regard themselves as 'artists' is another question entirely. The painter Francis Bacon said that 'Fashion is only the attempt to realize art in living forms and social intercourse.' For me, the process of dressing is to embrace a role, to explore an aspect of my own character, and the same could be said of the creation of a self-portrait. But there are designers who would argue that 'realizing art' has nothing to do with perfecting, say, the cut of a dress, and question why fashion should feel the need to validate itself as art.

The subject of art and fashion's dual identity has long divided designers. Karl Lagerfeld and Jean Paul Gaultier, for instance, are adamant they are categorically clothing designers and not artists. For them, the sole objective is to create wearable clothes. Elsa Schiaparelli's perspective differed entirely: her understanding of fashion was borne out of a philosophy that it should be treated as art. Alexander McQueen indisputably bound together the two spheres. His shows were not runways as we'd seen them before; they were spectacles: beautiful, yes – but also unnerving, provocative and haunting. Many now consider them performance art; indeed, my own experience was that to attend one of McQueen's shows was to re-examine the self, to somehow feel a part of what was playing out. Time and again McQueen challenged his audience to face themselves; literally so in the case of 'VOSS' (Spring/Summer 2001) where we were forced, uncomfortably, to look at our collective reflection in a square, mirrored box for nearly two hours prior to the show's opening (they were late starting, deliberately so). In the show's finale, this glass fell and shattered, and what it revealed – Michelle Olley reclining naked, be-masked and moth-ridden – left as profound an impact on me as anything I've viewed at the Tate Gallery.

Immanuel Kant declared that 'Fashion belongs under the title of vanity, because in its intention there is no inner value.' For Kant, the line between art and fashion was exact: there was no bridge between the sanctity of the former and the frivolity of the latter. As the years have passed, it has become acceptable, encouraged even, to attempt to rectify this. Increasingly museums are exhibiting clothing, elevating the status of the designer to that of an artist. Fashion is a form of self-expression that reflects the cultural zeitgeist. Art and fashion will continue to develop alongside each other, feed off each other, collaborate. Both reflect the tensions, sentiments and issues of the times. The question is not whether an item is created to be interpreted as art, but whether its designer is considered to be deserving of an artist's status. This book celebrates the work of those who, whether they like it or not, are revered as such.

Daphne Guinness

Opposite: Philip Treacy headpiece for
Alexander McQueen, Spring/Summer 2008.

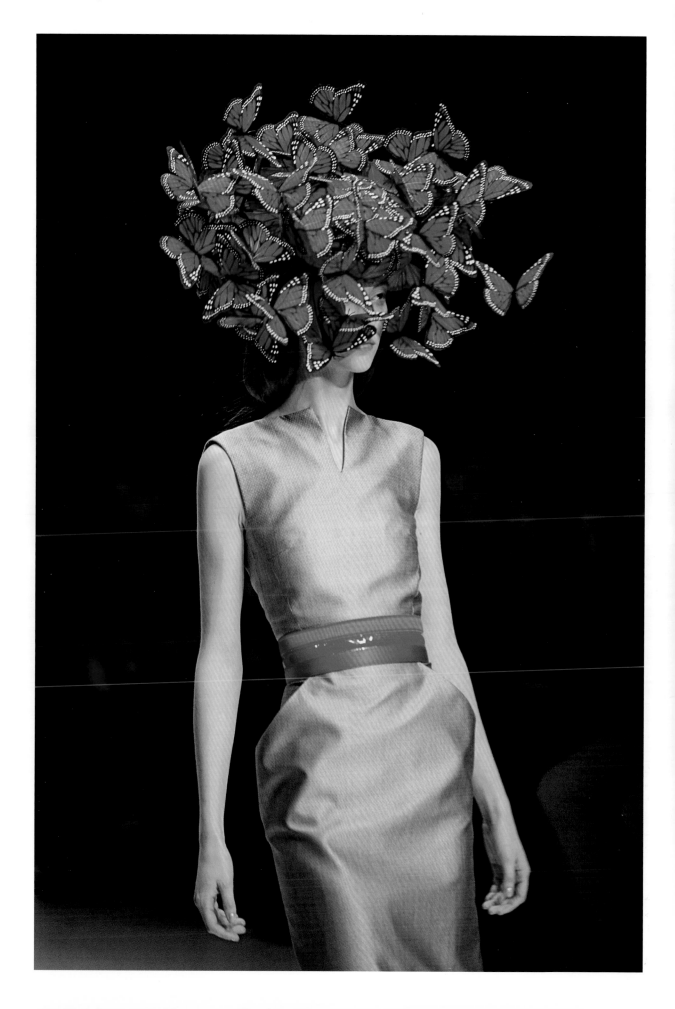

Introduction:
An artistic embrace

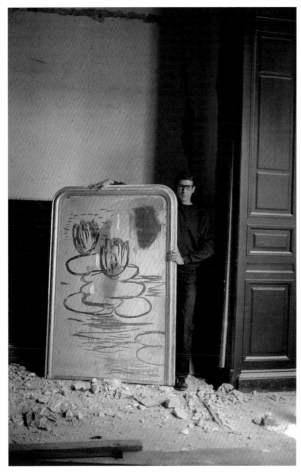

Yves Saint Laurent photographed by Lord Snowdon
(Antony Armstrong-Jones), 1980, part of a series reproduced in
Snowdon Blue, a monograph published by Acne Studios, 2012.

Since the turn of the millennium, the global fashion industry has increasingly looked to the art world for inspiration and information. Some of the larger luxury brands have taken a philanthropic approach, building relationships with artists by establishing foundations in support of the arts, or by funding projects and exhibitions independent of their own fashion businesses. Other brands have incorporated the fine arts directly into their products, inviting individual artists to collaborate. Such partnerships have encouraged and complicated the perpetual debate about whether fashion really is art to such an extent that it's almost impossible to discuss one without the other. Moreover, the start of the 21st century saw fashion staking a claim to the hallowed spaces of contemporary art galleries and traditional art museums via blockbuster exhibitions that have broken numerous attendance records and sparked further discussion about the role and place of fashion within an artistic context.

Much has been said about this topic in both art and fashion circles, yet at the same time there has been no systematic examination of the specific projects that have changed the nature of fashion as we know it. *Art/Fashion in the 21st Century* therefore aims to document and interrogate the creative work and theoretical significance of the most important artists, designers, fashion houses and museums that have participated in this aspect of contemporary fashion since the start of the new millennium.

Any dialogue about the relationship between art and fashion must begin with the recognition that, by any definition, not all art is 'Art with a capital A'. Similarly, not all fashion is 'capital-F Fashion'. Within each discipline there has traditionally existed a hierarchy of 'high' and 'low' forms. A discussion about art and fashion, then, is also a discussion about redefining the boundaries of both spheres in recognition of the fact that these traditional hierarchies have now all but collapsed. Mass-market (or 'low') fashion influences haute couture, and as early as the late 1950s Andy Warhol (and Marcel Duchamp before him) challenged notions of high art by turning images of supermarket fodder into financially viable, museum-collected artworks.

It is useful to explore these historical oppositions in order to better understand how and, perhaps more importantly, why, fashion and art have become co-conspirators and creative collaborators for mutual benefit.

On the face of it, art and fashion are philosophically opposed. Fashion is generally understood to be fickle, transient and largely driven by popular culture, whereas

'I think the way people dress today is a form of artistic expression. Saint Laurent, for instance, has made great art. Art lies in the way the whole outfit is put together. Take Jean Paul Gaultier. What he does is really art.'

Andy Warhol[1]

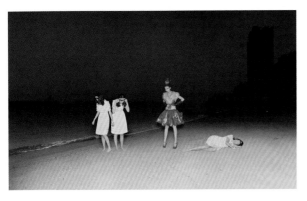

Quentin Shih, *No. 08*, from his *Hong Kong Moment*
photographic series created for Christian Dior, 2010.

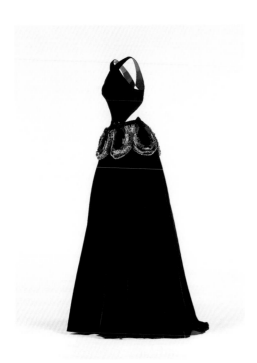

Azzedine Alaïa dress, Autumn/Winter 2011
haute couture collection, in the exhibition
'Azzedine Alaïa in the 21st Century' at the
Groninger Museum, the Netherlands, 2011.

fine art is viewed as timeless, considered and elitist. Art has historically been exalted as the more noble and intellectual pursuit in comparison to fashion, which was regarded as a primarily commercially motivated form of expression. Another historical argument for the supremacy of fine art over fashion was the privileging of the concept of 'originality' in contrast with the act of reproduction inherent in fashion. This argument was perhaps most concisely formulated in the seminal essay 'The work of art in the age of mechanical reproduction', written by Marxist theorist Walter Benjamin in 1936, in which he declared the pre-eminence of the original over its reproduction:

'Even the most perfect reproduction of a work of art is lacking in one element: its presence in time and space, its unique existence at the place where it happens to be. This unique existence of the work of art determined the history to which it was subject throughout the time of its existence. This includes the changes that it may have suffered in physical condition over the years as well as the various changes in its ownership. The presence of the original is the prerequisite to the concept of authenticity.'[2]

Benjamin's essay asserted the supremacy of the inherent 'aura' of authenticity – that intangible quality that makes something art – which he claimed disappears in the act of reproduction. His argument is curiously timely: authenticity seems to be precisely what is missing in the current 'fast' consumer culture. By the same logic, however, haute couture – defined as garments produced by hand for a specific body – should share the status of high art by virtue of being unique productions. Like limited-edition prints, haute couture pieces are individually numbered and catalogued, in contrast to mass-produced factory-sewn garments and even designer ready-to-wear collections, which by Benjamin's definition might be deemed to lack the aura of authenticity that allows them to be considered art.

In contrast to both ready-to-wear and 'fast' mainstream fashion, haute couture garments do not serve a practical purpose; they are not made for the primary function of 'clothing' the body. Although haute couture is typically associated with flights of fantasy, excess, theatrical runway shows and exorbitant prices, its allure resides not only in the folly it represents but also in the way in which it speaks to the idea of 'the handmade', characterized by hand sewing and pattern cutting.

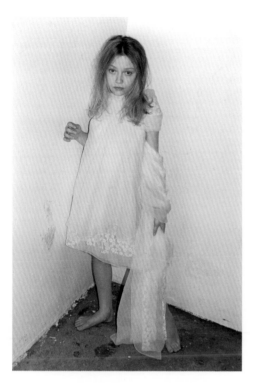

Actress Dakota Fanning photographed
by Juergen Teller for Marc Jacobs,
Spring/Summer 2007.

Haute couture is a combination of exemplary artisanship and craftsmanship that more profoundly fulfills a deeply held human desire for a haptic experience. These are clothes intimately imbued with a sense of touch – both that of the couturier and that of the wearer, whose body the bespoke garments describe. Although the demise of couture has been much mooted since the rise of ready-to-wear in the 1960s, it continues to prevail on a smaller but no less expensive scale, despite financial meltdown and ongoing questions about its relevance. The question of 'relevance' is in itself irrelevant, for it is debatable whether couture has ever truly been relevant – that is, fulfilled a practical function – since the advent of ready-to-wear. In this respect art and couture have a great deal in common: both exist because they can, and not because they serve a practical purpose.

The acknowledged commercial imperative at the heart of fashion, particularly in the case of ready-to-wear and mass-market labels, sets up a contrast between fashion as a whole and the traditional, ideal-istic vision of art as a pursuit wholly unmotivated by financial gain. Yet this trope is a romantic fiction. In the 21st century, art is openly recognized as a commodity like any other; it is often bought and sold as an invest-ment. Contemporary 'A-List' artists (to borrow a fashion phrase) such as Damien Hirst and Jeff Koons enjoy mil-lionaire status in their own lifetimes, often seeing their work appear on the secondary market several times over. Many artists, moreover, have become aware of this notion of art as a commercial pursuit and have embraced it in their work. Beyond such self-reflexive appropriations, art has become so wholly absorbed into the capitalist model that it now enjoys the status of a luxury item and appears alongside handbags, shoes, yachts and watches as an object of desire, the subject of 'status anxiety' as Alain de Botton describes it. To put it more plainly, art has become, like fashion, popular. Collectors of expensive contemporary art wear and buy expensive contemporary fashion; there exists a mutual audience for these two genres that seems to parallel the blurring of lines among other creative pursuits apparent in wider contemporary culture.

Although both fashion and art are more widely accessible to the masses than they were a century ago, and disseminated by radically different means, their collision is certainly nothing new. In the 1920s and 1930s Italian designer Elsa Schiaparelli collaborated with Surrealists such as Jean Cocteau and Salvador Dalí. In the 1960s, French designer Yves Saint Laurent

Fashion is popularly understood to be fickle, transient and largely driven by popular culture, whereas fine art is viewed as timeless, considered and elitist. Art has historically been exalted as the more noble and intellectual pursuit in comparison to fashion, which was regarded as a primarily commercially motivated form of expression.

Opposite: *Dissecting Waltz*, collaboration between designer Nicholas Kirkwood and artist Simon Periton for the exhibition 'Britain Creates 2012: Fashion + Art Collusion' at the Victoria & Albert Museum, London.

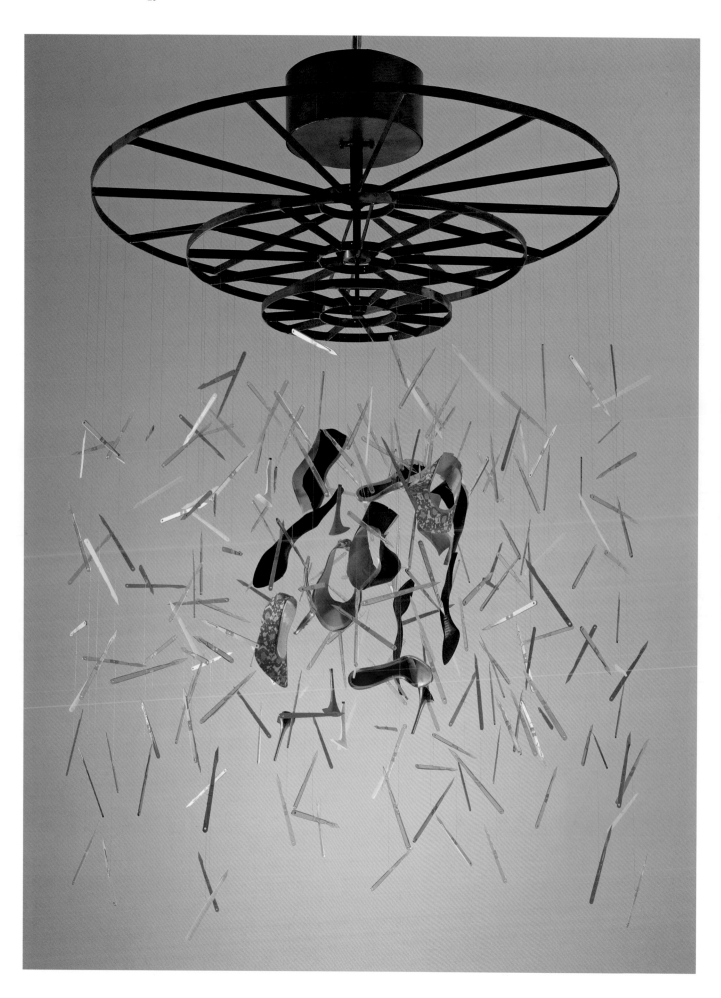

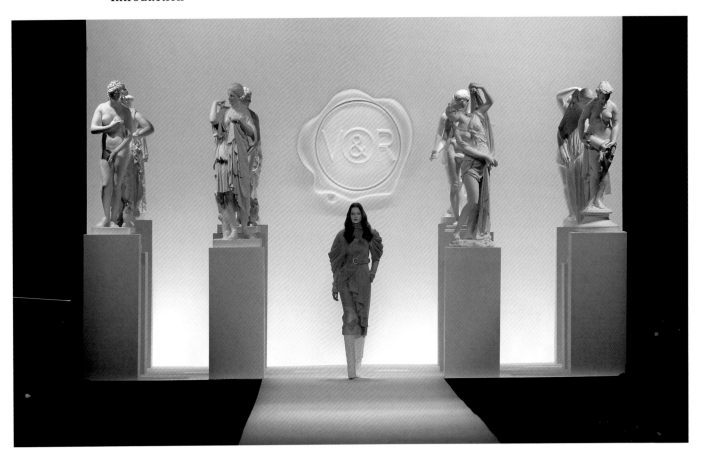

Above: Viktor & Rolf runway show, Paris,
Autumn/Winter 2009.

employed the then-radical shift dress, largely a flat, square surface, as a canvas for Piet Mondrian's famous colour-blocked works (Autumn/Winter 1965). As with all of the artists to whom Saint Laurent later paid homage – including Tom Wesselmann, Cocteau, Vincent van Gogh and Pablo Picasso – the designer's greatest accomplishment lay in his adaptation of the artwork to the human body, rather than simply adopting it wholesale. Today, established fashion houses such as Hermès, Louis Vuitton and Bally collaborate with artists to simultaneously reinvent their brands for existing clientele and make them relevant to new audiences in a contemporary context. When Japanese anime artist Takashi Murakami's cartoon prints of soft toys were printed over Louis Vuitton's feted monogram, a logo central to the house's closely protected authenticity, the result was both a radical artistic gesture and one of the house's greatest commercial successes. In what amounts to a calculated risk, a historic house such as Louis Vuitton can successfully thwart its own status quo while reasserting itself as the original tastemaker, thus assuming a position of cultural sophistication. By aligning with contemporary art, fashion affords itself a criticality that it lacks. This criticality can then be acquired, literally, by the buyer, in a knowing gesture of cultural and economic mastery, turning a shopper into a collector.

Collaboration in the commercial fashion sphere has become synonymous with the luxury-store experience, making it almost impossible to buy a shirt or bag or shoe

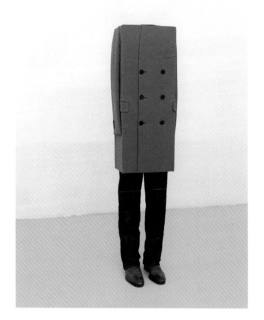

Erwin Wurm, sculpture from his *Untitled* series
created for Hermès, 2008.

that has not been given an artist's personal makeover. This form of collaboration, whereby a brand commissions an artist to reinterpret its signature products – or in certain cases, simply purchases an existing print with which to decorate them – has flooded the market since Louis Vuitton's head designer Marc Jacobs initiated the practice in 2001 with Stephen Sprouse, and these initiatives have proven so successful that the practice of artist-collaboration has also been adopted by mass-market high-street labels. Such collaborations result in the creation of something unique, albeit produced in multiple. The object – a handbag, scarf, shoe – bears the sign of the artist's hand at a remove and in many cases is still considered his or her intellectual property. This raises the question of whether such collaborations between artists and fashion houses actually produce 'artworks'. In a post-postmodern, post-art-historical critical context, Benjamin's 'aura' is located within the concept itself, and the physical execution of the artwork is but the expression of the original idea. From this perspective, the product of a collaboration is imbued with the 'aura' of the original artwork, even when the handbag or dress is commercially reproduced in large numbers. In the case of Murakami's collaboration with Louis Vuitton, the distinction between commercial product and high art was blurred in a truly Warholian gesture when the artist later incorporated the paintings and sculptures he had produced for the house into his solo gallery exhibitions.

There are also many designers who can be considered artists in their own right, whether they simply employ the body as a canvas or use it to create performance art in their runway shows. Alexander McQueen, Hussein Chalayan, Viktor & Rolf and MATERIALBYPRODUCT are just a few who have used the catwalk to convey deeper messages about transmutation, rooted in the fundamental notion that fashion seduces the wearer with its promise to transform, affording them the opportunity to become many different characters. These designers so fully integrate the body into the artwork that is the garment that in essence one cannot exist without the other, raising the question of whether the act of simply *wearing* fashion is itself a form of art, a performance.

Fashion also speaks to the notion of art as spectacle. In the early 20th century garments were shown to clients on models in a salon setting, but the continued rise of ready-to-wear in the 1980s and 1990s saw the development of some of the most lavish runway presentations in history. Fashion shows have since evolved to resemble, as Lydia Kamitsis argues, evocative museum presentations

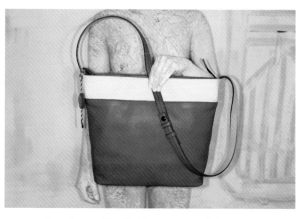

Bag designed by Olaf Breuning in collaboration
with Graeme Fidler and Michael Herz for
Bally Love #2, 2012.

with equivalent didactic labels and meanings.[3] As an example of this phenomenon, she cites Hussein Chalayan's 'One Hundred and Eleven' (Spring/Summer 2007) collection that featured a mechanical dress that shifted and expanded, taking the shape of one historical fashion style after another. The shows of designers such as Viktor & Rolf, John Galliano for Christian Dior, Alexander McQueen and Chanel have rivalled the scale and expense of the world's most ambitious operatic productions, yet are less than 15 minutes in length.

This is fashion as theatre, as live performance, the sheer speed of which meets the demands of a 24-hour news cycle. This in turn has seen a rapid shift in the way in which fashion is marketed, written about and, most importantly, sold. The proliferation of fashion bloggers since the beginning of the new millennium at one time looked set to render traditional fashion media (that is, magazines and newspapers, with their associated reporters, critics and journalists) obsolete. The general

The shows of designers such as Viktor & Rolf, John Galliano for Christian Dior, Alexander McQueen and Chanel have rivalled the scale and expense of the world's most ambitious operatic productions.

Opposite: Alexander McQueen runway show,
Paris, Spring/Summer 2010.

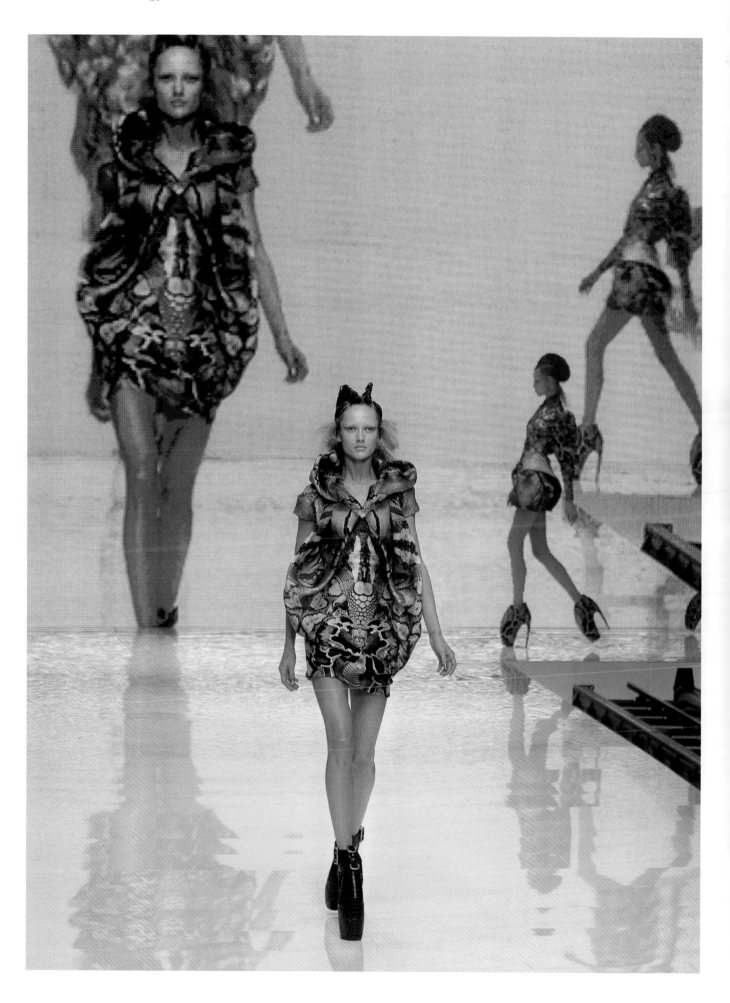

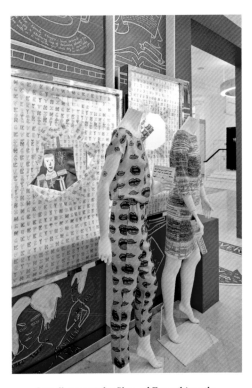

Installation at the Shop of Everything, the
retail component of the 'Museum of Everything'
exhibition at British retailer Selfridges flagship
Oxford Street store, London, 2011.

consensus is that there is still room in the market for both online and print content, yet the new media platforms have radically changed the fashion landscape they report. A growing number of fashion houses, for instance, now live-stream their seasonal runway shows, delivering the 'slow art' of haute couture as quickly as possible to an impatient global audience. The rapidly proliferating internet fashion blogs and discussion forums offer a constant stream of information with little mediation, raising the question of how much of this new fashion writing can truly be called 'criticism' in the classic sense. In this transformed media landscape, the art world lends fashion a much-needed cerebral element that is otherwise lost in fashion's interminable transience and lack of a formal, intellectual critical framework. Fashion magazines invite artists to serve as guest editors, working in a curatorial rather than commercial mode, and, like the leading fashion houses, seek out collaborations with fine-art photographers for shoots that break the traditional moulds. Film, too, has become an important medium for artist collaborations in the digital age, as fashion houses increasingly reach their customers via film shorts disseminated online.

The rise of the internet has radically changed the retail sphere of fashion as well. Since the turn of the millennium, fashion houses have successfully developed techniques for exploiting e-commerce, challenging the supremacy of the boutique and department store. Consumers can now browse for and buy garments online from the comfort of their own homes; Burberry, for example, has even introduced functionality for online customers to purchase looks directly from its live-streamed runway shows. Ironically, this technological economic revolution has been concurrent with the advent of architect-designed flagship stores for major fashion brands. These new, innovative, architecturally significant megastores are, in effect, the museums of the fashion world, and operate in a way that resembles the art museum model: the visitor is invited to view works of art and then make a purchase – either a financial donation to the building or a souvenir of its contents – on the way out. Some of the wealthier labels have taken this process a step further, building their own art museums and exhibition spaces, or sponsoring innovative public art projects.

In comparison, the art world has been somewhat slower off the mark in adapting to these new retail and media landscapes. It has proven difficult for art to move outside the 'white cube' of the gallery space. The art world is still reliant upon museum and gallery

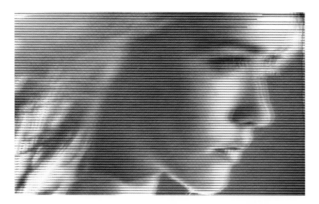

Still from an untitled short film created by Geoff Ang
for ck Calvin Klein, Spring/Summer 2010.

exhibitions to generate media exposure via magazine reviews and the publication of exhibition catalogues, and the success of an exhibition is still measured by its attendance figures. More fundamentally, however, art requires a viewer in the same way that fashion needs a wearer. Although art is now available to a wider audience via the internet (virtual tours of museums and galleries are now regularly offered), there is still the perception that art must be seen in the flesh. This face-to-face apprehension is part of the haptic experience that the artistic gesture demands, and a means of personally verifying the 'authenticity' of the artist's hand. Moreover, although art can be and is sold online, the traditional models of art gallery, dealer and auction house have survived largely unchanged, as these institutional structures are still necessary to secure and authenticate the status of the artist.

Fashion shares this need to establish the authenticity of a work. Luxury houses have always had to defend their brands in the face of widespread counterfeiting. Although brand identity is therefore especially important to fashion houses, many of the most successful artists – such as Murakami, Hirst or Cindy Sherman – are also brands in their own right; the reproduction of their work vigorously protected by copyright.

A discussion about art and fashion inevitably comes back to a concept of implied value and worth. We understand that fashion has a 'price' and art has a 'value'. Art typically appreciates in value, whereas fashion, despite the perpetual trend for vintage, typically depreciates. Very few items of fashion hold their price outside the world of haute couture and beyond the immediate desire that surrounds an 'It' bag or designer, because this desire is by its very nature fleeting. An 'It' bag is designed to be usurped by the next 'It' bag. This is the natural system of fashion, because fashion is, after all, *fashionable*, inextricably rooted in its immediate epoch. Perhaps one of the most interesting trends of the new millennium has been the rise of luxury retail in tandem with the global financial crisis that started in 2007. On the surface it would seem that consumers are turning to bespoke and luxury items for solace in a time of widespread austerity, and we might postulate that on a deeper level this is motivated by a desire for certainty in an era of upheaval. But certainty of what? That an object is well made, perhaps, but more specifically that it has been designed by an artist or handmade by an artisan; that it has taken time to make, and therefore has value beyond its monetary price. It seems that contemporary culture, in which time itself is the ultimate valuable commodity, has generated a global craving for 'authenticity' that the union of art and fashion is uniquely able to fulfill.

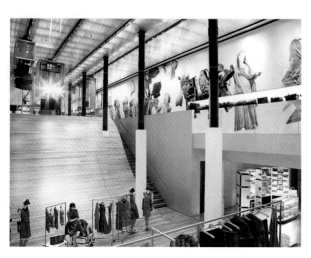

Interior of the Prada Epicenter, New York,
designed by Rem Koolhaas/OMA.

In this transformed media landscape, the art world lends fashion a much-needed cerebral element that is otherwise lost in fashion's interminable transience and lack of a formal, intellectual critical framework. Fashion magazines invite artists to serve as guest editors... and, like the leading fashion houses, seek out collaborations with fine-art photographers for shoots that break the traditional moulds.

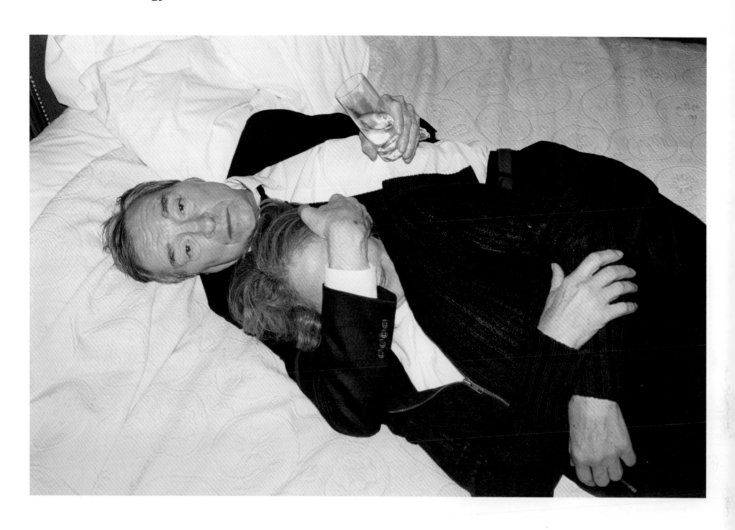

Above: William Eggleston and Charlotte Rampling photographed
by Juergen Teller for Marc Jacobs, Spring/Summer 2007.

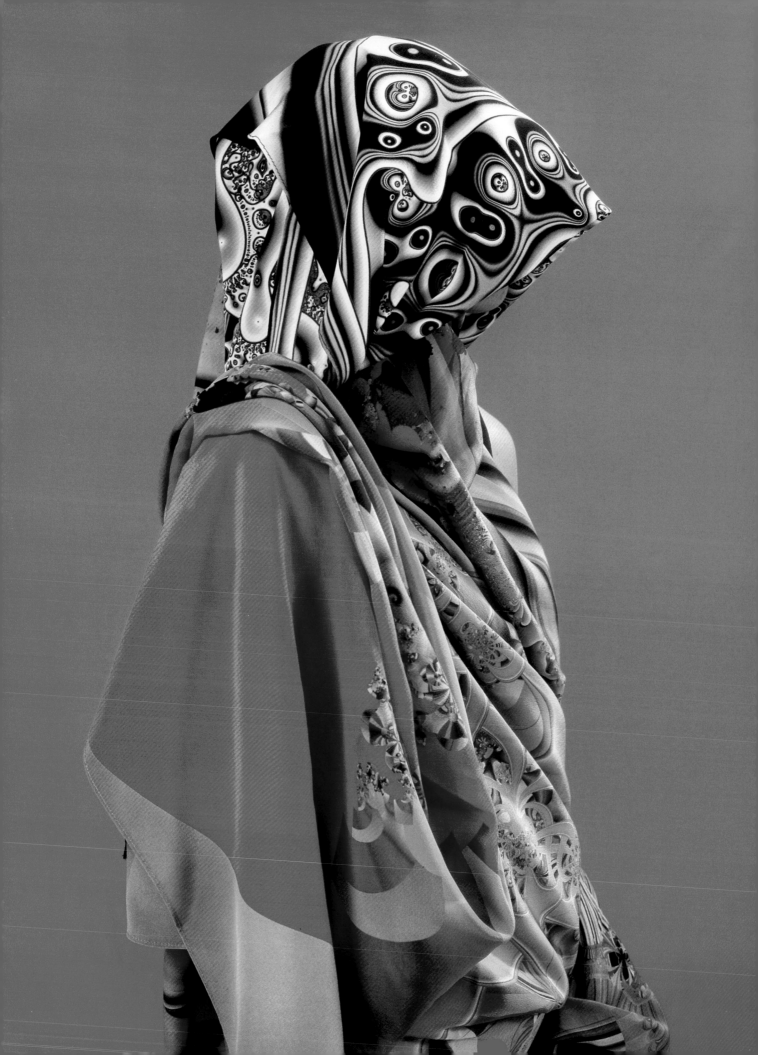

More than clothes: Fashion as art

Opposite: Tru$t Fun!, 'Glory' scarves, 2009.

Introduction:
More than clothes

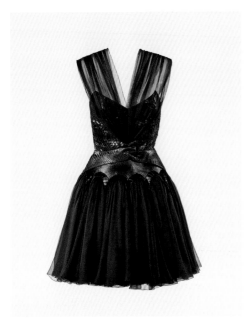

Azzedine Alaïa dress, Spring/Summer 2010
haute couture, in 'Azzedine Alaïa in the 21st Century'
exhibition at the Groninger Museum,
the Netherlands, 2011.

Given fashion's newly acquired status as a contemporary form of cultural entertainment, in large part due to the predominance of digital media, it is unsurprising that many visual artists have made a serious, critical engagement with it as a subject of their work. Swiss artist Sylvie Fleury, for instance, well known for her commentary on fashion, consumerism, art and brand culture, has produced a sculpture of a pair of chrome-plated bronze Prada shoes (*Prada Shoes*, 1998), an installation composed of shopping bags from luxury brands (*Insolence*, 2007), and an 'intervention' comprising one hundred bottles of Chanel Égoïste perfume packaged in small branded bags, which she displayed at the Cologne Art Fair in 1991. The work of Italian performance and installation artist Vanessa Beecroft similarly maintains a dialogue with fashion's construction and manipulation of beauty, perhaps most memorably in a performance in which naked models, selected to resemble the artist and signed and numbered like limited-edition prints, were assembled in the atriums of art museums and directed to stand silent and unmoving for several hours while viewers mingled around them. Both Beecroft and Fleury have collaborated with Louis Vuitton, reflecting fashion's new self-criticality. Fleury created a series of metallic monogrammed embossed Keepall bags (the 'Miroir' collection) that resembled a chromed-bronze sculpture she had made of Vuitton's iconic handbag in 2000. For Vuitton's launch of its flagship store on the Champs-Élysées, Beecroft reimagined the house's logo using naked models, drawing inspiration from an iconic *Vogue* magazine alphabet from the 1940s (based in turn on an Art Deco alphabet by the famous illustrator Erté).

Other contemporary artists who have made work about fashion in relation to the body include Beverly Semmes, Tom Sachs, Lucy Orta, Karen Kiliminik, Elizabeth Peyton, Hélio Oiticica, Michael Zavros and Leigh Bowery. In 1987 Jana Sterbak made a dress of meat and documented herself wearing it as it decomposed, a gesture famously echoed by fashion icon Lady Gaga's notorious 'meat dress' by Argentinian artist and fashion designer Franc Fernandez that she wore at the 2010 MTV Video Music Awards. The mutual inspiration of art and fashion operates in two directions: outside of their officially commissioned commercial collaborations with contemporary artists, many fashion designers have looked to the fine arts for inspiration, from John Galliano's homage to painter John Singer Sargent to Yves Saint Laurent's famous 'Mondrian' dress or Rodarte's 'Fra Angelico' collection.

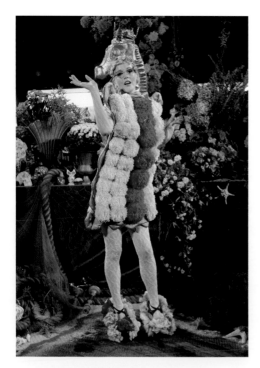

Romance Was Born, 'Iced Vovo' dress,
Spring/Summer 2009.

As sociology professor Diana Crane notes: 'Artists who design clothes as works of art are not interested in the utilitarian or commercial aspects of this activity. Some of these artists deliberately create dresses that cannot be worn.'[1] A criticism often levelled at haute couture is that it is 'unwearable', as though this were a negative quality. Certainly, this unwearability would seem to negate the commercial viability of fashion, challenging its reason for existing. Like many haute couture garments, however, Fleury's bronze Prada heels, too, are not wearable; they are transitory fashion given longevity and a value outside of the immediate financial transaction. In this context, might we not then view the work of some fashion designers as art?

An obvious shared platform is performance: the art of dressing can be performative, and many designers present their work in ways that resemble contemporary performance or conceptual art. We might call this 'fashion theatre'. For Maison Martin Margiela's solo exhibition at Museum Boijmans van Beuningen, Rotterdam, in 1997, garments from the label's archive were reproduced in neutral tones and then treated with various strains of bacteria, yeast and mould so that the colours of the fabric altered over the course of the exhibition: a case of fashion meets science as mediated by art. In 1999 Alexander McQueen concluded the presentation of his seminal 'No.13' collection with an epic finale in which model Shalom Harlow spun slowly on a turntable in a white dress as she was spray-painted by a robot. British designer Hussein Chalayan is especially well known for the performative aspect of his presentations: 'Before Minus Now' (Spring/Summer 2000), which featured a dress that changed shape by remote control; 'Afterwords' (Autumn/Winter 2000) in which clothing transformed into furniture; and several collaborations with Swarovski in which garments decorated with crystals and thousands of LEDs created spectacular light shows on darkened runways.

Whereas the work of artists engaging with fashion is generally considered in more intellectual terms (that is, favorably), fashion is often criticized for what is perceived as its lack of content; judged for its speed, commerciality and ephemeral, 'throwaway' nature, despite the clear artistic rigour exhibited in the design process and the presentation of garments. There is too often the assumption that fashion is easy to understand, as opposed to art, which is popularly perceived as intelligent by virtue of its complexity. There are, however, several contemporary designers who maintain a conceptual approach

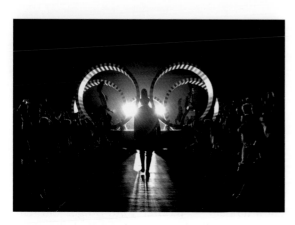

Henrik Vibskov, runway show, 'The Human Laundry Service'
collection, Autumn/Winter 2009.

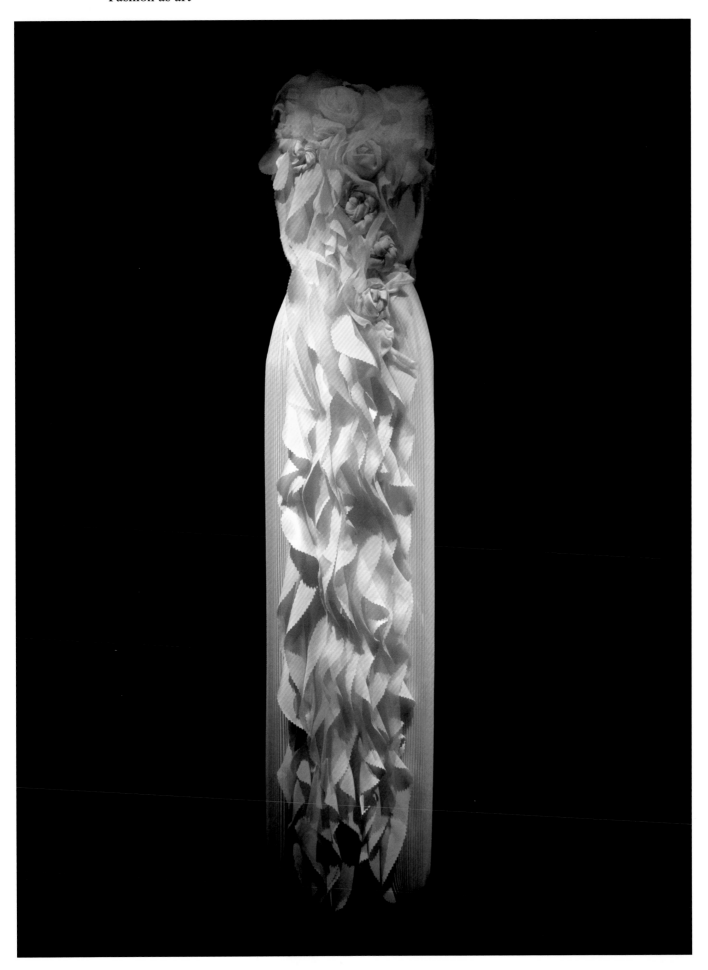

'One should either be a work of art, or wear a work of art.'

Oscar Wilde[2]

to fashion, and aspects of whose work could be deemed art, because clothing is used as a physical representation of their ideas. Chalayan, Bernhard Willhelm, Henrik Vibskov, Maison Martin Margiela, Viktor & Rolf and Walter Van Beirendonck all create clothing that is not primarily about following trends for commercial gain, and that challenges definitions of what fashion is and how it functions. Interestingly, these designers are predominantly European and Japanese. One reason for this may be that European fashion historically developed as part of a broader aesthetic culture that included art, music, film and architecture: what theorist Karin Schacknat calls *Gesamtkunstwerk* (literally, 'total work of art') or multimedia, evidenced in movements such as Arts and Crafts or those of the Belle Époque.[3] Similarly, as Valerie Steele emphasizes 'traditionally in Japan, there existed no hard-and-fast distinction between art and craft.'[4]

As a measure of the respect accorded such designers' work, it is often curated into group and solo exhibitions and collected by private galleries and public museums where it is displayed alongside the great masterpieces of art.

It is here – the museum – that fashion's validity as an art form is questioned, prompting countless discussions and debates in recent decades. As with similarly culturally and economically accessible contemporary media such as photography, film, graffiti or street art, fashion has struggled to achieve the status accorded to more traditional artistic forms, a challenge furthered by its connection to capitalist culture. Perhaps questions, and answers, about fashion's cultural, social, economic and aesthetic worth should ultimately remain with the viewer, or consumer.

Opposite: Rodarte evening dress, Autumn/Winter 2006, displayed in the 'blog.mode: addressing fashion' exhibition at the Costume Institute, Metropolitan Museum of Art, New York, 2007.

Hussein Chalayan

Named British Designer of the Year in 1999 and 2000, Hussein Chalayan's intellectual approach to fashion sees him frequently described as an artist. He is well known for his non-conventional approach to materials and for his inclusion of technological elements within designs that meld the languages of fashion, furniture, architecture, theatre, music and cinema. His collection presentations typically take the form of performances or installations. As Karin Schacknat writes: 'His aesthetic relies on intellectual concepts that are often related to social engagement and where the boundaries between fashion, architecture and art become blurred.'[5]

Cypriot-born Chalayan's work can be understood as a response to his childhood experiences living in a fractured country. To that end, his clothing has a political agenda of sorts and references his 'uprootedness'. One of his most celebrated collections, 'Afterwords' (Autumn/Winter 2000), empathized with the experience of political refugees, exploring the idea of having to flee, via furniture that could be turned into clothing. He frequently references the concept of travel and speed, in terms of both distance and time: another seminal presentation, 'One Hundred and Eleven' (Spring/Summer 2007), involved a single dress that mechanically changed shape, taking the form of a series of historical fashion styles.

In 2005 Chalayan represented Turkey at the Venice Biennale, one of the key events in the international contemporary art world, with a film entitled *Absent Presence*, starring Tilda Swinton. His work has been the subject of exhibitions at the Victoria & Albert Museum, London; the 21st Century Museum of Contemporary Art, Kanazawa, Ishikawa, Japan; the Tate Modern, London; the Museum of Modern Art, New York; and the Groninger Museum, the Netherlands.

'The boundaries between fashion, architecture and art become blurred.'

Karin Schacknat

Opposite: Hussein Chalayan, LED electronic dress,
Autumn/Winter 2007.
Overleaf: Hussein Chalayan, 'Inertia' collection,
Paris Fashion Week runway show, Spring/Summer 2009.

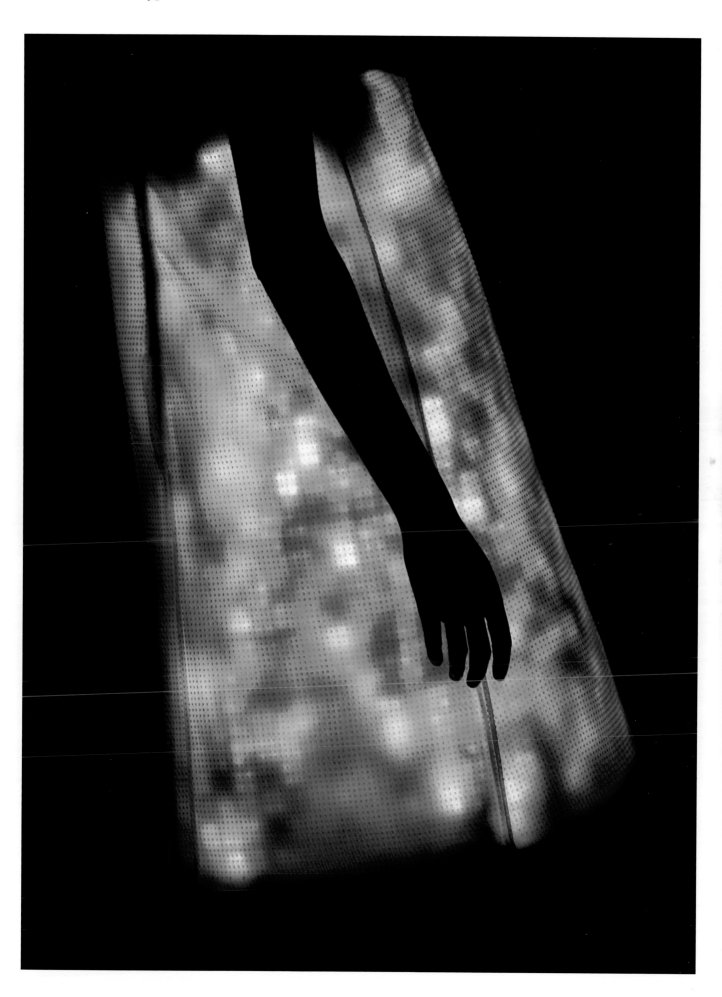

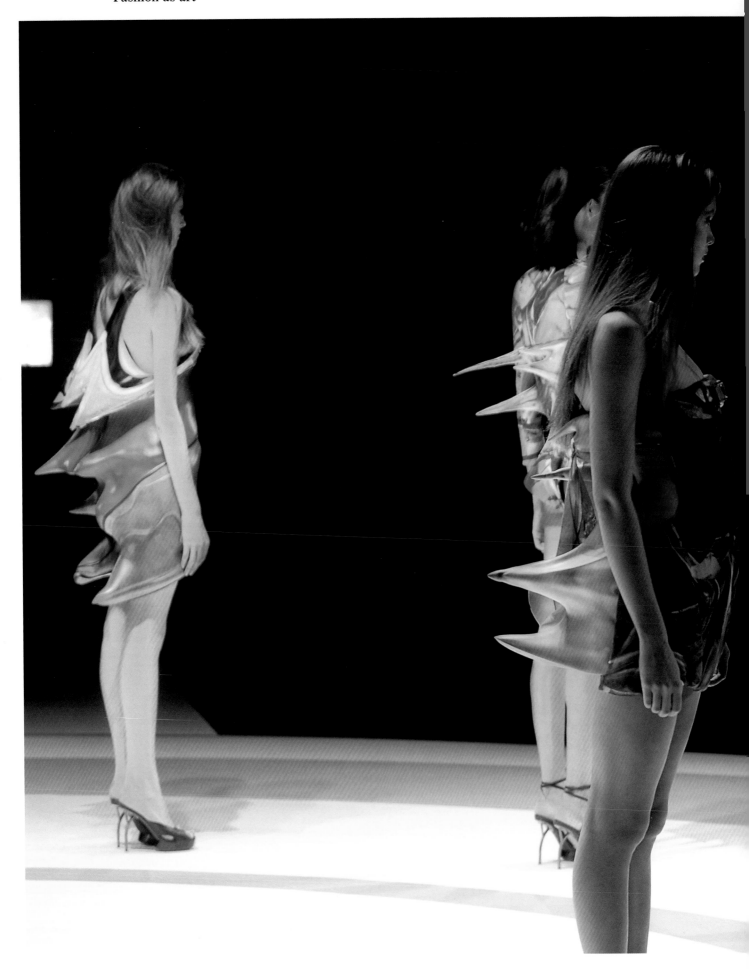

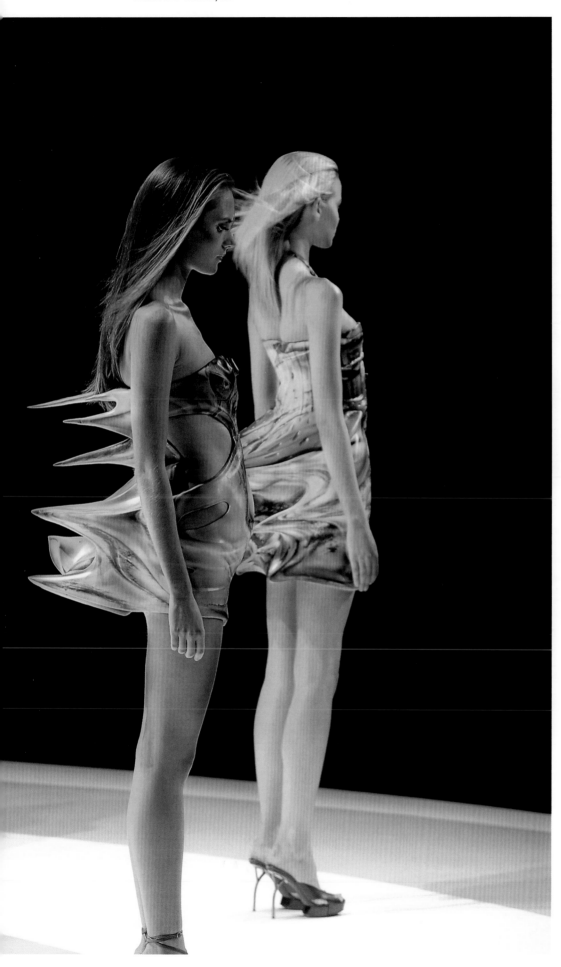

In conversation:
Anna Plunkett & Luke Sales,
Romance Was Born

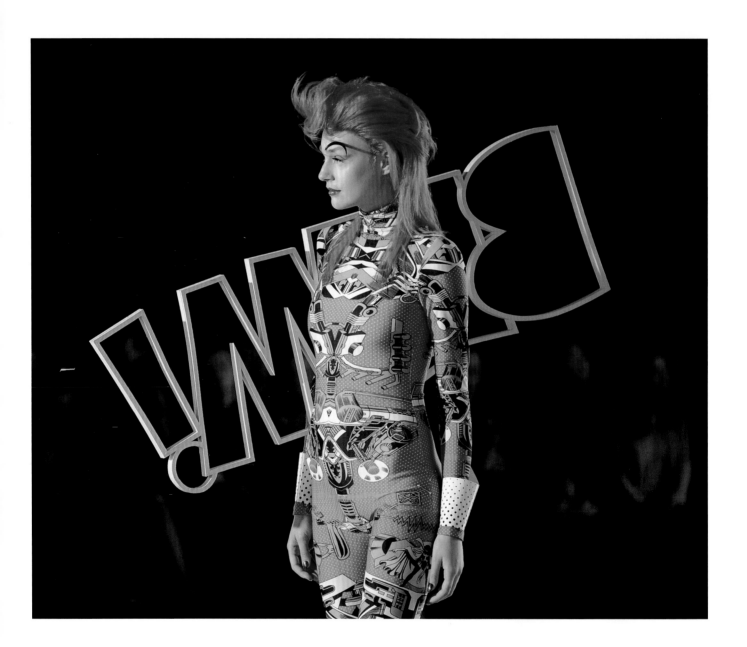

Above and overleaf: Romance Was Born,
'Berserkergang' collection, Spring/Summer 2013.
Pages 38–39: Romance Was Born, 'Doilies and Pearls,
Oysters and Shells' collection, Spring/Summer 2009.

An important part of Australian label Romance Was Born's commercial and critical success has come from its collaboration with visual artists, perhaps most notably 2008 Archibald Prize-winning painter Del Kathryn Barton. Founding designers Anna Plunkett and Luke Sales have also engaged collaborators from the performing arts, including the bands The Presets and Architecture in Helsinki, and the Sydney Theatre Company under the artistic direction of Cate Blanchett, a longtime supporter of the label. Another important collaborator has been the artist Kate Rohde, with whom Plunkett and Sales created an exhibition of sculptures, wallpaper and accessories inspired by their collection. Sydney-based artist Nell was responsible for the digital prints featured in the label's Spring/Summer 2011 collection, most notably the black-and-white text-based prints made up of collages of images from her paintings.

MITCHELL OAKLEY SMITH *Your work is often described as art rather than fashion. But can fashion – that is clothing – ever really be art?*

ANNA PLUNKETT If the idea behind the clothing hasn't come from a commercial place, I don't see why not. I think art spaces are a great place to showcase clothing. When we were in Europe recently we saw a presentation by Bernhard Willhelm, which was held in a tiny art gallery and it just had the greatest energy. There was performance and the clothes were bright and graphic, [so] that it made sense in this space.

LUKE SALES One of our first shows was staged at Kaliman Gallery [Paddington, Sydney] because it was a celebration of the prints we had created over three seasons with Del Kathryn Barton. Kaliman was Del's gallery, her environment, so it really lent itself to what we were doing.

MOS *Do you view yourselves as artists in the same way Del does?*

AP It's a really fine, blurry line. At the end of the day we are fashion designers who make commercial collections to be sold in retail stores, but we also make one-off pieces that are worn for performances and shown in exhibitions. I guess these pieces can be considered art, as they don't serve a commercial purpose, but for us it's just about storytelling.

MOS *You've also integrated contemporary artists such as Del and Nell into your practice. Is collaboration important to what you do?*

LS We want to work with special, creative people, as I think it keeps the ready-to-wear seasons – which you need to keep churning out to keep up with the fashion cycle – interesting. We only work with people who we feel are appropriate to the story we want to tell.

MOS *Does fashion become art because of the way it is made, like couture, or because of the way it communicates a message?*

LS I guess it depends on the original thought process and motivation behind the piece, but both of these points are valid. That said, we aren't the greatest fans of very conceptual fashion. We believe fashion should evoke an emotional response, and that's what we strive for in our work.

MOS *And yet, like an artwork, much of what you create is one-off.*

AP What we like and enjoy making and sampling isn't always what will be ordered by stores, and we know that, but those particular pieces really speak to us and communicate the ideas behind the collection, and often inspire the rest of the ready-to-wear collection. Without them our practice wouldn't be as special or relevant to us.

MOS *Those pieces are usually the ones photographed and circulated in the press, which explains where the theatricality tag that follows your label comes from.*

AP We like to create a world for the pieces to belong to. It helps to communicate the feelings and ideas behind them to the audience. You can walk down the street and see ready-to-wear clothing at any time, so what then is the point of having a show that's no different to what you see everyday?

LS We don't necessarily aim to make our presentations showy or theatrical, as they seem to be perceived – it's just a natural extension of the clothes we make in our studio. The theatrical side of our presentations is just the cherry on the cake for us. We feel so strongly about the theme and mood of the collection, having lived and breathed it for months, that it's just a final celebration and communication of all these ideas.

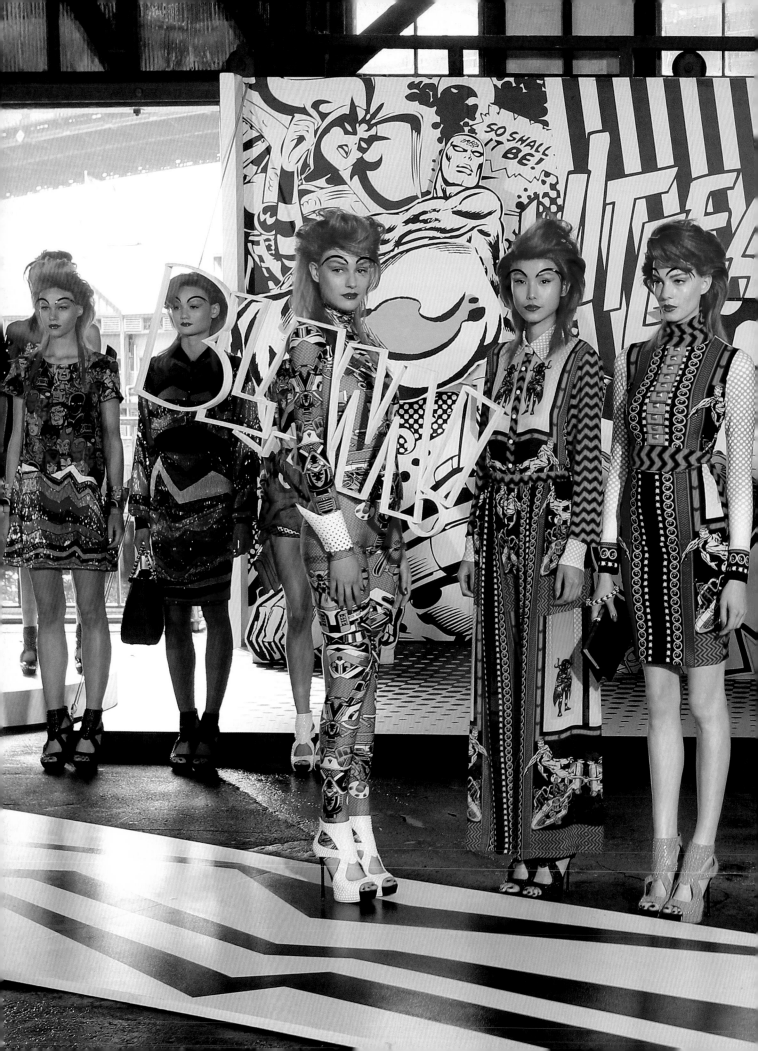

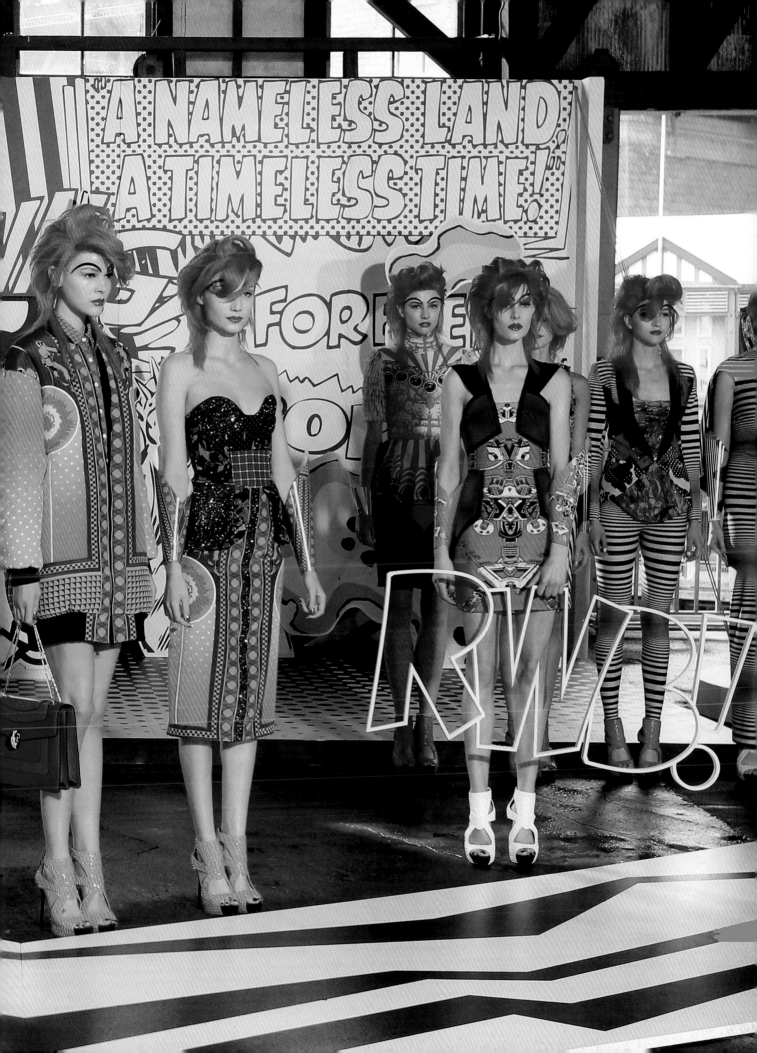

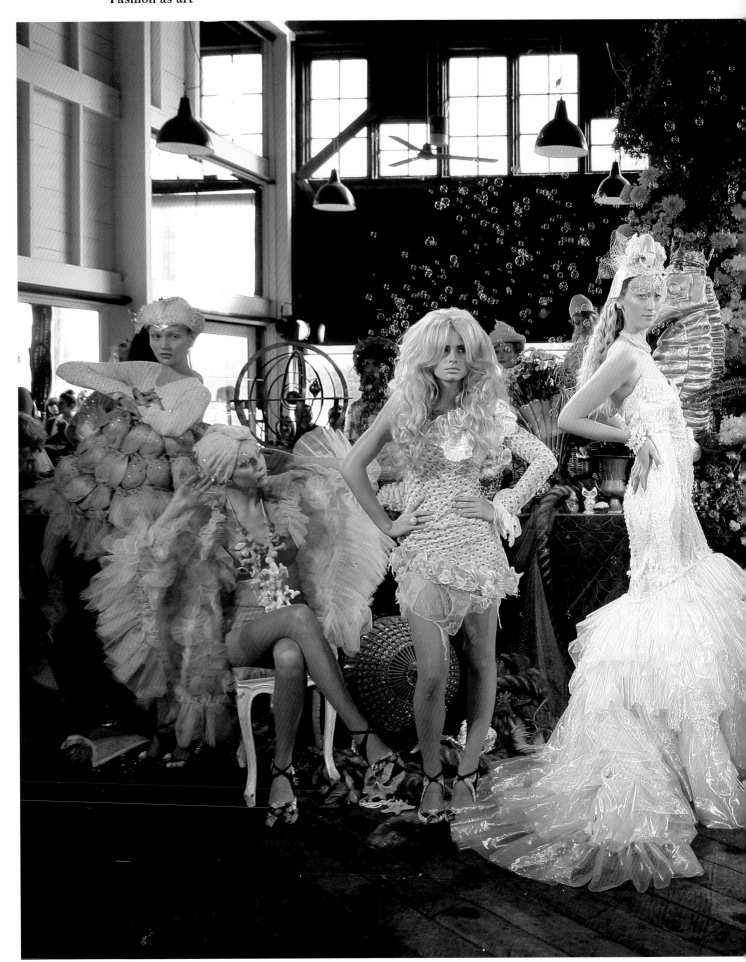

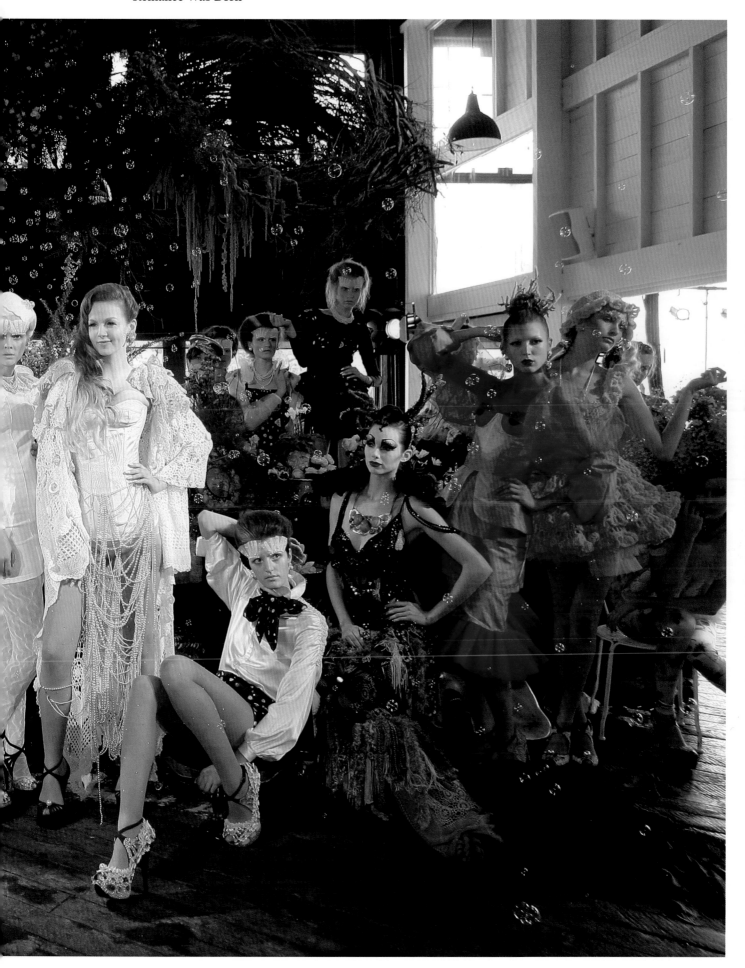

Maison Martin Margiela

The French contemporary fashion house Maison Martin Margiela is renowned for both its intellectual platform and its wit. Belgian-born Margiela founded the label that still bears his name, although he retired as creative director in 2009. Margiela has always played with the notion of personality and visibility in his work, however, and allowed speculation to swirl in the lead-up to his retirement about whether he was still in the role. He is never photographed, and has never appeared on the catwalk – a rare thing in the personality-driven fashion world where a brand is so often confused with a person – yet, despite his anonymity, he enjoys considerable fame and critical acclaim, and his loyal fans frequently describe themselves as 'collectors' of his work.

Margiela's critical engagement with fashion could be described as absurdist or surrealist. His collections regularly employed non-traditional materials (lining as outerwear, for example) and questioned notions of what constitutes a finished garment. This conceptual approach resulted in improbable, surreal pieces including jackets made of collaged gloves or belts, and his notorious 'Hair Coat', which incorporated wigs resembling human hair. Another important aspect of Margiela work involved upcycling vintage clothes: in 1994 he made an entire collection out of pieces from his past collections. Some designs also played with shape and volume, becoming surrogate bodies that could be either inflated to grotesque proportions or divided so that they included only one arm and one leg. Margiela's agenda was not about celebrating conventional notions of beauty; indeed, at times his style seemed more about the suppression of the female form.

Such extreme, conceptual pieces are the showstoppers that thematically underpin the more wearable garments in each collection. In making something ludicrous, Margiela both hinted at the inherent folly of fashion and avoided the possibility that the garment could be re-created and mass produced. Following Margiela's retirement, however, in 2012 the label collaborated with high-street retailer H&M, the epitome of global mass-produced fashion, to produce a capsule collection of more wearable and affordable versions of some of the founder's signature designs. Some observers branded the H&M collaboration an insult to Margiela's original creative vision; others, such as fashion correspondent Fiona Duncan, saw it as a deliberate act of performance, 'a continuation of Margiela's funhouse-mirror reflection of the fashion system, an inside joke and an insidious proposal of protest, a statement on authenticity and mechanical reproduction.'[6]

Opposite: Maison Martin Margiela patchwork coat, Autumn/Winter 2005.
Overleaf: Maison Martin Margiela dress, Spring/Summer 2009.

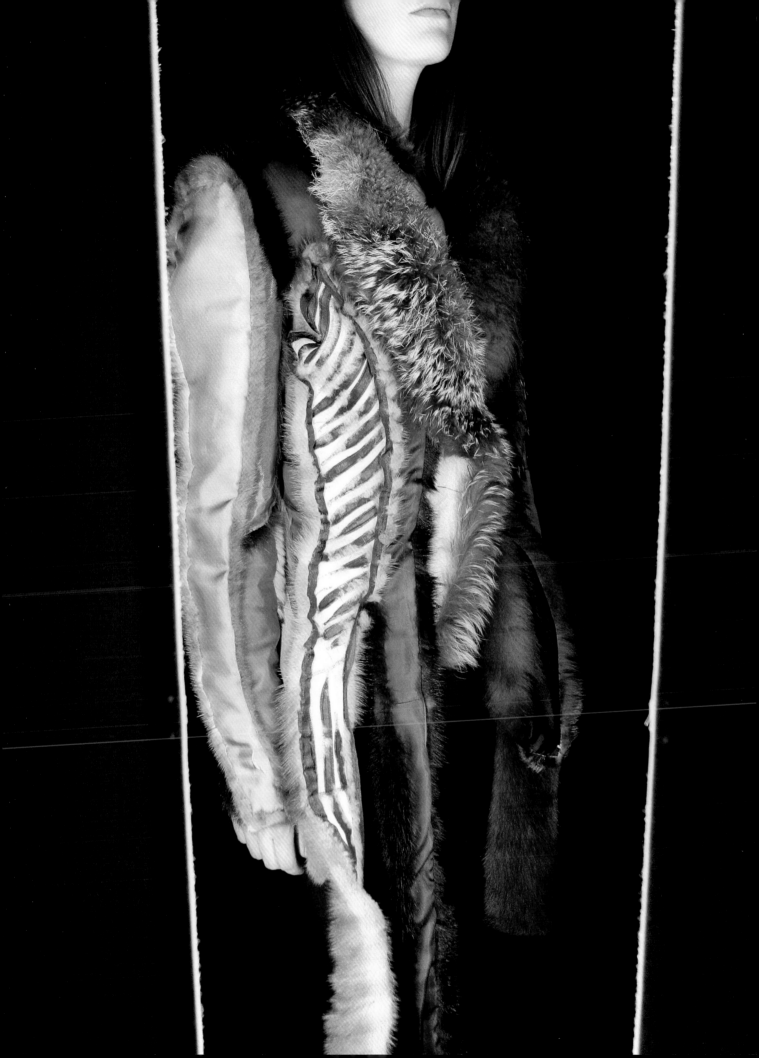

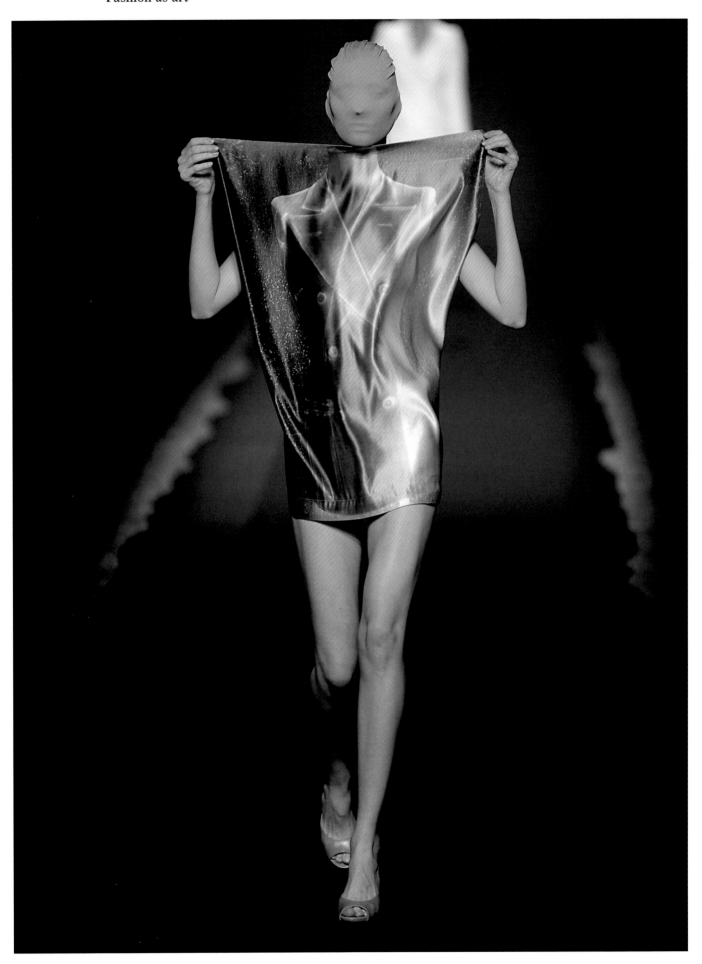

In making something ludicrous, Margiela both hinted at the inherent folly of fashion and avoided the possibility that the garment could be re-created and mass produced.

Bernhard Willhelm

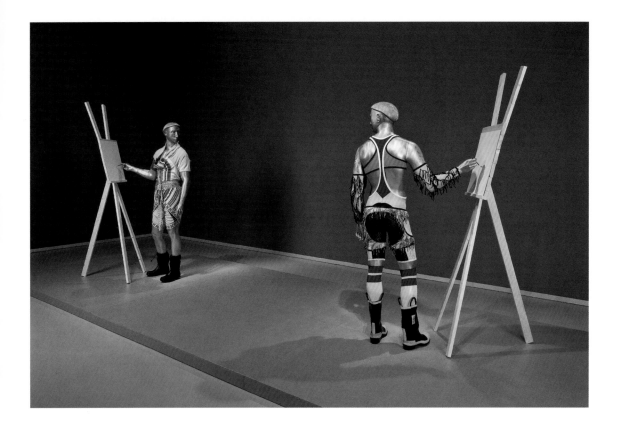

German fashion designer Bernhard Willhelm graduated from Antwerp's Royal Academy of Fine Arts a decade after the famed avant-garde design group the Antwerp Six, but during his studies he worked with several of its members, including Walter Van Beirendonck and Dirk Bikkembergs, and his work has been lauded for possessing a similar sensibility of thwarting the norm. That said, Willhelm should be judged on his own merits, and since launching his namesake label with business partner Jutta Kraus in 1999, he has developed a singular reputation for his continued subversion of established modes of dress, which earned him a place in several exhibitions, including the solo exhibition 'Bernhard Willhelm & Jutta Kraus' at the Groninger Museum on the occasion of the label's tenth anniversary in which the designer's work was presented in tableaux created by scenographer Žana Bošnjak.

What makes Willhelm's creative output worthy of critical discussion in the context of art is, as the Groninger Museum noted in its introduction to the exhibition, how he gives expression to the grotesque, childish and fantastic in a way that draws on both the current pop culture and the traditions of haute couture. Willhelm's seasonal ready-to-wear shows at Paris Fashion Week are recognized for the artistry of their performances, which not only contextualize the inspirations behind his collections, but also, by removing fashion from its natural environment – the runway – give greater voice to the power of fashion to communicate ideas.

Above, opposite and overleaf: Bernhard Willhelm designs from Spring/Summer 2010 (above), Spring/Summer 2008 (opposite) and Autumn/Winter 2007–8 (overleaf) collections, displayed in the exhibition 'Bernhard Willhelm and Jutta Kraus' at the Groninger Museum, 2009–10.

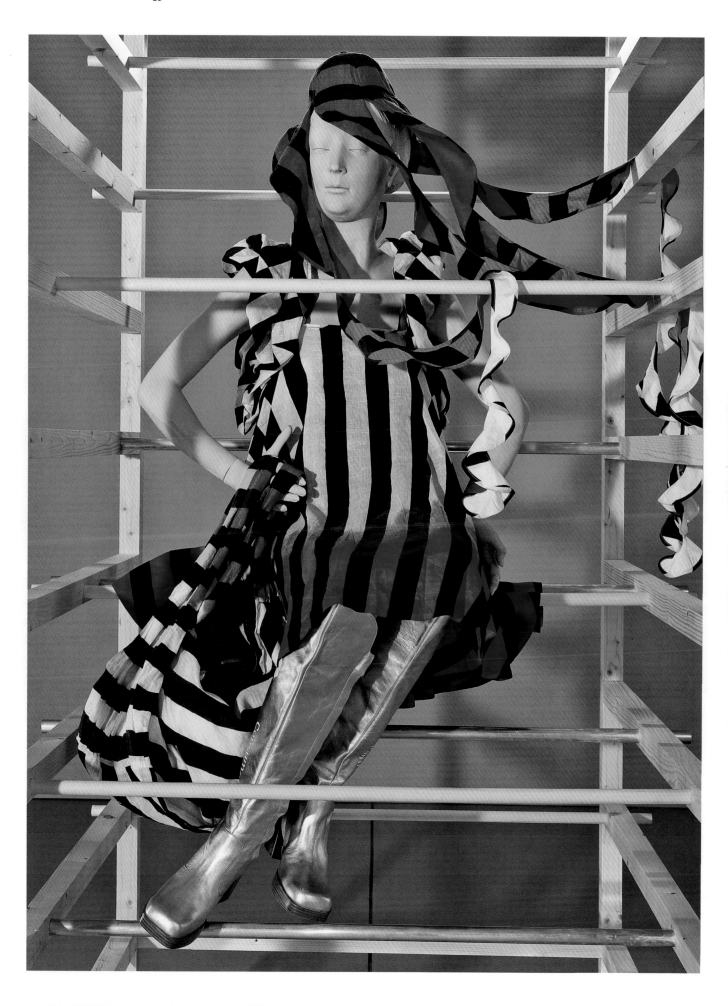

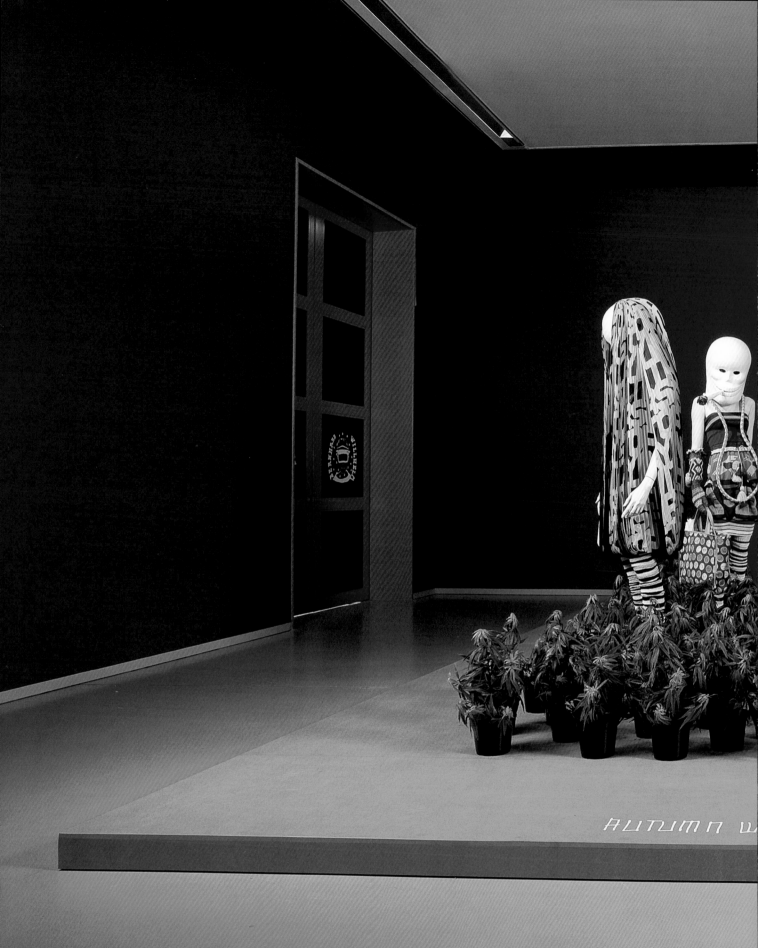

AUTUMN W

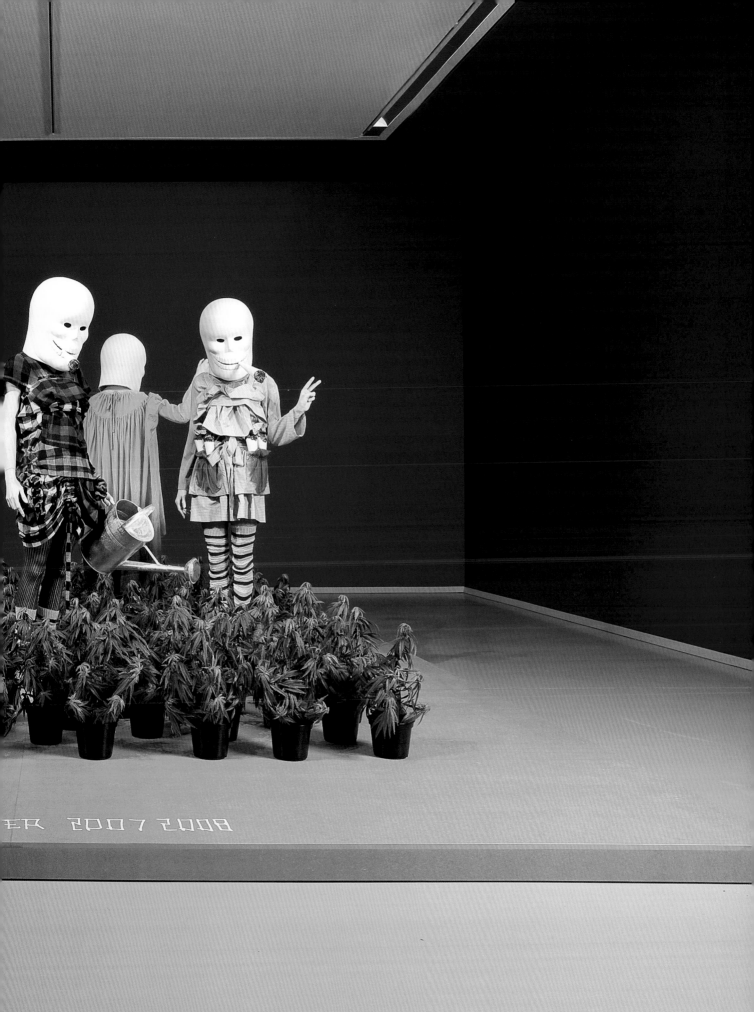

Alexander McQueen

When Lee Alexander McQueen committed suicide in 2010 the fashion world reeled. At just forty years old he was arguably the most important designer of his generation, famed for his heady mix of classic couture techniques, punk sensibility and futuristic vision of fashion. Both McQueen's design legacy and the near-mythic story of his rise from humble origins to head designer at Givenchy and founder of his own eponymous label were much celebrated in the immediate aftermath of his death, and the remarkable and unexpected popularity of the posthumous survey exhibition 'Alexander McQueen: Savage Beauty' at the Metropolitan Museum of Art, New York, in 2011 has cemented his place, already firmly established, in the cultural archives of the 21st century. Yet even during his lifetime, the designer was often labelled an artist.

McQueen particularly enjoyed the tension between light and dark, taking inspiration from all things macabre, which found expression in his moody, romantic collections. He was well known for his spectacular, sometimes provocative, fashion collection presentations that blended theatrical art, music and film to unforgettable effect. Some of his most memorable shows also incorporated a strong conceptual thread. His infamous 'Highland Rape' collection (Autumn/Winter 1995), featuring ravaged tartan shown on dishevelled models, was popularly misunderstood as a misogynistic gesture when in fact the designer was making a serious comment about the troubled relationship between Scotland and England. McQueen dressed women to empower them, and he spoke about the clothing he made as a kind of armour for the contemporary woman, featuring epaulets in the form of bird skulls, prints of writhing poisonous snakes, improbable shoes that resembled an armadillo, or feathered layers that transformed the wearer into an exotic bird.

Art was important to McQueen, both for its own sake and as a source of inspiration. His personal art collection featured the work of Jake and Dinos Chapman, Sam Taylor-Johnson (formerly Taylor-Wood) and Francis Bacon, as well as Victorian and Byzantine art (his final fashion collection explored Byzantine icons). McQueen's Spring/Summer 2001 collection show, 'VOSS', was inspired by a Joel-Peter Witkin photograph entitled *Sanitarium*, which depicts an obese woman connected to a monkey via an archaic breathing apparatus. McQueen engaged fetish writer Michelle Olley to play the role of the woman, concealed within a gigantic mirrored box. The audience was forced to look at its own reflection for over an hour before the show began, setting up an unease that the designer enjoyed. As the presentation began the lights went on inside the box and the tableau of the woman and the monkey became visible; the glass walls fell away and shattered. McQueen explained: 'In this collection the idea was to turn people's faces on themselves. I wanted to turn it around and make them think, "Am I actually as good as what I'm looking at?"...These beautiful models were walking around in the room, and then suddenly this woman who wouldn't be considered beautiful was revealed. It was about trying to show...that beauty comes from within.'[7]

Opposite and overleaf: Alexander McQueen runway show, Paris, Autumn/Winter 2009.

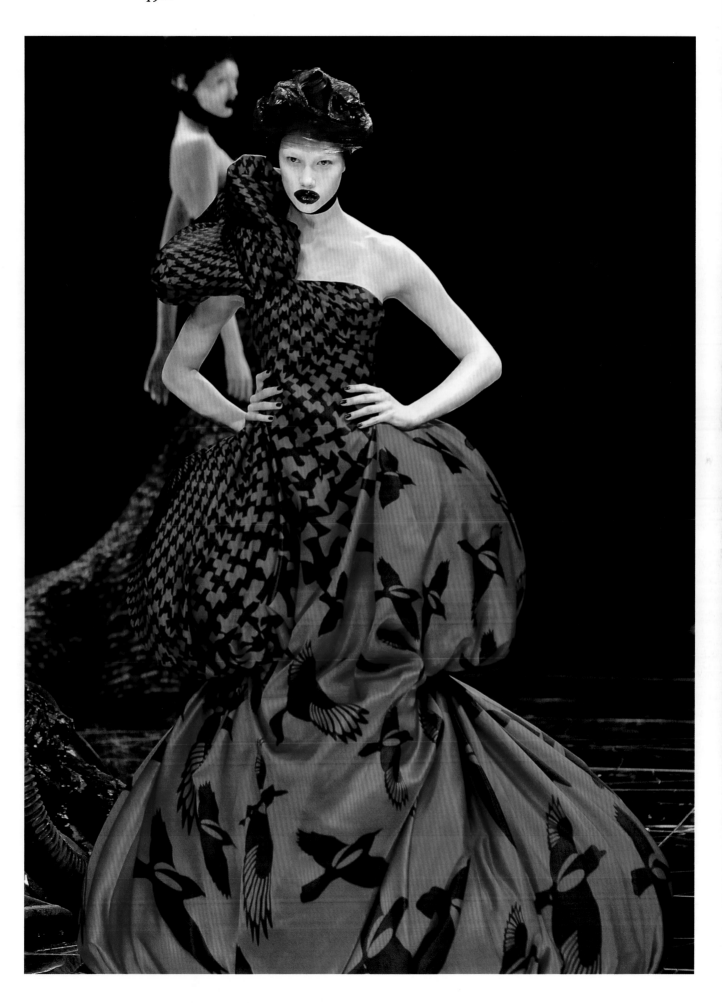

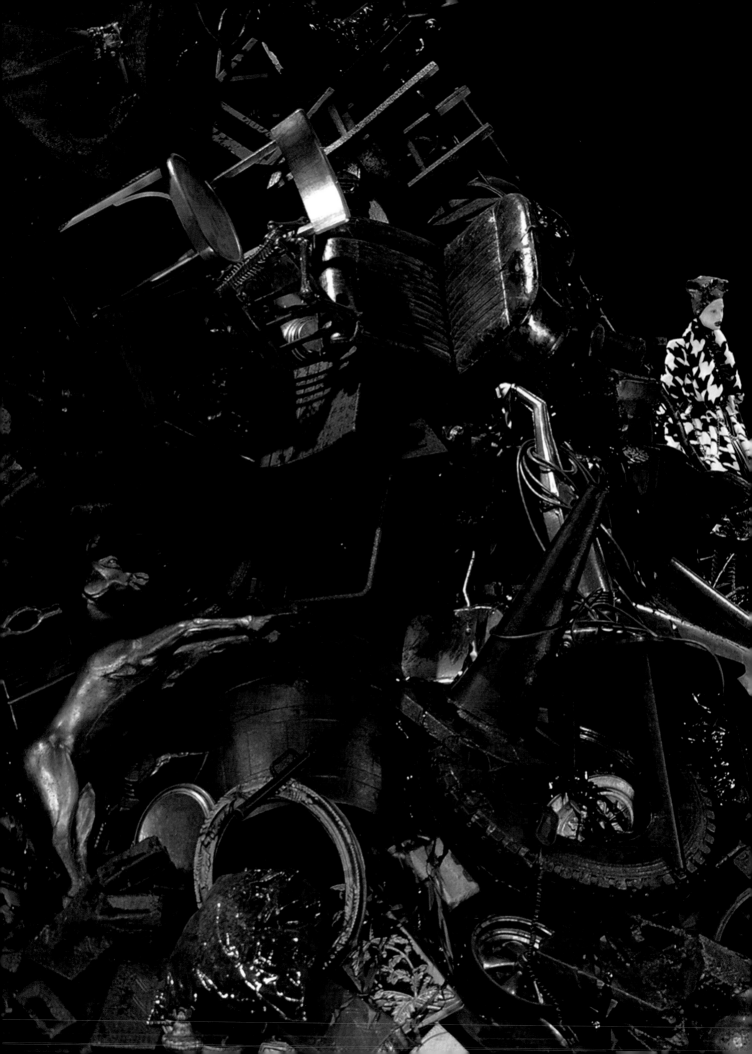

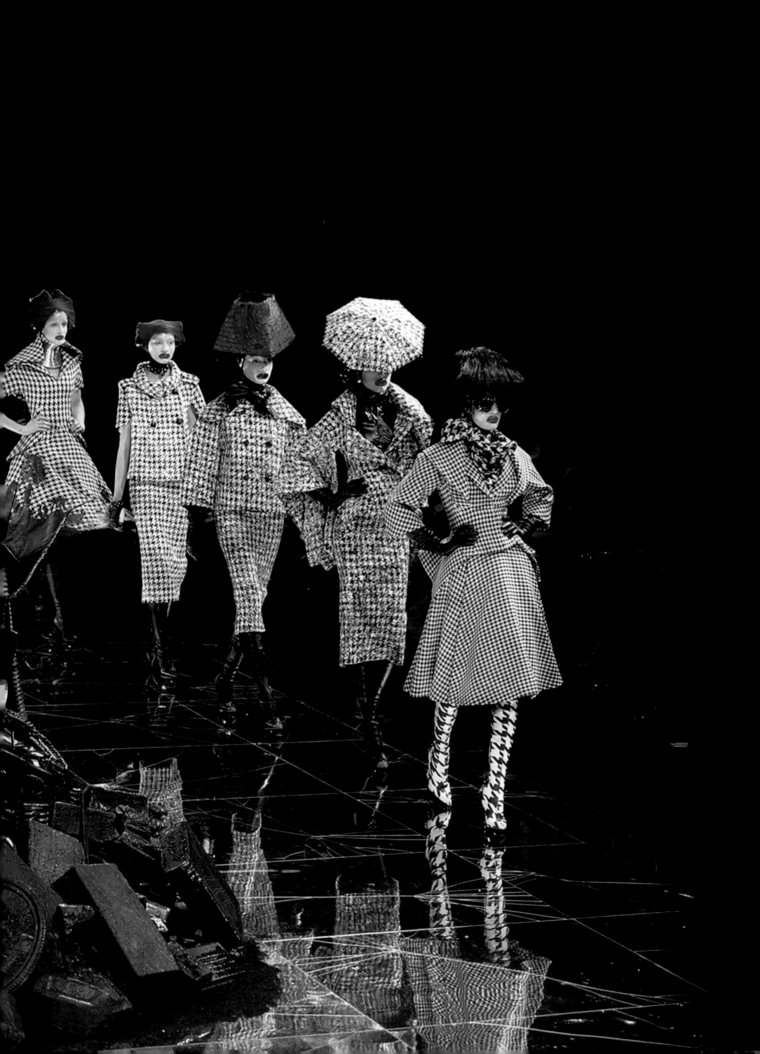

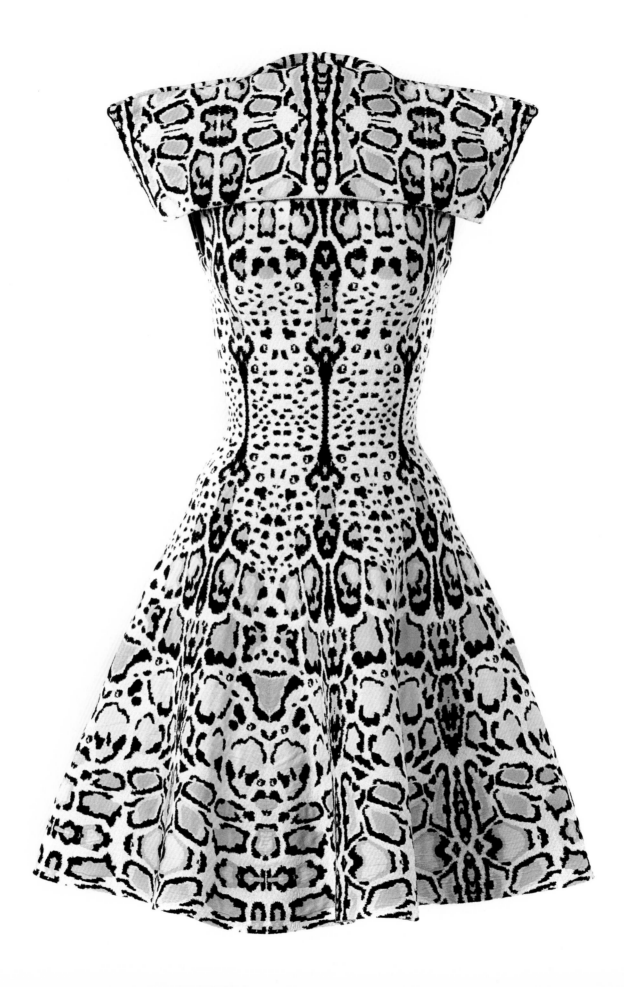

Azzedine Alaïa

Tunisian-born designer Azzedine Alaïa is disinterested in the cyclical nature of fashion. He eschews advertising, preferring to present new collections to his loyal clientele in his atelier whenever the clothing is ready, rather than in observance of the established fashion calendar. He does not court celebrity endorsements, although his clothing is worn by a litany of famous names, among them Michelle Obama. The longevity of his career – he has been designing since the 1960s – and his critical approach to fashion as a sculptural extension of the body have contributed to his reputation as an artist. His work has been the subject of several major solo exhibitions, including 'Azzedine Alaïa in the 21st Century' at the Groninger Museum in 2011, and has been included in numerous group exhibitions. In 2000 Alaïa's label was partially acquired by Prada with the tacit agreement that the Italian company would create a museum to house the Alaïa archive, which also boasts works of important vintage couture by designers such as Cristóbal Balenciaga and Madeleine Vionnet.

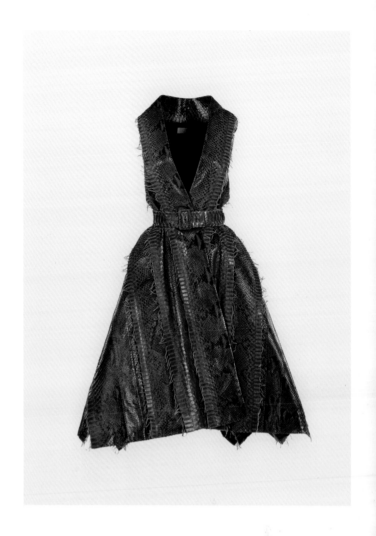

Alaïa's critical approach to fashion as a sculptural extension of the body has contributed to his reputation as an artist.

Above, opposite and pages 54–55: Azzedine Alaïa pieces from Spring/Summer 2009 (above), Autumn/Winter 2010 haute couture (opposite), Autumn/Winter 2011 haute couture (page 54) and Autumn/Winter 2008 haute couture (page 55).

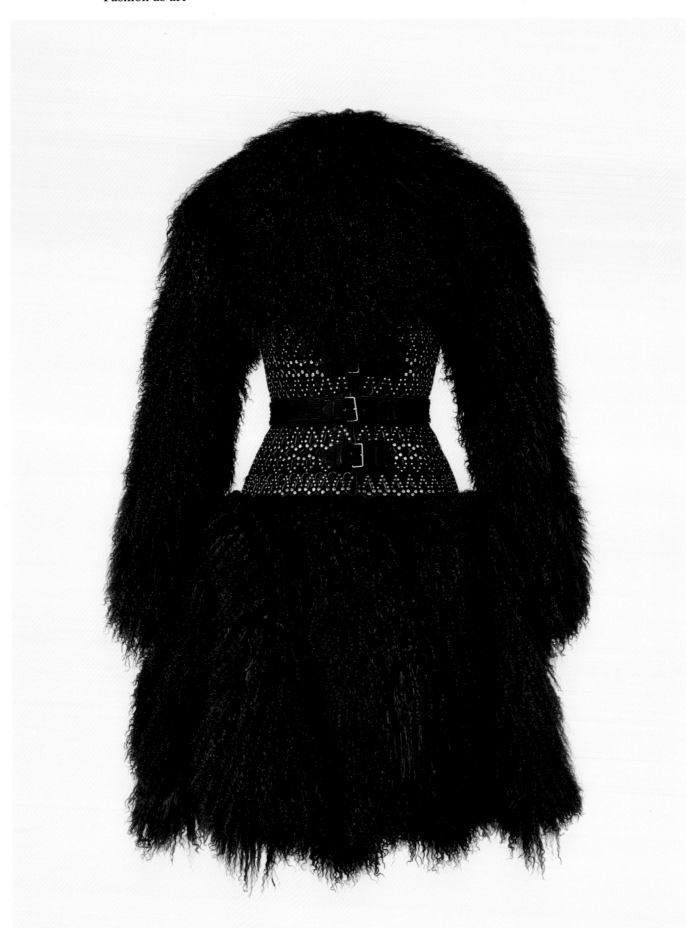

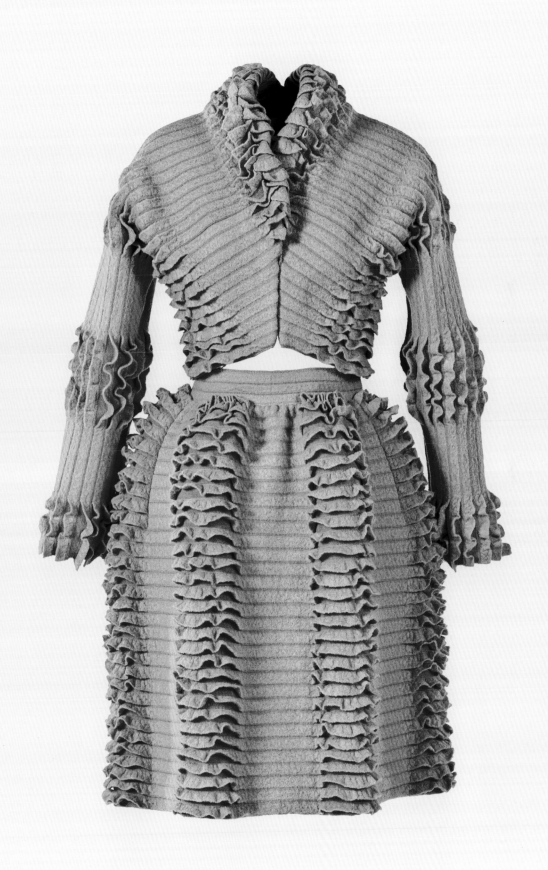

Rodarte

Rodarte, the Los Angeles fashion house established by sisters Kate and Laura Mulleavy in 2005, has achieved considerable success despite its youth. In 2010 the Mulleavys became the first fashion designers to be awarded the prestigious Americans for the Arts National Arts Award. They have quickly made a name for themselves with their cross-disciplinary approach to fashion, working on projects as diverse as the ballet costumes for the Oscar-winning film *Black Swan* (2010) and their work with artist Brody Conden on a performance piece for the exhibition 'MOVE!' at New York MoMA PS1, also in 2010.

In 2011 Rodarte was the subject of a major exhibition 'Rodarte: States of Matter' at Los Angeles County Museum of Art (LACMA), featuring the sisters' collection inspired by the Renaissance painter Fra Angelico, which they showed at the Pitti Immagine Uomo show in Florence the same year and later donated to LACMA's Costume and Textiles Department. The chiffon and satin gowns, in hues of orange, soft pink, light blue, pale green and gold that emulated Fra Angelico's palette, were installed in the museum's Italian Renaissance gallery alongside the artist's own paintings and sculptures.

In 2011 the sisters also collaborated on a handsome art book, *Rodarte, Catherine Opie, Alec Soth,* a collection of photographs of their work by artists Catherine Opie and Alec Soth, both of whom have reputations for making challenging documentary work that tackles issues of sexuality and difference (Opie), and race and class (Soth). Opie photographed models wearing Rodarte's more 'difficult' designs in everyday scenarios, while Soth's Polaroids and larger photographs depicted an array of apparently unconnected objects such as 'a torn rubber tire, a curving staircase, a depressing wooden cot with a cross on the pillow in unidentified California locations said to have inspired the Mulleavys' designs'.[8]

Fashion reporter Deidre Crawford described the duo's artistic process as reminiscent of that used by painters: 'Usually the pair start with an idea, then choose the colors and select about 100 images that they feel tell the story of what they're trying to convey and then they go about designing the collection. The images they choose could be anything from pictures of tornadoes to blades of grass, pieces of art, or varying degrees of sunlight...They created "wheat print" dresses that captured the colors from a wheat field during dusk, dawn, midday and stormy weather. Yet another collection was influenced by Van Gogh's starry skies and views from Pasadena's Mt Wilson Observatory.'[9] The sisters cite a wide spectrum of the arts as influences (at university Kate studied art history, and Laura literature) with past collections inspired by everything from the work of abstract expressionist painter Helen Frankenthaler to 1980s horror films.

Opposite: Rodarte runway show, Spring/Summer 2010.
Overleaf: Rodarte runway show, Autumn/Winter 2011.

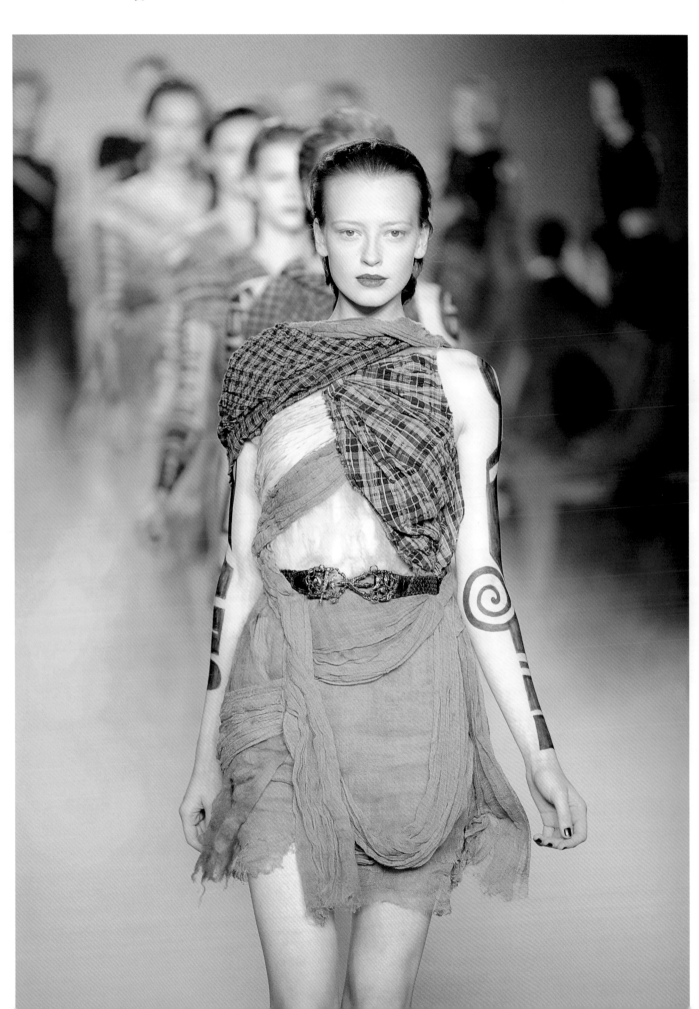

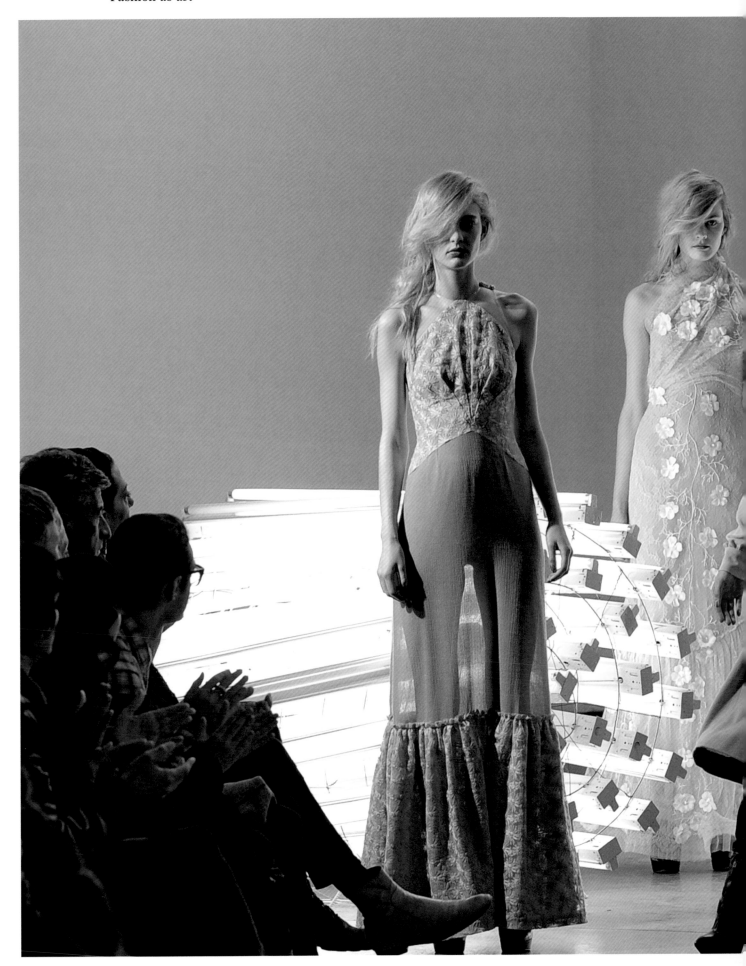

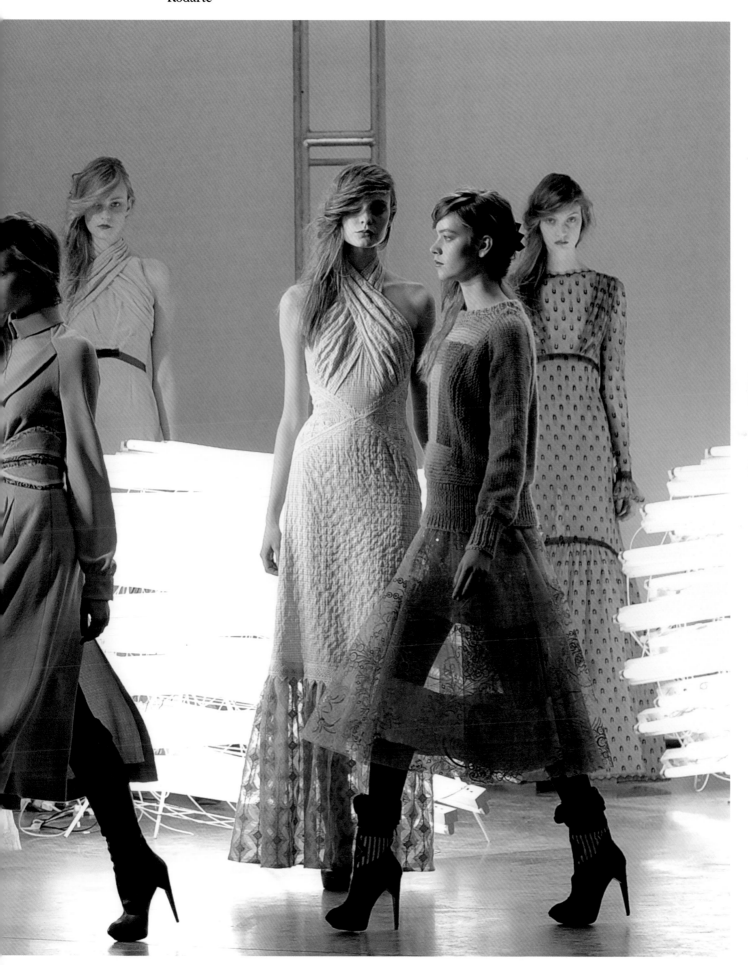

In conversation: Walter Van Beirendonck

Belgian Walter Van Beirendonck is known as one of the Antwerp Six, a group of influential avant-garde fashion designers, including Ann Demeulemeester and Dries Van Noten, who graduated from Antwerp's Royal Academy of Fine Arts between 1980 and 1981 and showed as a group at London Fashion Week in 1988. Van Beirendonck is the former member of the group most closely involved with the art world by virtue of his innovative designs and his continued presence in both individual and group museum exhibitions. In 2011 he collaborated with Austrian artist Erwin Wurm on a series of sculptures shown at the Middelheim Museum, Antwerp. In 2012 Van Beirendonck was the subject of a large-scale retrospective, 'Dream the World Awake', at the ModeMuseum, Antwerp, showcasing over three decades of his work and including a specially commissioned film with director Nick Knight and stylist Simon Foxton.

MITCHELL OAKLEY SMITH *Do you see your work as art?*

WALTER VAN BEIRENDONCK The way I work on a fashion project is completely different to how I approach an art project, but the end results have something in common – you can see a fashion show as a performance, in many ways. On the other end, it's very important for me that the fashion collections can be bought and worn and have a link to reality and the consumer. So I think there's a great distinction between the two [worlds]. I still feel very much a fashion designer. Since the very beginning [of my career] there has been a lot of interest from the art world in my shows, but despite this, and maybe because of my active presence in the fashion world, I feel more like a designer. It's the field through which I choose to communicate. I could

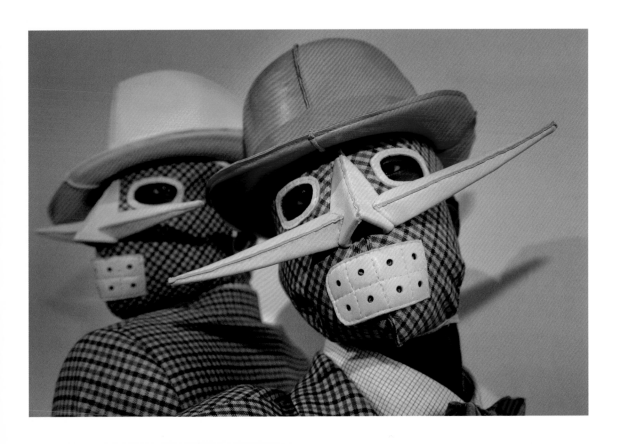

have chosen to be a painter or a sculptor, but I chose fashion, not because I saw it as more commercial, but because it gave me more opportunities to communicate.

MOS *What makes the end results of fashion and art similar?*

WVB Well, of course, it's all about communication, and that's something that fashion and art have in common – we communicate messages through what we create.

MOS *Do you prefer one over the other?*

WVB I like that fashion has a quick pace, and every six months you can reflect on what is happening in the world – it's an advantage for a fashion designer that your pace is faster than other artists, and that's interesting for me. But I enjoy both [art and fashion]. I only started to make art by invitation – it wasn't that I desperately wanted to become an artist. A gallery that followed my work came up with an idea for me to do an installation. It was a very spontaneous way to enter the art world and I really enjoyed it. The power of being in a gallery is a really different energy to the fashion world.

MOS *Is how a collection is communicated important to the way it is received?*

WVB Every collection has a very clear topic or subject. Not so much that it's more prominent than the actual clothes, but it's something very important to me. The names [of the collections] always reflect something I want to express in that moment. It's not a necessity that everyone who sees the clothes in the shops gets the message. It's great the shopkeepers can explain certain slogans and ideas, but it's not important to me. I like that people can just buy the clothes because they love them.

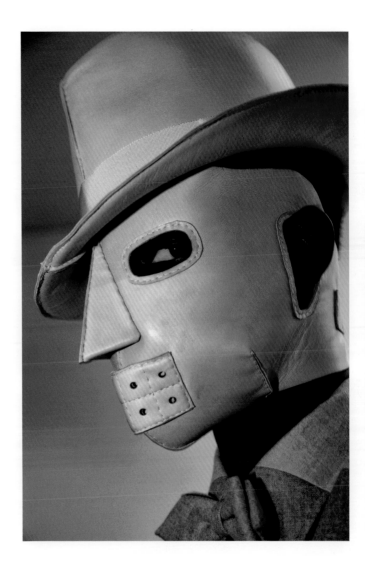

Above and opposite: Walter Van Beirendonck,
Autumn/Winter 2012.
Overleaf: Walter Van Beirendonck, Spring/Summer 2013.

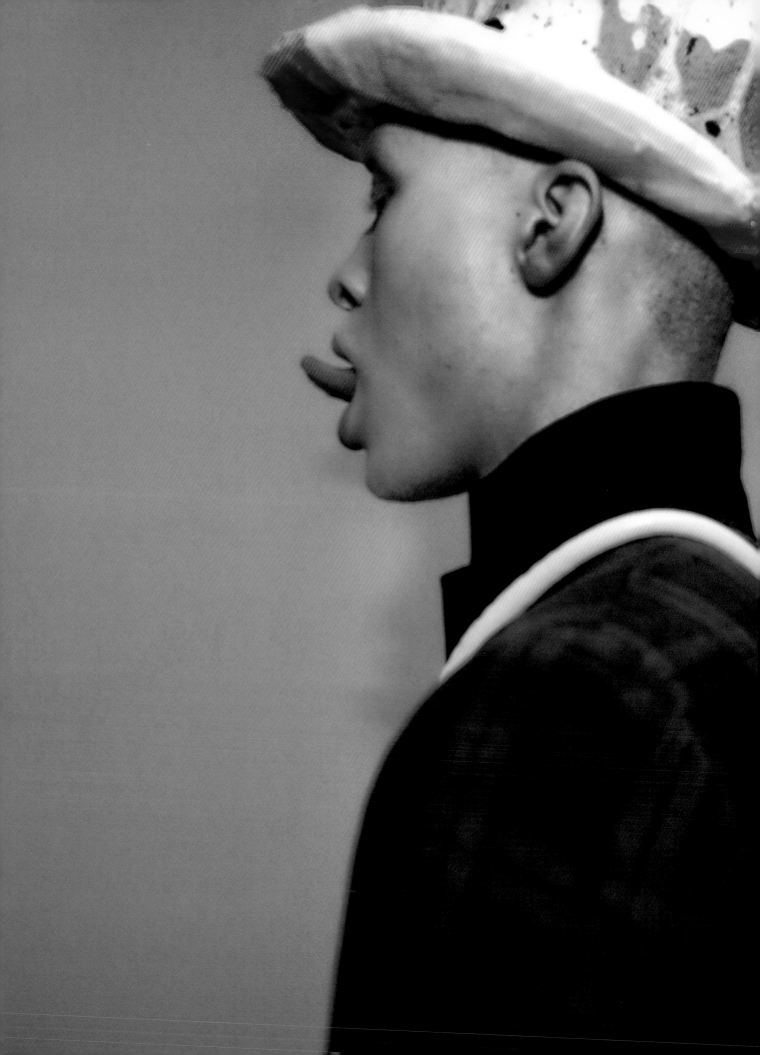

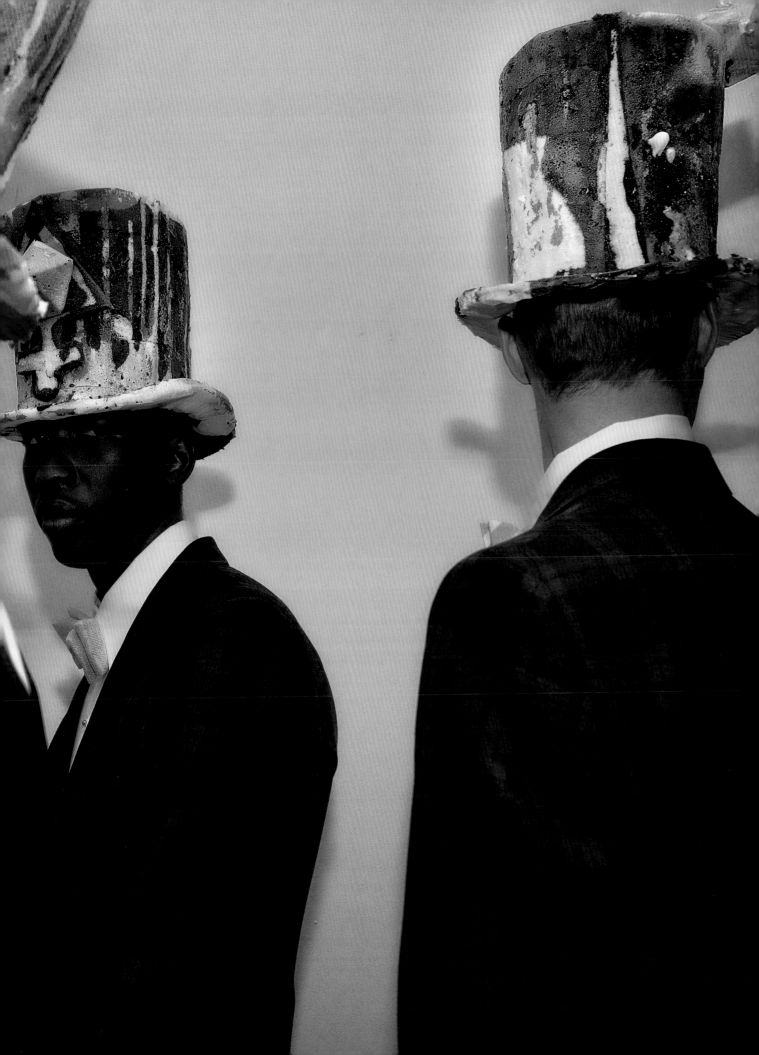

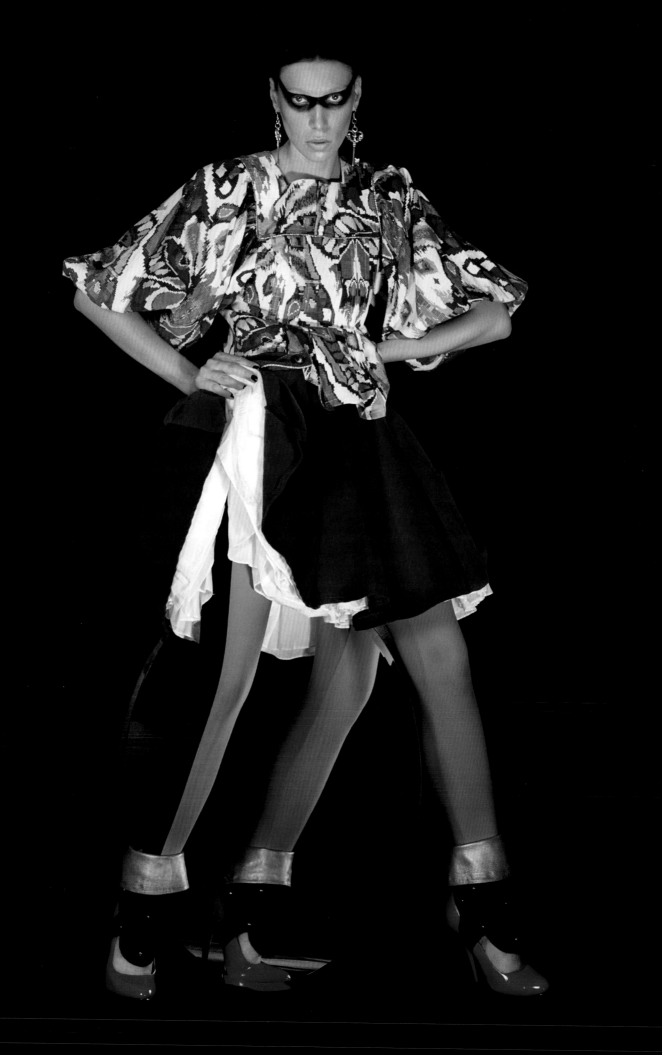

Birthday Suit

While Australian label Birthday Suit is a commercially rooted venture like much of the fashion business, the creative output of its founding designers, Técha Noble and Emma Price, has a much greater artistic value. Born from their decade-old performance group The Kingpins, which was formed in the Sydney drag king scene of the early 2000s, Birthday Suit explores the varying elements of costume - gender, culture, sexuality and race - that subvert traditional ideas of beauty and challenge perceptions of the norm. 'It always harks back to costume,' explains Price. 'What we end up making is conceptually driven, but is often informed by something we find: a readymade wig or costume, for example. In a way, this creates a more complex conversation because what we make is inspired by something of the same medium.'[10]

Price part-owns Sydney vintage clothing emporium Zoo and lectures in performance art at the College of Fine Arts, Sydney, while Noble works as a graphic artist, often in the fashion industry. To launch their fashion label then seemed like a natural progression. Founded in 2007, Birthday Suit remains intrinsically connected to Price and Noble's art, yet it allows them to engage with their audience in a more direct way. As Price explains: 'We struggled with and debated the validity of the commercial space [with The Kingpins' work], trying not to fall into making souvenirs or work that is softened or watered-down for a domestic space.' As well as wardrobe staples, the label also creates one-off accessories: a safety-pin-and-bead wig resembling that worn by Elizabeth Taylor in *Cleopatra*; a cape that wryly incorporates hand-stitched images of the characters in the film *Picnic at Hanging Rock*; or catsuits made from crocheted cobweb fabric.

'For me, fashion was always about dressing up,' explains Price. 'I have a nostalgic approach to fashion, as opposed to a forward approach. It's collective. It's from a memory and of a time.' While fashion references the past cynically, recycling period designs at regular intervals, it rarely acknowledges the present as a product of history. Birthday Suit's approach is therefore the antithesis of the concept of historical fashion held by the majority of commercial designers. The designers list the Art Deco era as a strong influence on their work, not for its style of clothing but for its historical significance as 'a movement that really changed the figure and form of the female – it was revolutionary and about female liberation,' referring to the removal of corsetry. Perhaps, then, Birthday Suit is revolutionary and liberating in the way it approaches the machine-like global fashion industry with an alternative approach to clothing.

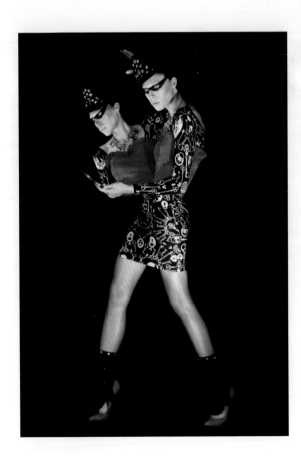

Above, opposite and pages 66–67: Birthday Suit, 'Smoke & Mirrors' collection, Autumn/Winter 2010.

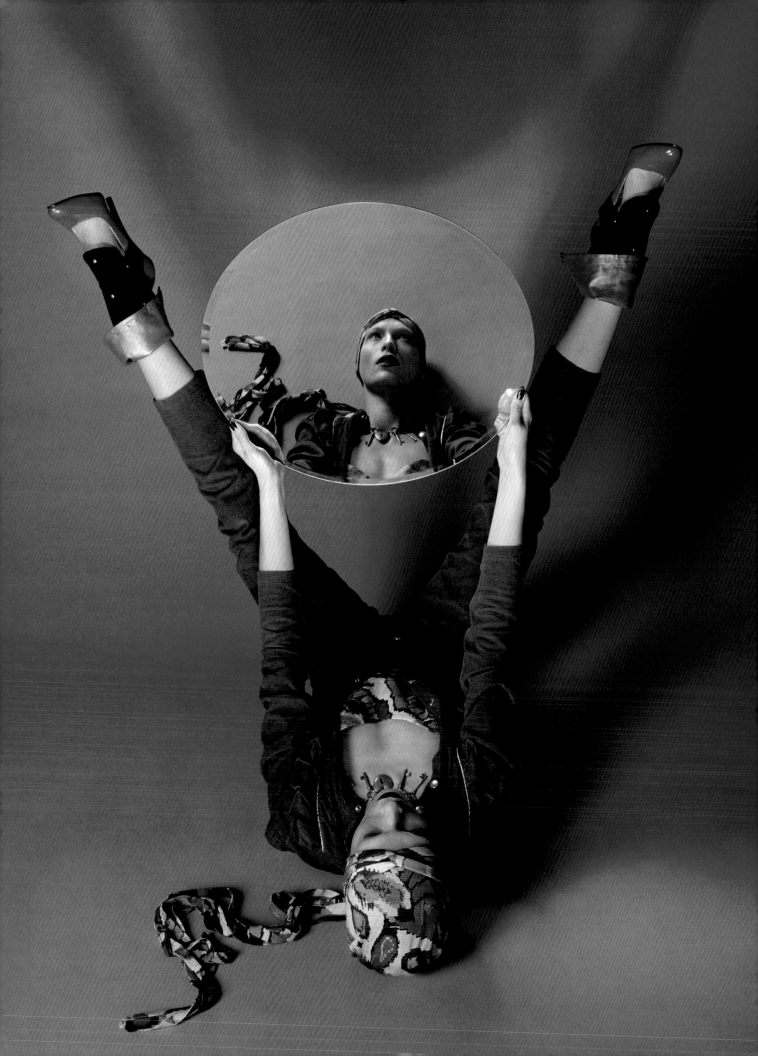

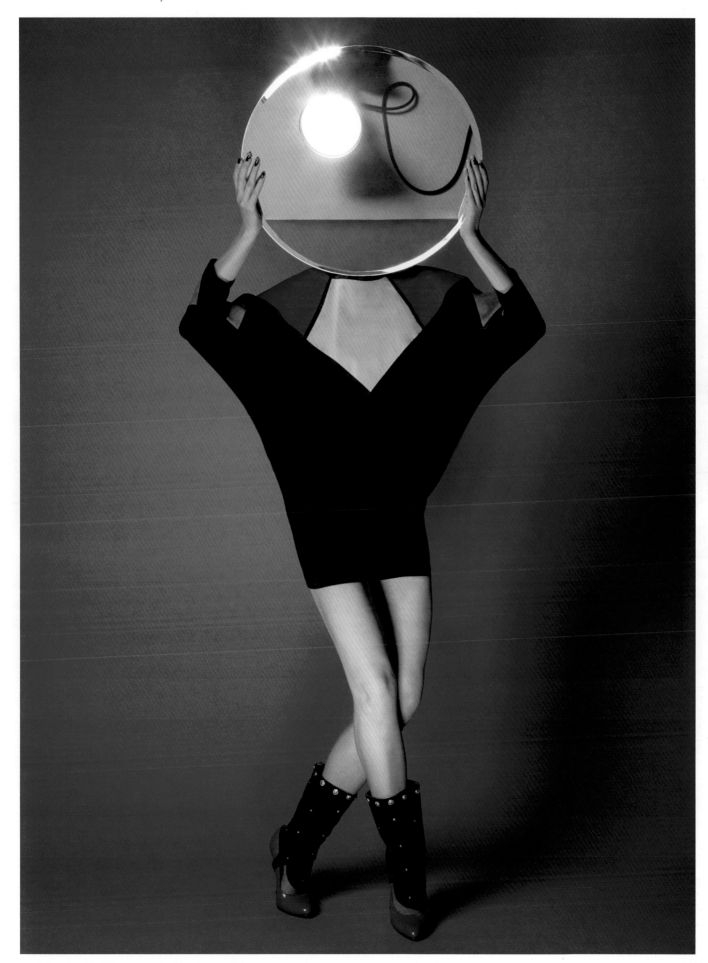

In conversation: threeASFOUR

threeASFOUR is the creation of designers Gabi Asfour, Angela Donhauser and Adi Gil, who formed the New York-based fashion label in 2005. Their work has been collected and displayed by the Victoria & Albert Museum, London; the Cooper–Hewitt Museum, New York; and the Costume Institute at the Metropolitan Museum of Art, New York, where it featured in the 2008 exhibition 'Superheroes: Fashion and Fantasy'. The label is favoured by the innovative musician, artist and fashion maverick Björk, who the designers have dressed on several occasions, notably for her music video *Moon*. threeASFOUR's Spring/Summer 2010 collection was the result of a collaboration with conceptual artist Yoko Ono. The collection, based on Ono's dot drawings, was presented at Milk Studios, New York, accompanied by a loose reenactment of Ono's seminal 1964 performance *Cut Piece*.

MITCHELL OAKLEY SMITH *Why do you show your work in both fashion and art worlds?*

THREEASFOUR threeASFOUR has, from the very beginning, been involved in fashion and art. Along with the show we do during New York Fashion Week we have participated in numerous exhibitions at museums and galleries around the world. The result has been always surprising and rewarding as the pieces find new life in their new temporary homes. It is always inspiring to see people's reactions to our work in different contexts: on a mannequin, on a rack, worn on the body or displayed in an art venue or museum.

MOS *Is it important for you as fashion designers to engage in projects outside the regular commercial presentations of the fashion world?*

TAF It is important for us to have a variety of creative projects as it keeps our creative juices flowing. Sometimes the routine of the fashion cycle, with its fashion shows, showroom period and manufacturing, gets repetitive and predictable. It is nice to break the ice before it freezes you.

MOS *The way you present your collections differs greatly from the standard runway show. Why is this?*

TAF In the case of threeASFOUR, we feel the clothing is part of the environment it resides in, and the performative aspect [of our shows] is necessary as it brings [the clothes] to life. In conveying the language of our garments, presentation is key, like a book with its corresponding cover and graphics.

MOS *Do you consider what you do art or design?*

TAF Some people call us artists; others call us designers. All we know is that we are in the art of the communication of ideas and through our clothing.

Opposite and overleaf: threeASFOUR, Autumn/Winter 2012.

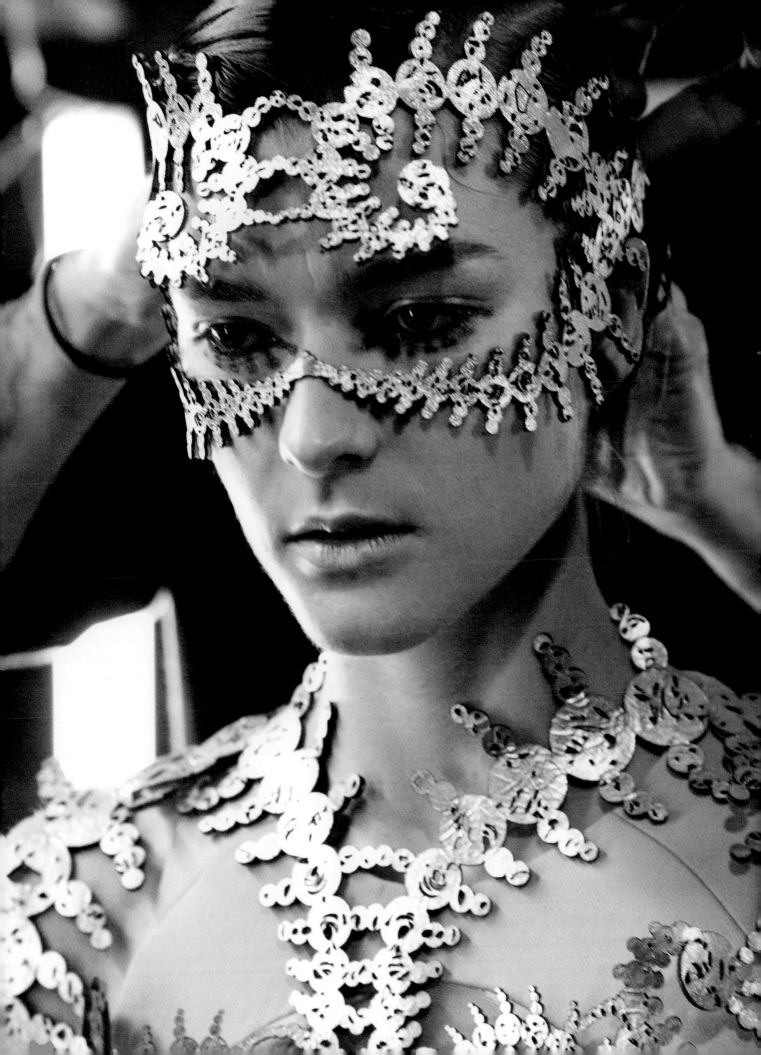

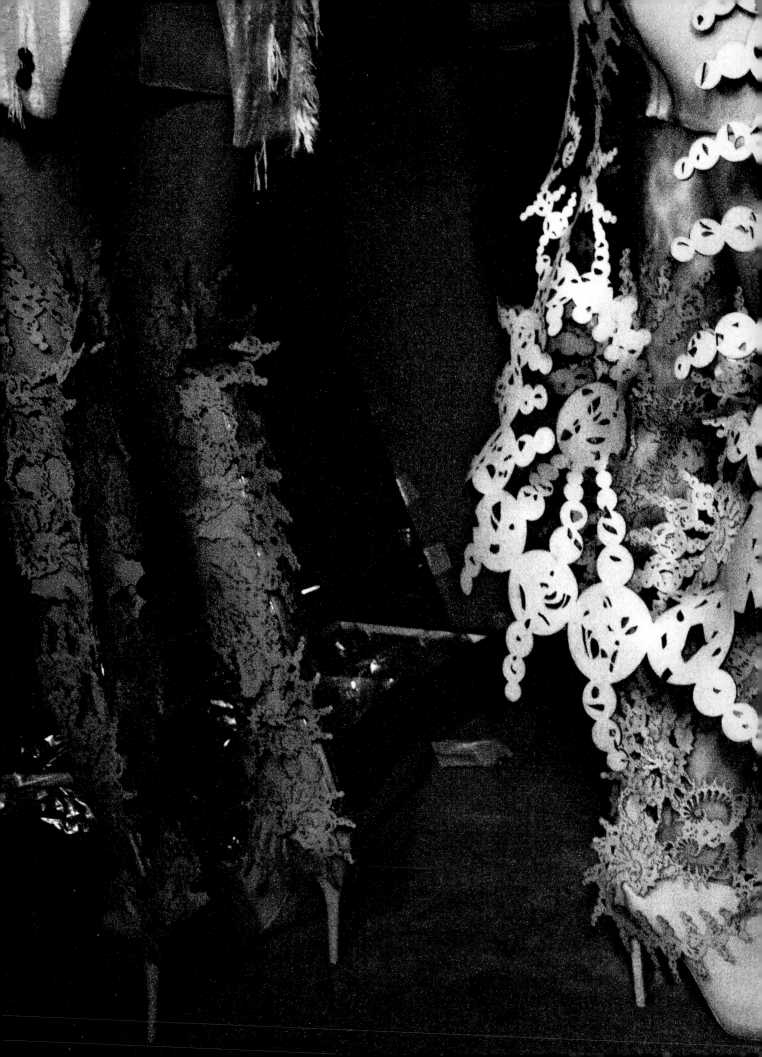

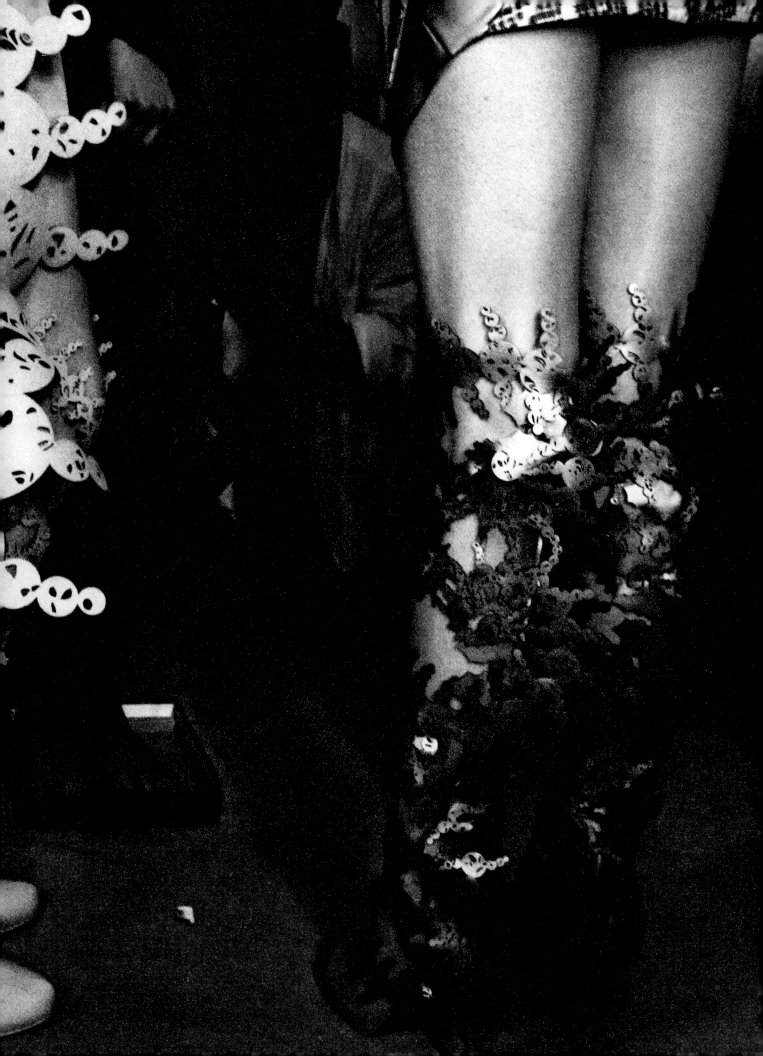

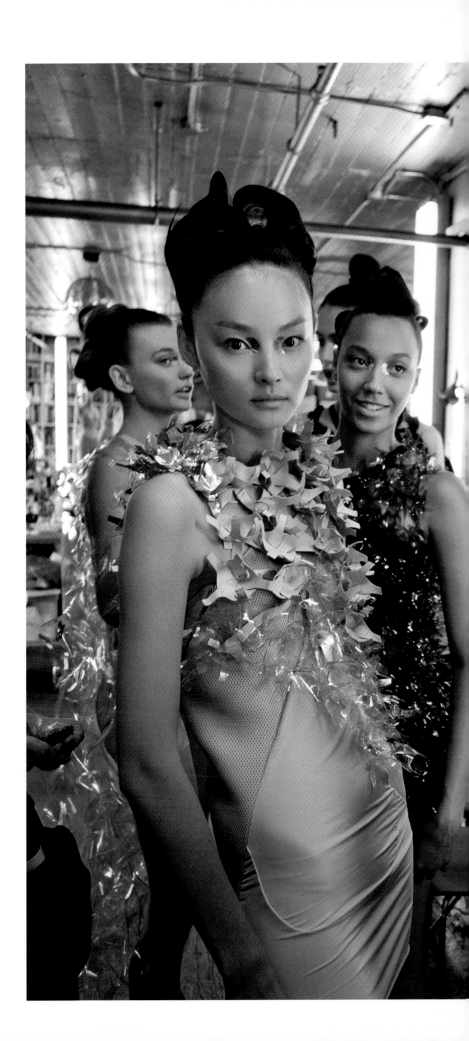

threeASFOUR, Spring/Summer 2011.

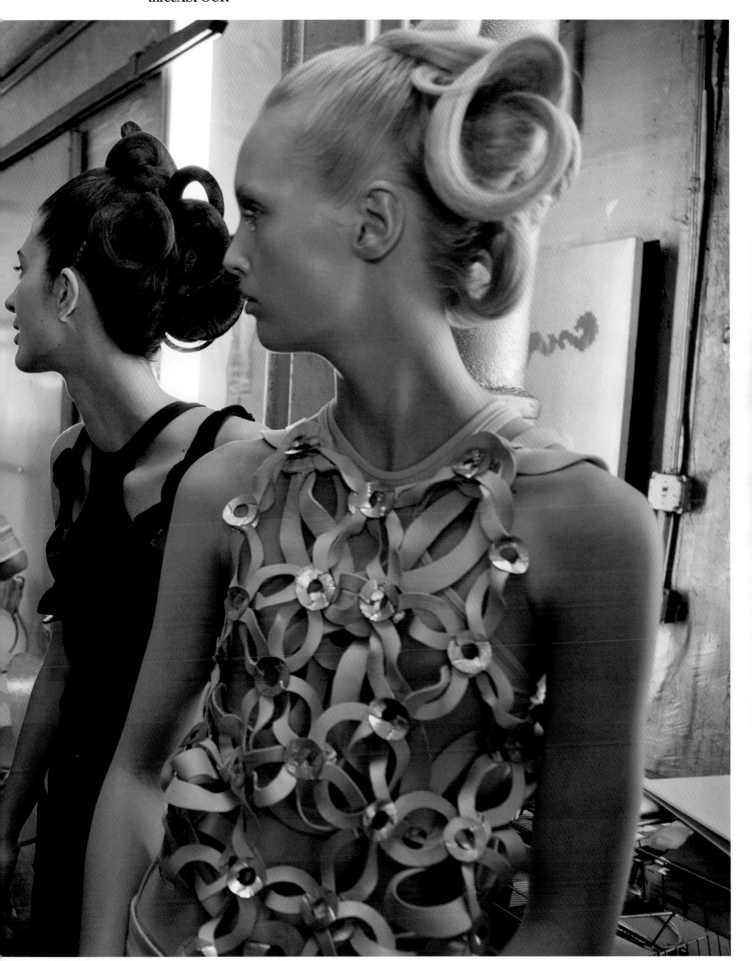

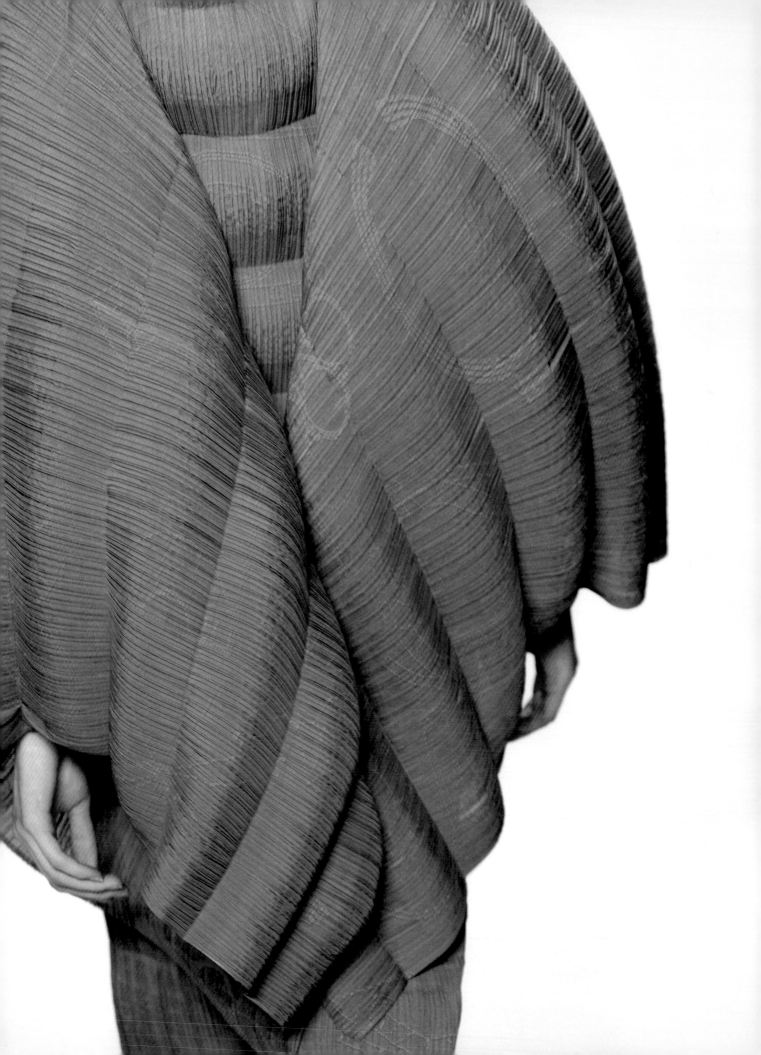

Issey Miyake

Issey Miyake is part of a seminal group of 20th-century Japanese fashion designers, including Rei Kawakubo (of Comme des Garçons) and Yohji Yamamoto, whose work is considered revolutionary for its use of materials and its iconoclastic, conceptual approach to fashion. Their creative output is frequently described as art by virtue of its contribution to a larger dialogue about what fashion is and what it could become.

Miyake blends traditional, historical elements of Japanese fashion (such as wrapping and folding) with cutting-edge technological innovations that have revolutionized fabric manufacturing. His designs demonstrate a desire to expand the potential for clothing outside of the purely functional. Some showcase the development of new materials that have a sculptural quality when worn on the body; others feature clothing that is installed and exhibited in absence of the body. He is best known for his technique of permanently pleating silk via a heat treatment, first used in his iconic, long-running 'Pleats Please' collection in 1993, which payed homage to legendary early 20th-century couturiers Madame Grès and Fortuny while taking fashion into the future with technological advances. The fruits of this project formed part of the exhibition 'Issey Miyake: Making Things' at Fondation Cartier in Paris in 1998.

A-POC (A Piece of Cloth), another long-running project developed with designer Dai Fujiwara in 1998, further exemplifies Miyake's conceptual and technologically innovative approach to clothing. Essentially a cutting-edge take on the notion of bespoke tailoring, A-POC allows clients to custom-make clothing by cutting material at their desired length from one continuous roll of machine-woven fabric, produced from a single piece of thread. A-POC represents an economy of means articulated as a utopian model of no wastage. The Museum of Modern Art in New York collected examples of the project in 2006, confirming both its conceptual merit and Miyake's artistic longevity.

Miyake has collaborated with numerous contemporary artists, including Japanese appropriation artist Yasumasa Morimura, whose reenactments of classic paintings were reproduced as fabric prints in 1996, and Chinese artist Cai Guo-Qiang, whose trademark gunpowder drawings were transferred onto delicate printed dresses in 1999. Japanese Superflat movement artist Takashi Murakami collaborated on a Kaikai Kiki/Issey Miyake series that was introduced in 2000, and in 2004–5 Miyake collaborated with Aya Takano, another Japanese artist associated with the movement, using her *kawaii* ('cute') pop-inspired images for a range of rain wear including jackets and boots. Other collaborators have included Japanese contemporary artists Chiho Aoshima and Mr. In late 2004, anime-inspired heads by Mr. were dressed in Issey Miyake clothes and installed in the label's boutique in Roppongi Hills, Tokyo's largest shopping complex.

Miyake's presence in the art world dates back to 1982, when one of his gowns appeared on the cover of *Artforum,* the first time a fashion designer had been featured in the magazine. This endorsement by one of the world's leading contemporary art journals was met with a derision and approbation that seems absurd in hindsight. Since then his work has been included in innumerable exhibitions and surveys at art galleries and museums and is held in the permanent collections of many fashion museums and costume institutes. The Miyake label hosts changing art exhibitions and installations in its own retail spaces, such as the boutique designed by Frank Gehry in New York's Tribeca neighbourhood.

Although Miyake officially retired in 2007, he retains a directorial vision for his namesake company, overseeing its many brand 'project' strands. He also remains active in the Miyake Issey Foundation, established in 2004 with four other Japanese designers; among its many projects is 21-21 Design Sight, a design museum that opened in Tokyo in 2007.

Opposite: Dai Fujiwara for Issey Miyake, garment from the A-POC project, Spring/Summer 2008.

Tru$t Fun!

Tru$t Fun! is an accessories-based collaborative venture initiated in 2007 by Shane Sakkeus, Jonathan Zawada and Annie Wright-Zawada, all of whom work predominantly in graphic design, illustration, typography and art direction in addition to exhibiting their work as solo artists. Sakkeus and Zawada had both previously worked in collaboration with fashion houses – Sakkeus creating prints for Sydney-based designer Josh Goot, and Zawada providing prints, art direction and graphic design for Australian labels Tina Kalivas, Insight and Ksubi – but Tru$t Fun! marked their first independent practice in a commercial fashion sphere. Zawada explains the origins of their emphasis on the

'It goes against the grain of commercial fashion because each piece is different.'

Jonathan Zawada

individuality of each piece: 'I had been doing a hell of a lot of T-shirt prints...I thought that the idea of printing the same T-shirt in multiple quantities was really archaic, and Shane felt the same way.'[11] In response, the trio employed manufacturing processes that other brands were not interested in at the time, such as tie-dye and digital printing, to create limited-edition, individually numbered scarves, bags, kimonos and jewelry. 'It goes against the grain of commercial fashion because each piece is different,' explains Zawada. This anarchic spirit also guides *Petit Mal!*, Zawada and Sakkeus's fashion comic, and *Fashematics!*, their fashion–maths blog.

Opposite and pages 78–79: Tru$t Fun!, 'Glory' scarves, 2009.

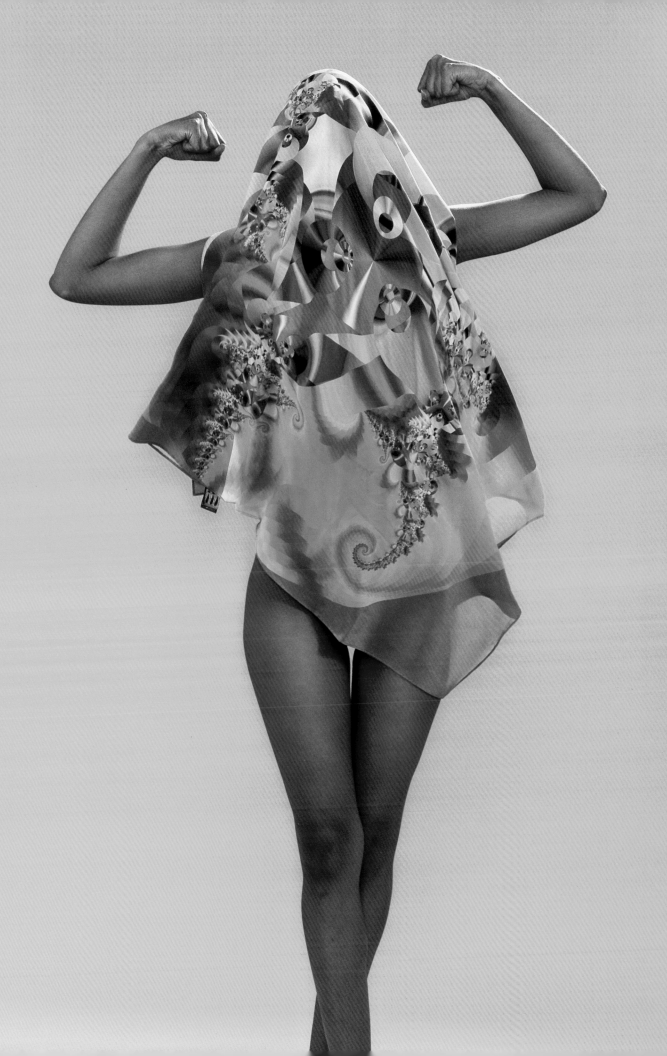

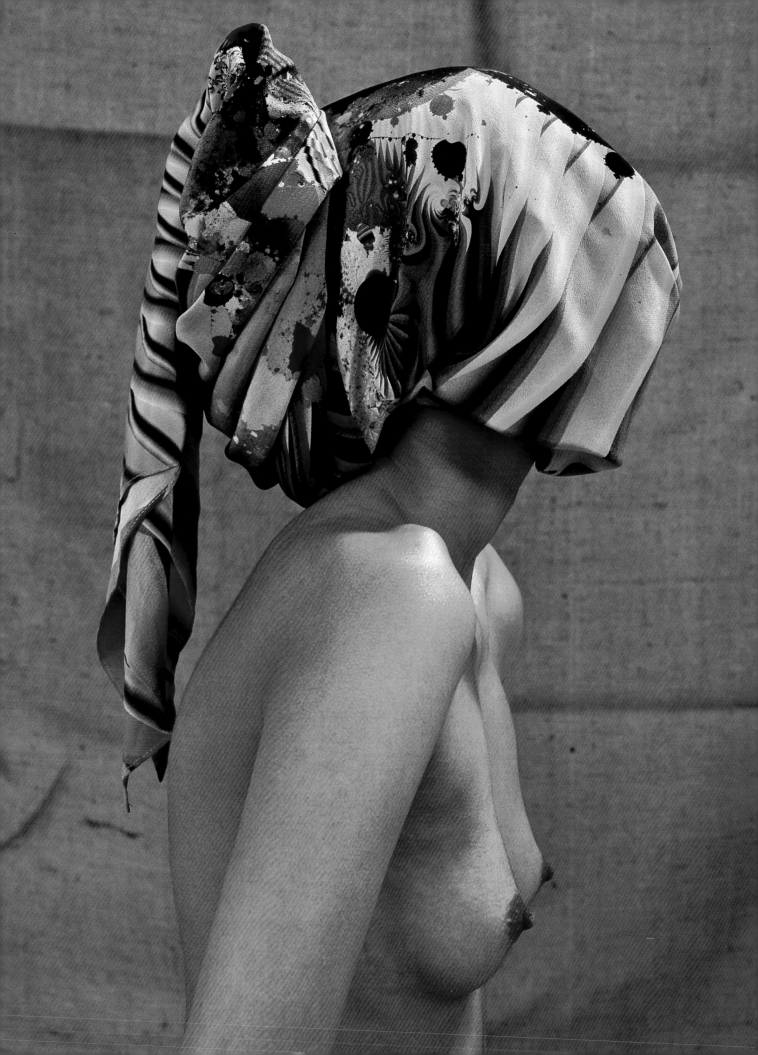

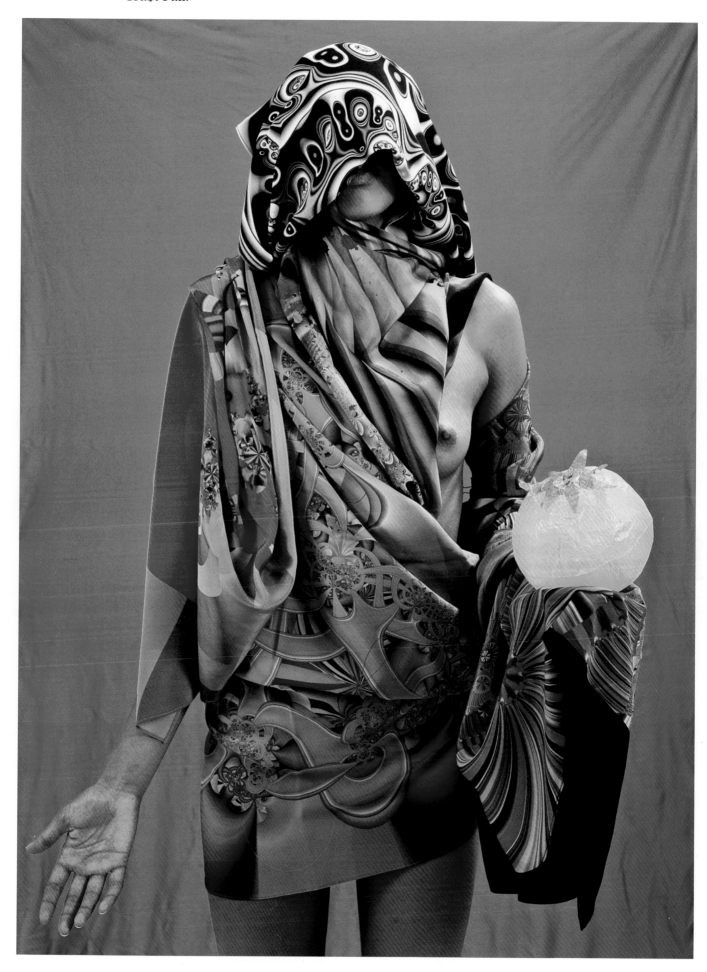

In conversation:
Adrian Mesko,
Temps Des Rěves

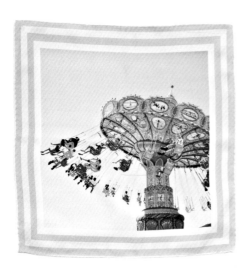

Czech-born, Sydney-raised, New York-based photographer Adrian Mesko has, since 2010, produced a series of photographic prints on silk-satin scarves under the label Temps Des Rěves as a creative aside to his career as a fashion photographer for magazines such as *Vogue, GQ* and *Harper's Bazaar*. The project, which is based on a philosophy of providing wearers with an intangible 'feeling', is sold at stores such as Liberty of London and has quickly gained global recognition.

MITCHELL OAKLEY SMITH *Why did you begin Temps Des Rěves?*

ADRIAN MESKO While I was living in London [1999–2005] I experimented a lot with printing my photographs onto different fabrics and sold this work in a couple of galleries in Notting Hill. When I moved back to Australia I stopped for some reason, but later I made a photographic print for a friend on silk/lycra. The left-over fabric from that project had been lying around the house for three years when the scarf idea presented itself. The whole story of the brand came to me almost immediately: the name Temps Des Rěves means 'Dreamtime' in French; the logo represents me and my greyhound Yves during the summer of 1988, which is when I first emigrated to Australia [from Czechoslovakia] and my Dreamtime began. The yellow packaging is the colour of my portfolio. It's all quite personal, including the photographs that I release to print onto the silks. There is a story woven into each one of them.

MOS *Some artists or critics feel that it devalues an artist's work to apply it to a fashion garment – do you share this view, or simply see fashion as a different form in which to show your work?*

AM Fashion is a means of expression. The way someone puts together what they choose to wear is a form of creativity, an expression of how they might be feeling before they step out the door or a projection of who they'd like to be. Even someone who wears a utilitarian form of clothing, such as a suit, five days a week can make the smallest gesture by choosing a certain tie. They might not even realize why they are reaching for it as they rush out the door, but this sort of expression on a subconscious level is still important. At the end of the day I don't see anything wrong with bringing art into people's lives, even if it is through an accessory. The first time I received a sample [printed scarf] and showed it to my girlfriend, there was a magic moment while she and her flatmate played with the floating photograph: throwing it into the air; wearing it on their heads, as skirts and as wrap-around dresses.

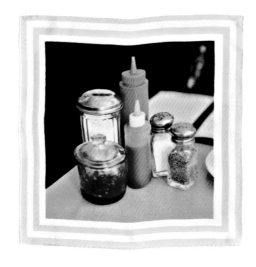

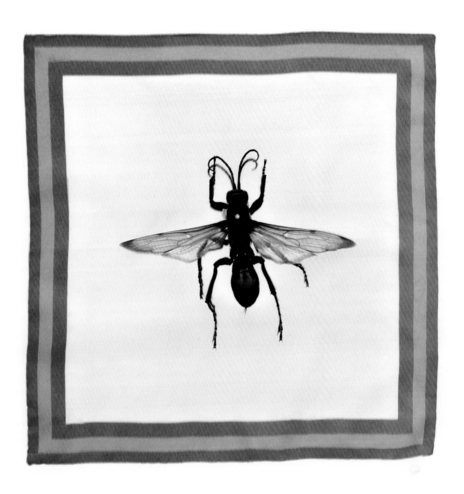

Above: Temps Des Rêves, 'Stanley' scarf, 2012.
Opposite: Temps Des Rêves, 'Santa Cruz' (above)
and 'Americano' (below) scarves, 2012.

MOS *If a fashion accessory such as a scarf bears the mark of an artist's hand, is it then an artwork in its own right?*

AM In my opinion art's main purpose is to be a sign of its times, a representation of what it means to be alive in this time, this place. Temps Des Rêves was never intended to be a commercial project. It was a personal project, a biographical one – the name, the symbolism of the boy – it's all my story. Although I'm not calling it art, I don't think it's any less worthy of the name simply because I'm not bringing it to the people via the traditional gatekeepers of the industry: galleries. I recently went to the Frieze Art Fair in New York, and I couldn't help feeling like I had just walked into a shopping mall. The whole building was divided into cubicles, and there were grim-looking gallerists staring at their laptops, looking more like bored, worried retail staff than guardians of the arts.

MOS *Is it pleasurable to see people 'wearing' your art, so to speak?*

AM There is a difference between seeing people wearing them, and the initial moment when the photograph is revealed as they unfold the silk. To be honest, while that first moment is quite special, seeing people wearing my photographs makes me feel a little embarrassed.

Henrik Vibskov

Danish design is globally recognized for its fine craftsmanship, use of natural materials and innovation, but beyond the work of a handful of artists such as Olafur Eliasson, the country is rarely associated with avant-garde eclecticism. It's precisely this incongruence, however, on which Copenhagen-based menswear designer Henrik Vibskov thrives, with a cross-disciplinary practice that extends to film, music and visual art.

Vibskov has operated his namesake label since he graduated from Central Saint Martins, London, in 2001. His designs interrogate and explore the established traditions of men's tailoring, challenging and updating existing styles for the contemporary customer. In 2003 Vibskov became the first Danish designer to show his collection at Paris Fashion Week. His experimental and experiential approach to presentation has earned him a reputation as an artist working within the established fashion system. His work has subsequently been included in numerous exhibitions, including shows at the V1 Gallery in Copenhagen, Sotheby's Gallery in New York and the Millbank Gallery in London. In addition to his fashion work, Vibskov participates in a collaborative art project, Vibskov & Emenius, with Swedish artist Andreas Emenius, a former classmate. Their *The Fringe Projects* – a series of installations, objects, performances, videos and self-portraits exploring illusion, surface and movement – was exhibited at the Zeeuws Museum in Middelburg, the Netherlands, in 2009.

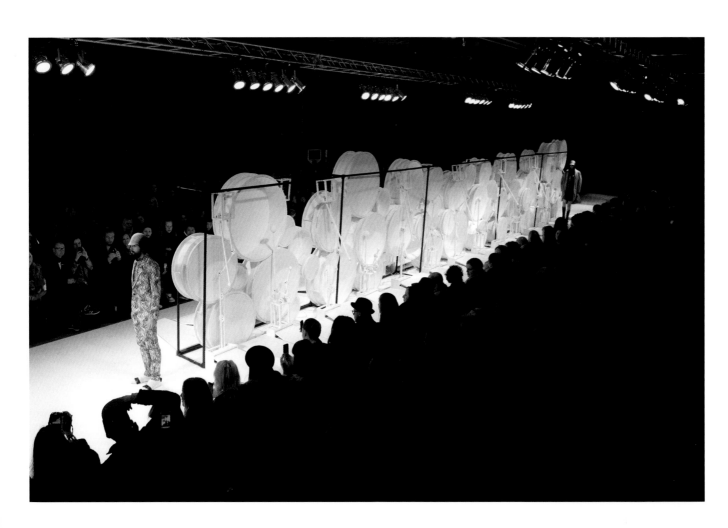

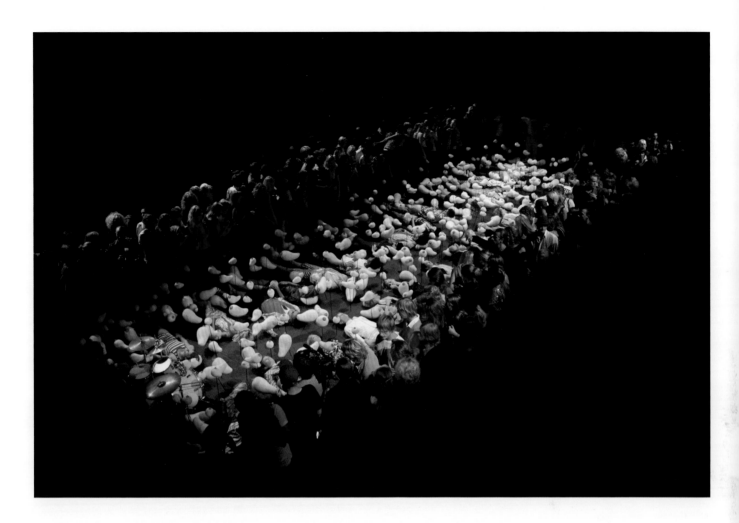

Vibskov's experimental and experiential approach to presentation has earned him a reputation as an artist working within the established fashion system.

Above: Henrik Vibskov, 'The Big Wet Shiny Boobies', Spring/Summer 2007.
Opposite: Henrik Vibskov, 'The Shrink Wrap Spectacular', Autumn/Winter 2012.
Overleaf: Henrik Vibskov, costumes for *Recollection Quartett*, installation
commissioned for the Mercedes-Benz Fashion Festival Berlin in collaboration
with MoMu, Antwerp and art director Frederik Heyman, 2010.

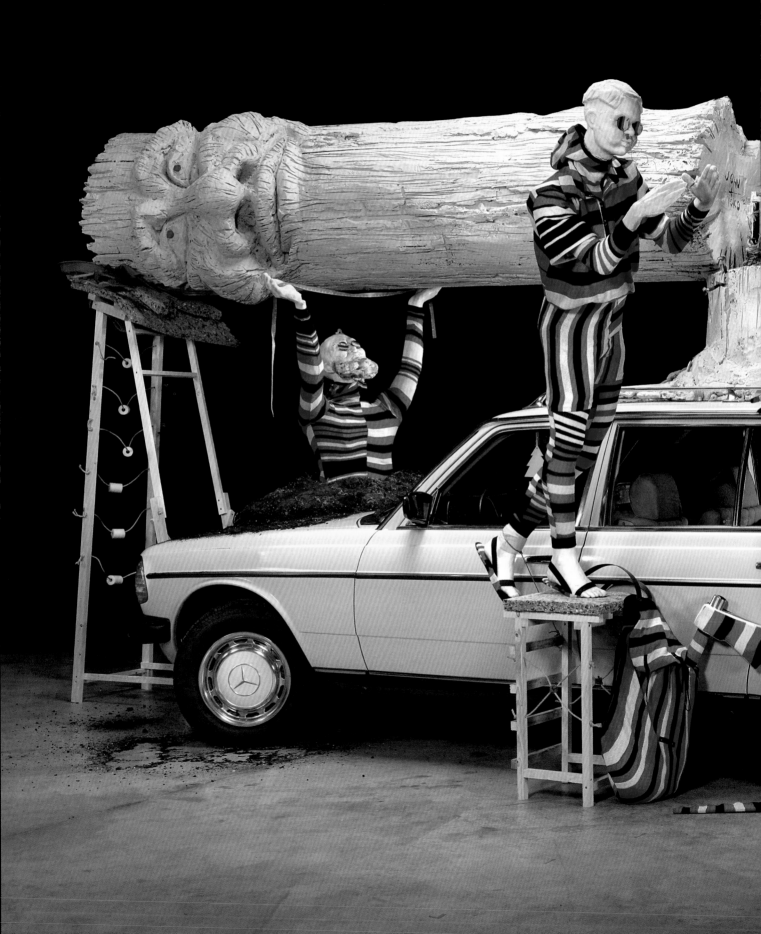

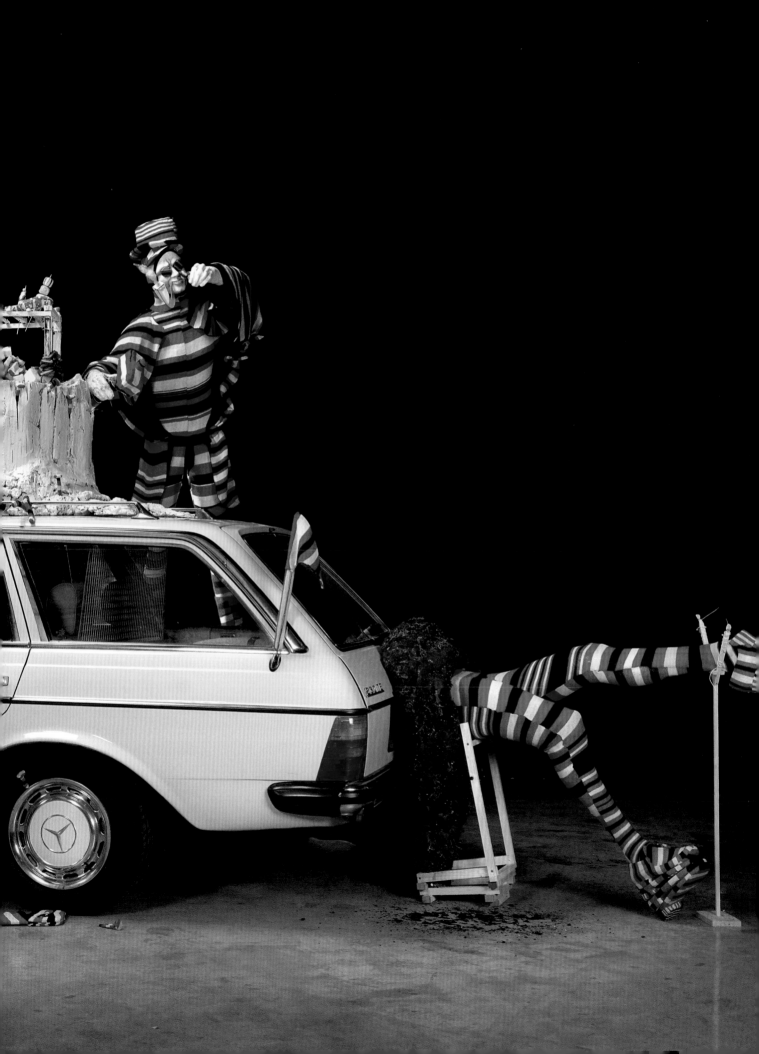

MATERIALBYPRODUCT

The French fashion industry maintains its own set of rules, determined by the Chambre Syndicale de la Haute Couture, regarding the authenticity and practice of haute couture, but Australian designer Susan Dimasi, founder of Melbourne-based **MATERIALBYPRODUCT**, has crafted her own approach: 'I am, in some way, trying to reinvent haute couture by drawing on artistic systems and methods to make it relevant and accessible in a contemporary age. Where I differ from Parisian haute couture is in that that system is a preserved tradition; I'm not preserving tradition, I'm creating my own, because I don't come from that tradition, I didn't train in it, and I'm not based in it. My concept is of a laboratory of invention of ideas [that are] relevant to me and my audience.'[12]

Each aspect of a MATERIALBYPRODUCT garment has been developed, perfected and continuously evolved by Dimasi as an entire concept, referred to by names such as The Mark, The Cut and The Join. The Mark is the textile pattern, also known as a template; it takes the form of a multi-sized grid, which is then labelled with a series of dots by Dimasi. Like a musical score, the markings on the template are functional as well as beautiful and guide pleating and cutting to manipulate cloth into garments. The Cut – that is, the cutting of the fabric – typically engages an entire length of cloth in a play with positive and negative shapes, resulting in little or zero waste. The Join highlights and finishes the cut with silk binding that joins the edges with a fine diagonal hand stitch. Dimasi's latest development of her couture system is called the Bleed Project; it involves hand-stamped coloured marks on the garment that evolve uniquely with each wearer's body as the ink bleeds due to body heat, perfume and washing. Clients are invited to bring garments back for a further evolution of the dots and marks. 'Each visit and wear makes the garment more customized and unique,' says Dimasi. 'The system is cumulative and gives people access to a demi-couture type of experience.' Dimasi sees the Bleed Project as working on multiple levels: conceptually, it straddles a line between commodity and art, suggesting to the fashion industry that its future lies in service rather than manufacturing; culturally, it creates a rare opportunity for client and designer to engage directly.

'I am...drawing on artistic systems and methods to make [haute couture] relevant and accessible in a contemporary age.'

Susan Dimasi

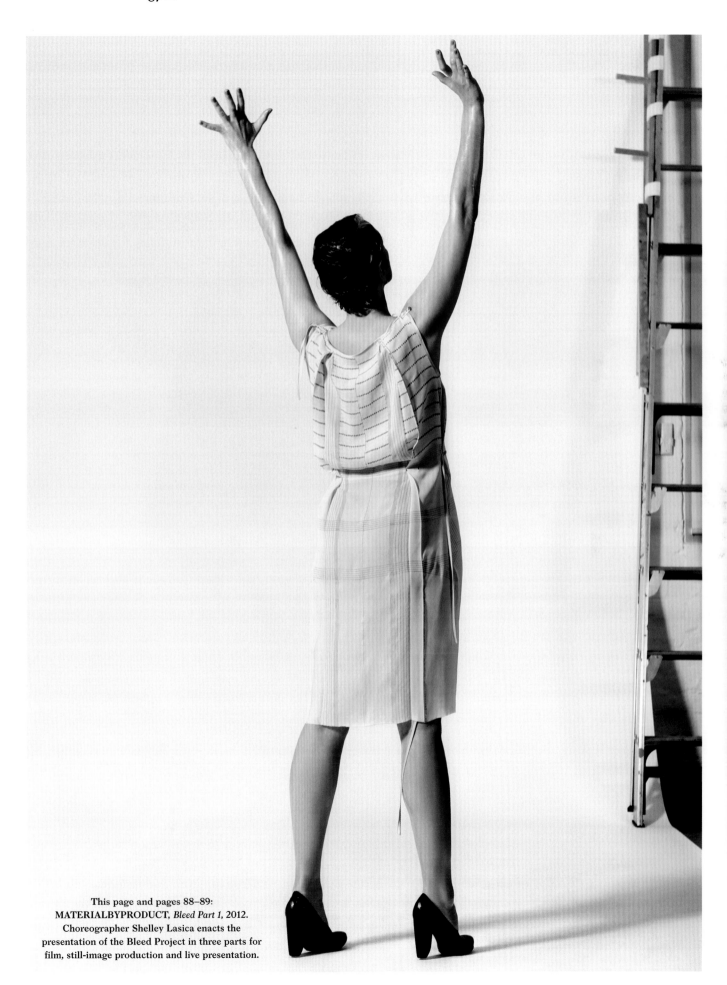

This page and pages 88–89:
MATERIALBYPRODUCT, *Bleed Part 1*, 2012.
Choreographer Shelley Lasica enacts the
presentation of the Bleed Project in three parts for
film, still-image production and live presentation.

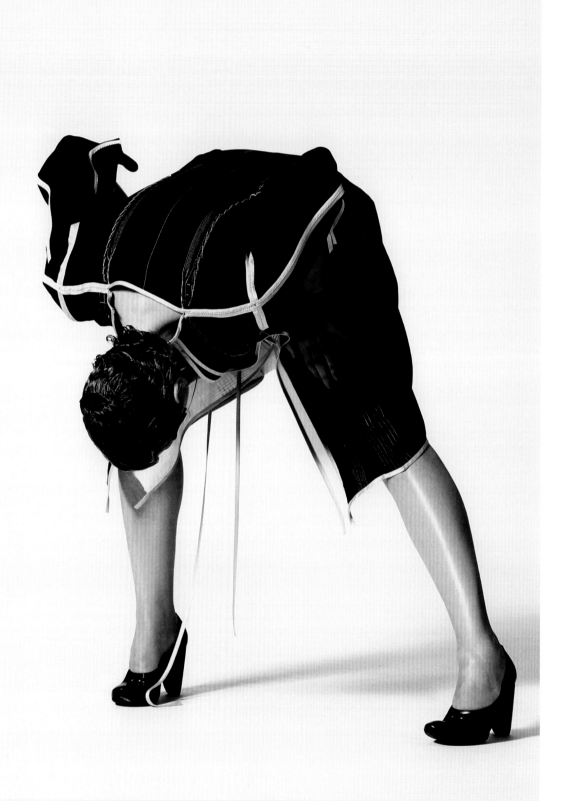

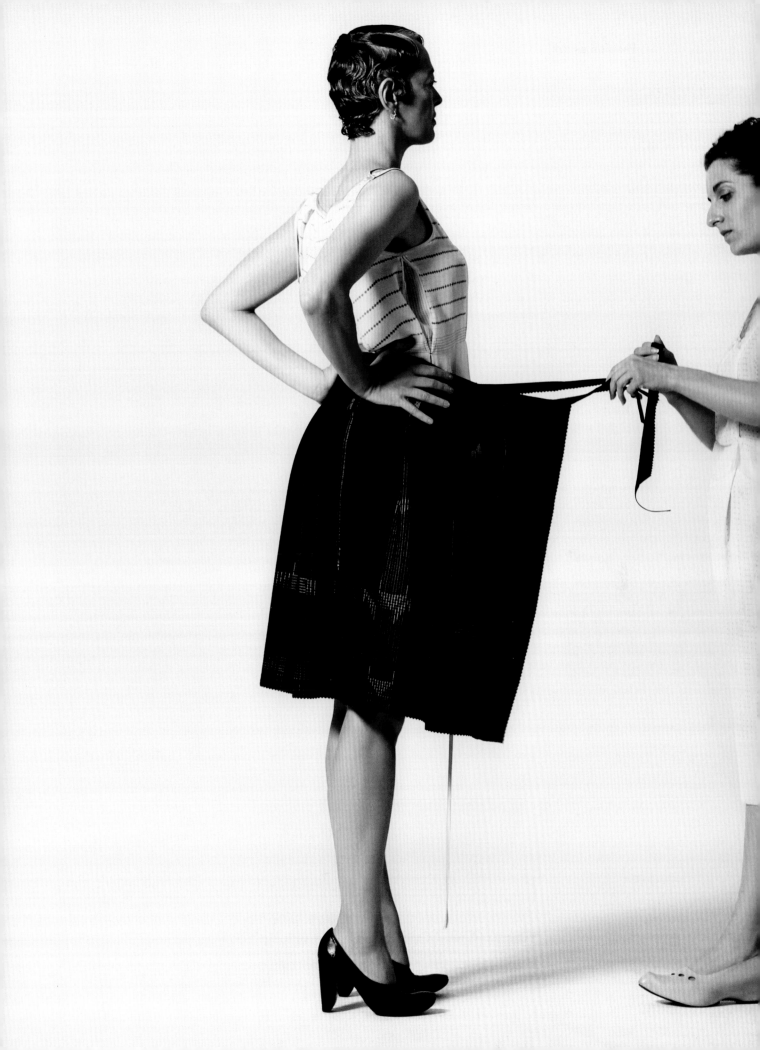

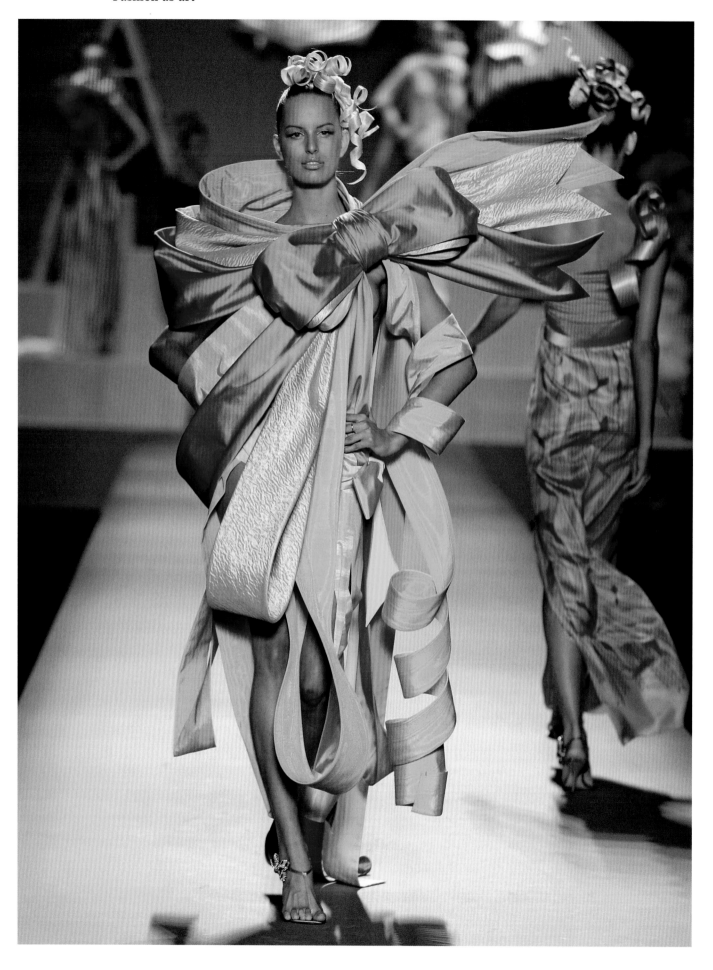

Viktor & Rolf

Masters of couture, Dutch duo Viktor & Rolf (Viktor Horsting and Rolf Snoeren) have often been described as artists by virtue of their complex and technically ambitious couture designs as well as their theatrical and performative collection shows. They have also crafted a public persona that is as much a part of the label as the clothes they create, presenting themselves as fashion's answer to quirky collaborative artists Gilbert & George, and appearing in specially commissioned photographs for collections.

'Art is very important. We have always treated our shows and our collections as a means of self-expression', explain the designers of the performance art for which their shows are renowned.[13] For the presentation of their first menswear collection the pair modelled the designs themselves, changing on the catwalk. Subsequent shows included 'Russian Doll' (Autumn/Winter

'We have always treated our shows and our collections as a means of self-expression.'

Viktor & Rolf

1999), a parade that featured a single model (Maggie Rizer) on a turntable wearing the entire season's collection, which was then revealed to the audience piece by piece; 'Black Hole' (Autumn/Winter 2001), a completely black collection in which even the models were painted black; 'Bedtime Story' (Autumn/Winter 2005), a collection of elaborate gowns that each resembled a bed complete with pillow; and 'Upside Down' (Spring/Summer 2006), an entirely upside-down collection reflecting the label's iconic upside-down store in Milan. For Autumn/Winter 2003 they built the entire collection 'One Woman Show' around the actress Tilda Swinton, their muse, and selected models who resembled her, sending a parade of red-haired doppelgangers down the runway. For Autumn/Winter 2007 they staged 'The Fashion Show', one of their most conceptually complex presentations, in which the parading models wore scaffolding and lights that transformed each into a self-contained fashion show. The Autumn/Winter 2008 collection 'NO!' was intended as a statement of disapproval at the nature of fast fashion. Models wore clothes with three-dimensional fabric or embroidered words such as 'DREAM', 'WOW' and 'NO'.

The duo's artistic reputation is demonstrated by the more than thirty fine-art exhibitions in which they have featured since 1998, including the major survey 'The House of Viktor & Rolf' at the Barbican Art Gallery, London, and the Centraal Museum, Utrecht, in 2008.

Opposite: Viktor & Rolf, Spring/Summer 2005.
Page 92: Viktor & Rolf, Spring/Summer 2010.
Page 93: Viktor & Rolf, Autumn/Winter 2009.

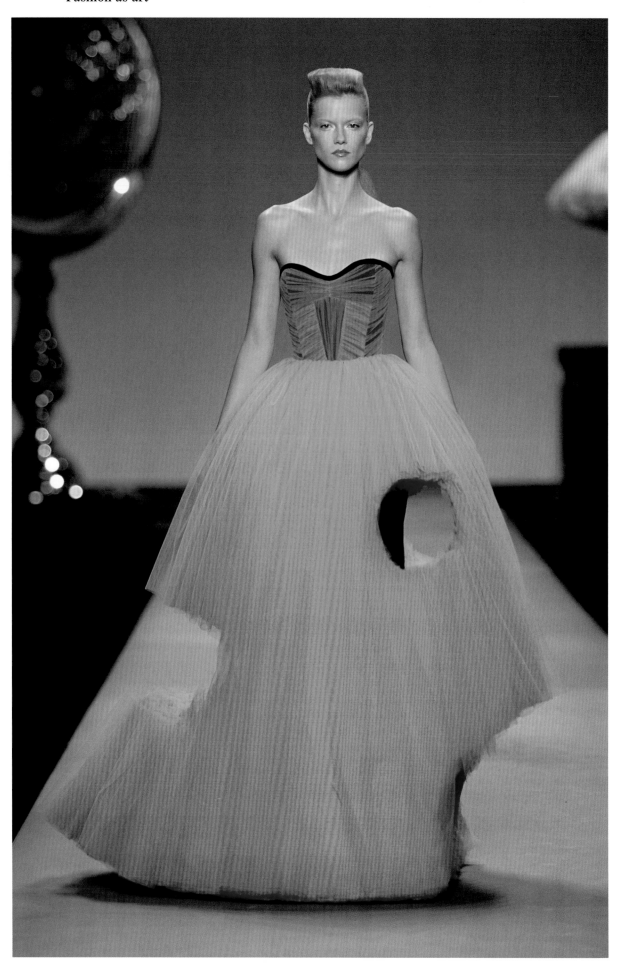

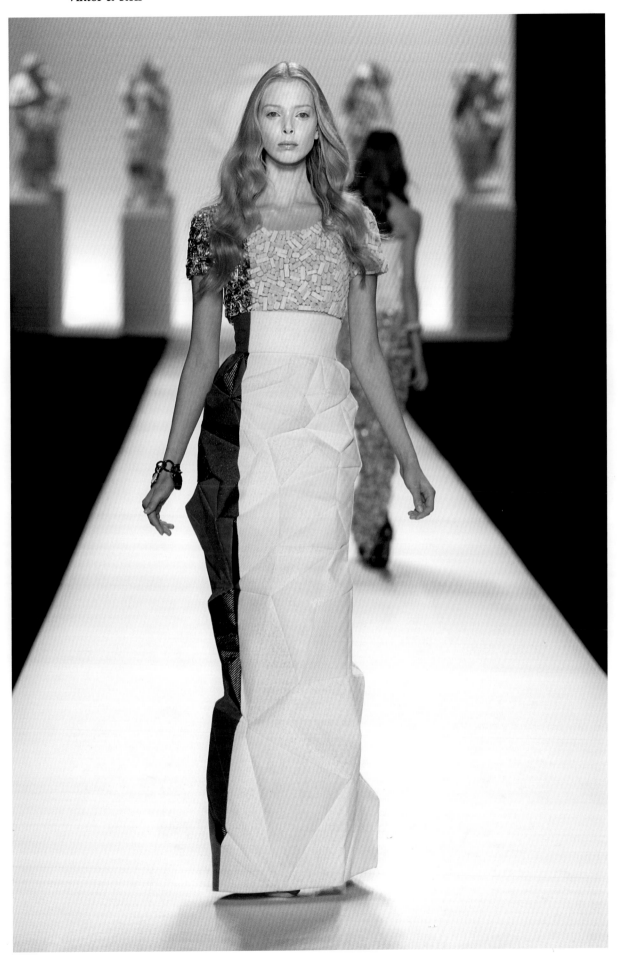

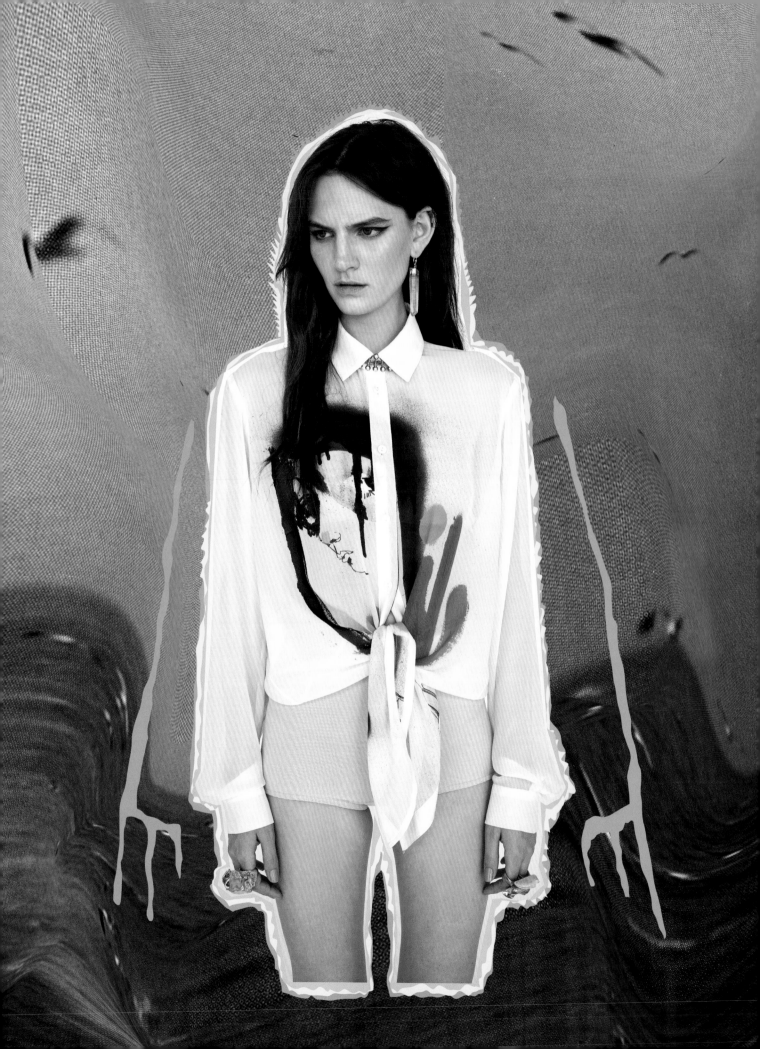

Art meets fashion: Collaboration

Opposite: Something Else, shirt reproducing an illustration
by Julie Verhoeven, Spring/Summer 2012.

Introduction:
Art meets fashion

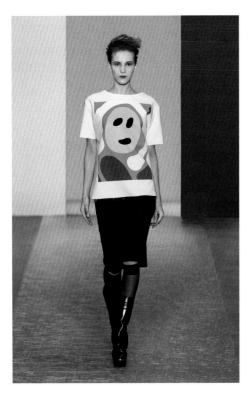

Marni, shirt reproducing artwork by Gary Hume,
Autumn/Winter 2010.

At its most basic level, the notion of collaboration in fashion is evident in the way a house employs an artist's work for the purpose of decorating its signature or staple products, such as leathergoods, accessories and fabrics.

The level of collaboration varies: while in some instances an artist is invited to alter a product's physical proportions, construction and style, or indeed imagine an entirely new product, most collaborations merely involve a print that is sold or licensed for a negotiated price based on the status of the house and the size of the production, and then applied to the brand's existing products. Whatever the level of creative involvement on the part of the artist, however, such collaborations between art and fashion represent an important meeting of the two worlds.

Such collaborations are not a new phenomenon: artists and art movements have been stylistically influencing fashion designers for centuries. In the early 20th century, for instance, the couturier Paul Poiret employed graphic artists such as Paul Iribe and Erté to create textile prints for his creations. A generation later, the Italian fashion designer Elsa Schiaparelli initiated the modern practice of collaborating with contemporary artists via her informal partnerships with Jean Cocteau, Salvador Dalí and Alberto Giacometti between 1927 and 1954. In Schiaparelli's day, far less emphasis was placed on the concept of 'collaboration' – a 21st-century buzzword – and she did not prominently credit her artists in the same way as is common practice now, but the publicity this work received, particularly the 'Lobster' dress designed with Salvador Dalí and famously worn by Wallis Simpson, set the trend for future collaborations between contemporary artists and fashion houses. Schiaparelli's influence in this respect was celebrated by the exhibition 'Schiaparelli and Prada: Impossible Conversations' at the Metropolitan Museum of Art, New York, in 2012, in which her work was curated alongside that of contemporary Italian designer Miuccia Prada, also known for her collaborations with visual artists. In 2010, MoMA PS1 in New York recognized the modern-day proliferation of fashion–art collaborations with 'Move!', a series of performances and temporary installations by fourteen designers paired with artists, including Marc Jacobs and Rob Pruitt, Cynthia Rowley and Olaf Breuning, and Proenza Schouler and Dan Colen.

In the intensely profit-driven modern fashion industry, however, the fact that so many collaborative projects with artists result in the creation of actual products indicates that, whatever their artistic ambitions, these initiatives are regarded as commercially viable by the international conglomerates who own the major luxury brands. A fashion

Collaborations are not a new phenomenon: artists and art movements have been stylistically influencing fashion designers for centuries.

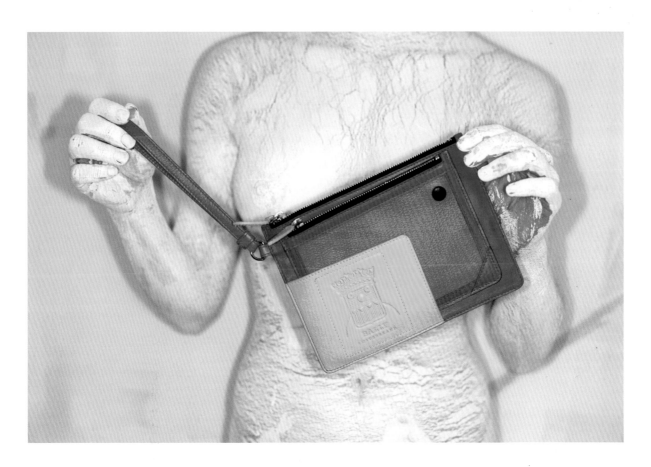

Clutch bag designed by Olaf Breuning in
collaboration with Graeme Fidler and Michael Herz
for Bally Love #2, 2012.

'Collaborating with contemporary artists brings a new kind of creative fecundity to the product. It forces creativity that is different from that typically found in fashion.'

Yves Carcelle, President and CEO, Louis Vuitton[1]

Opposite: Artist Yayoi Kusama photographed wearing
a handbag and shoes she designed in collaboration with
Marc Jacobs for Louis Vuitton, 2012.

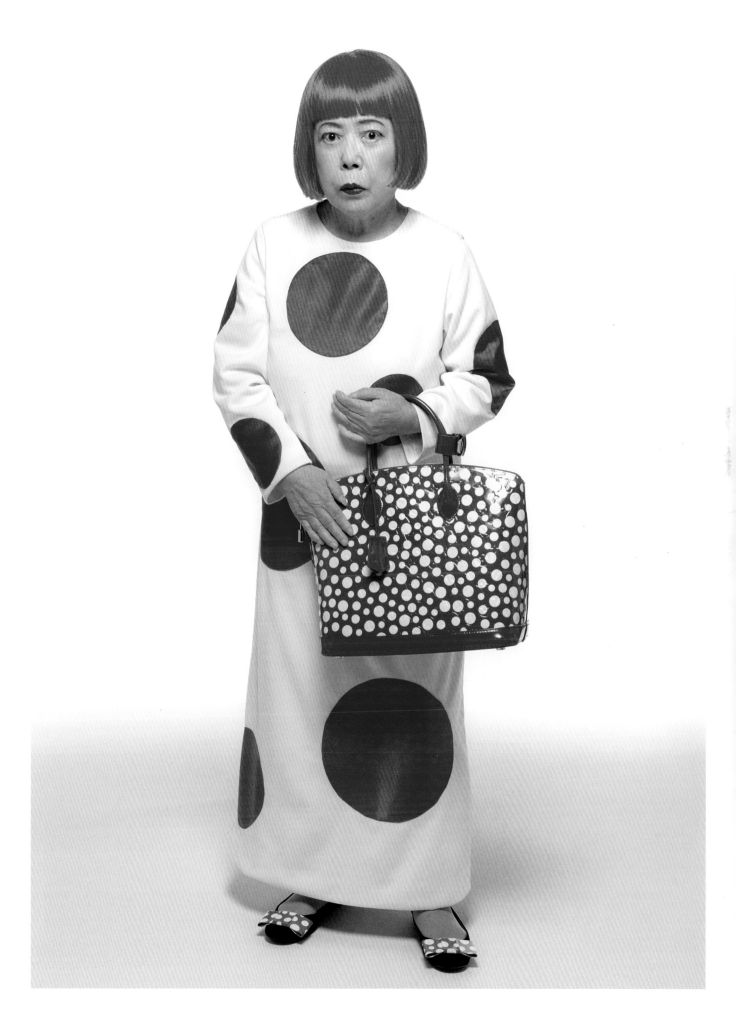

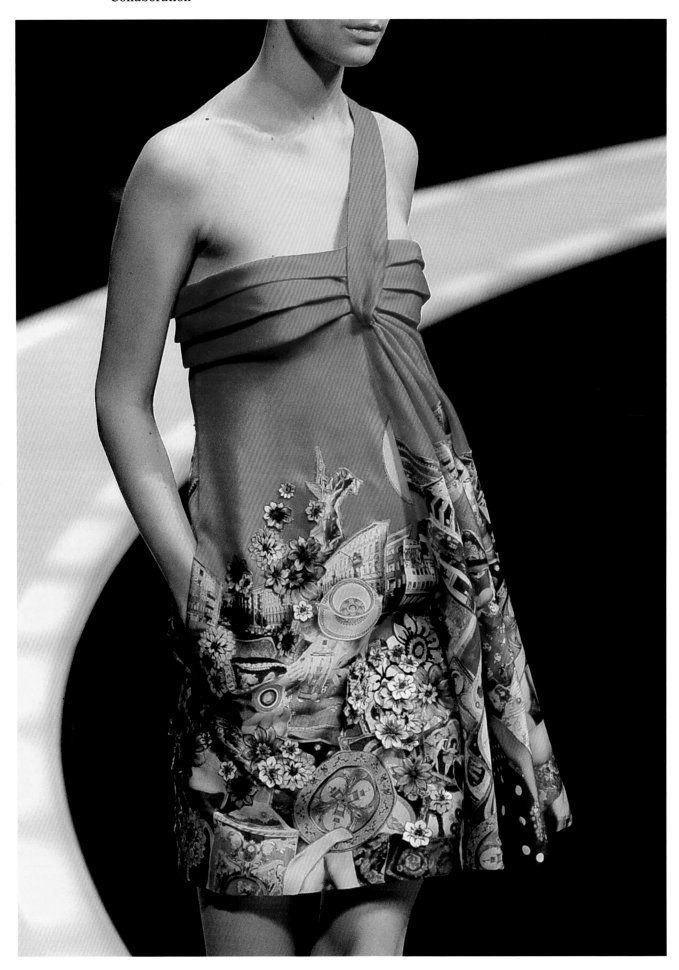

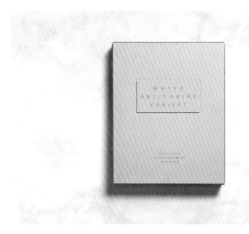

Packaging of the Acne *WHITE ART / T-SHIRT PROJECT*, Edition 2 by Lucy Skaer, 2011. Opposite: Versace, dress reproducing artwork by Tim Roeloffs, Autumn/Winter 2008.

collection created in collaboration with an artist is almost always a one-off capsule, whose status as a limited edition gives it the aura of authenticity normally associated with works of art. For fashion consumers, moreover, exclusivity is equated with luxury, and nothing is so desired as that which has sold out. The reception of Takashi Murakami's 2003 collection for Louis Vuitton – one of the house's most commercially successful special projects to date – indicates this desire from consumers for something 'extra'.

Aside from potential profits, collaborations offer other benefits for a fashion label. As the introduction of this book notes, many houses rely on their history as a powerful marketing tool, emphasizing notions such as tradition, authenticity and brand recognition to survive the fluctuating global economy, while simultaneously trying to remain relevant in the contemporary market. In addition to the prestige associated with collecting contemporary art, the incorporation of a visual art element into a fashion item adds an of-the-moment relevance that is especially important for historic luxury brands, and can bring both a fresh irreverence and additional gravitas to functional product lines such as leathergoods.

The relationship is a collusive one: mutual risk for mutual reward. Just as fashion houses risk the substantial financial outlay required to produce an experimental capsule collection, the artists who collaborate with them risk being branded 'sellouts' by their colleagues in the art world as they benefit from the increased publicity. However, this potential for wider exposure benefits not only the individual artist, but society at large. For many consumers, a collaborative fashion project is the channel through which they are first introduced to a particular artist's work, in a form that – unlike contemporary art – is not seen as requiring a strictly defined body of knowledge in order to be engaged with and discussed, and is open to anyone with the financial means to buy the products or a willingness to explore them via the media. In this way fashion collaborations perform the essential role of widening public access to contemporary art, and are able to enact a cultural education via the cash register.

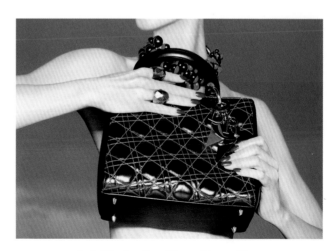

Lady Dior handbag, Mise en Dior necklace and Rock in Dior rings redesigned by Anselm Reyle for Christian Dior, 2012.

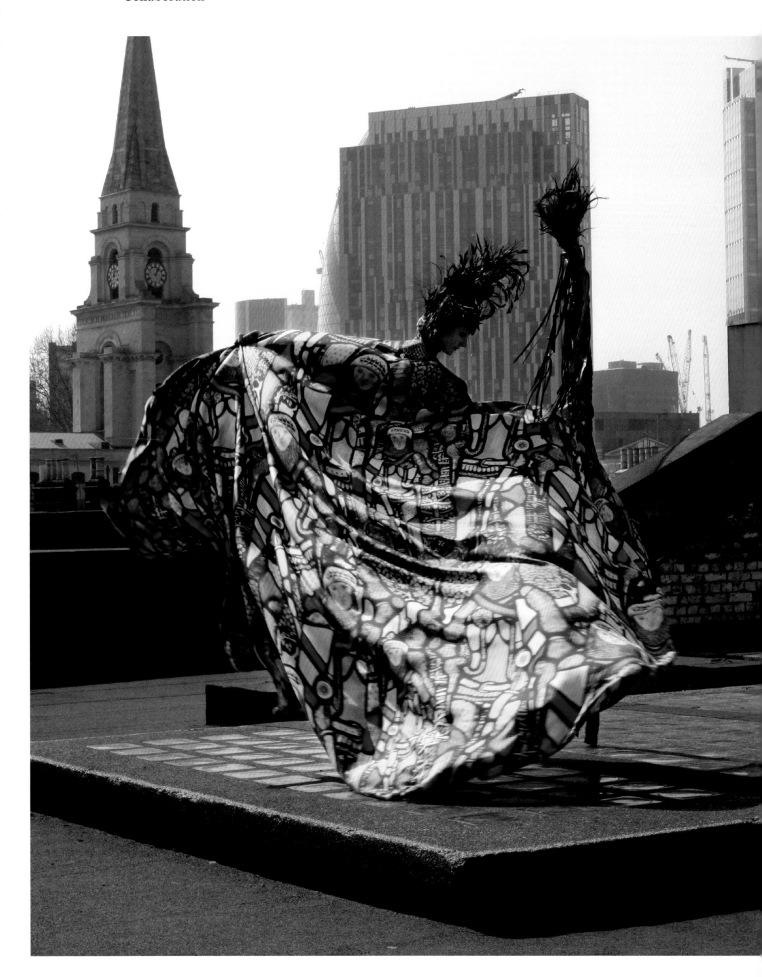

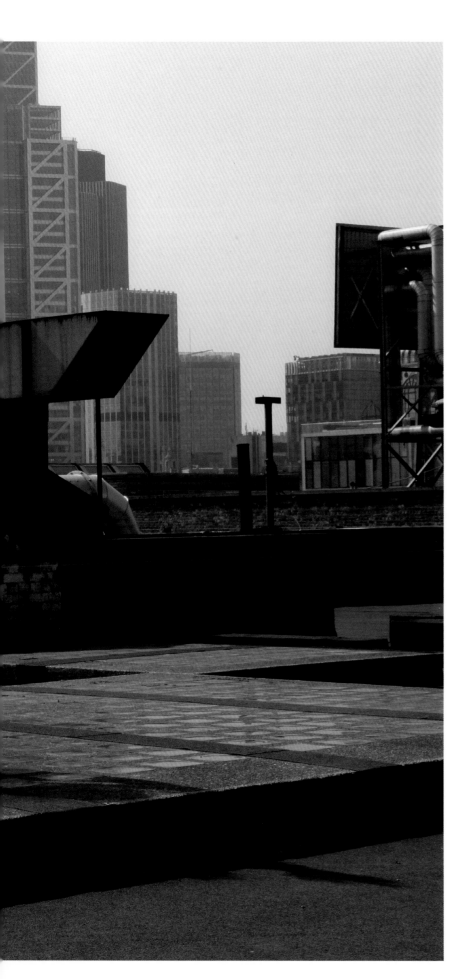

'Britain Creates 2012'

'Britain Creates 2012: Fashion + Art Collusion' was an initiative of the Fashion Arts Foundation set up by the British Fashion Council and *Harper's Bazaar* in order to foster connections between the world of fashion and opera, theatre, dance, cinema and visual art. The project celebrated the strength of British fashion and contemporary art as London prepared to host the 2012 Olympic Games. The programme, which was curated by Susanna Greeves, brought together nine prominent contemporary designers and artists: Giles Deacon and Jeremy Deller, Hussein Chalayan and Gavin Turk, Jonathan Saunders and Jess Flood-Paddock, Mary Katrantzou and Mark Titchner, Matthew Williamson and Mat Collishaw, Nicholas Kirkwood and Simon Periton, Sir Paul Smith and Charming Baker, Peter Pilotto and Francis Upritchard, and Stephen Jones and Cerith Wyn Evans. Each of the collaborative pairs was given free reign to create, in any medium that represented their dual practices and aesthetics, a one-off piece that was then displayed at the Victoria & Albert Museum, London. Says Greeves: 'We wanted to do something quite new in inviting this kind of genuine co-authorship, right from concept through to execution, and by giving them such an open brief so that they could take their conversation in any direction... Some saw it as a chance to make something completely different from their normal practice, others felt they wanted to bring something they were essentially known for, but all were ambitious in scope.'[2]

Untitled collaboration between designer
Giles Deacon and artist Jeremy Deller for the exhibition
'Britain Creates 2012: Fashion + Art Collusion'
at the Victoria & Albert Museum, London.

'We wanted to do something quite new in inviting this kind of genuine co-authorship, right from concept through to execution, and by giving them such an open brief so that they could take their conversation in any direction.'

Susanna Greeves

Opposite: *Arch*, collaboration between designer
Peter Pilotto and artist Francis Upritchard for the
exhibition 'Britain Creates 2012: Fashion + Art Collusion'
at the Victoria & Albert Museum, London.

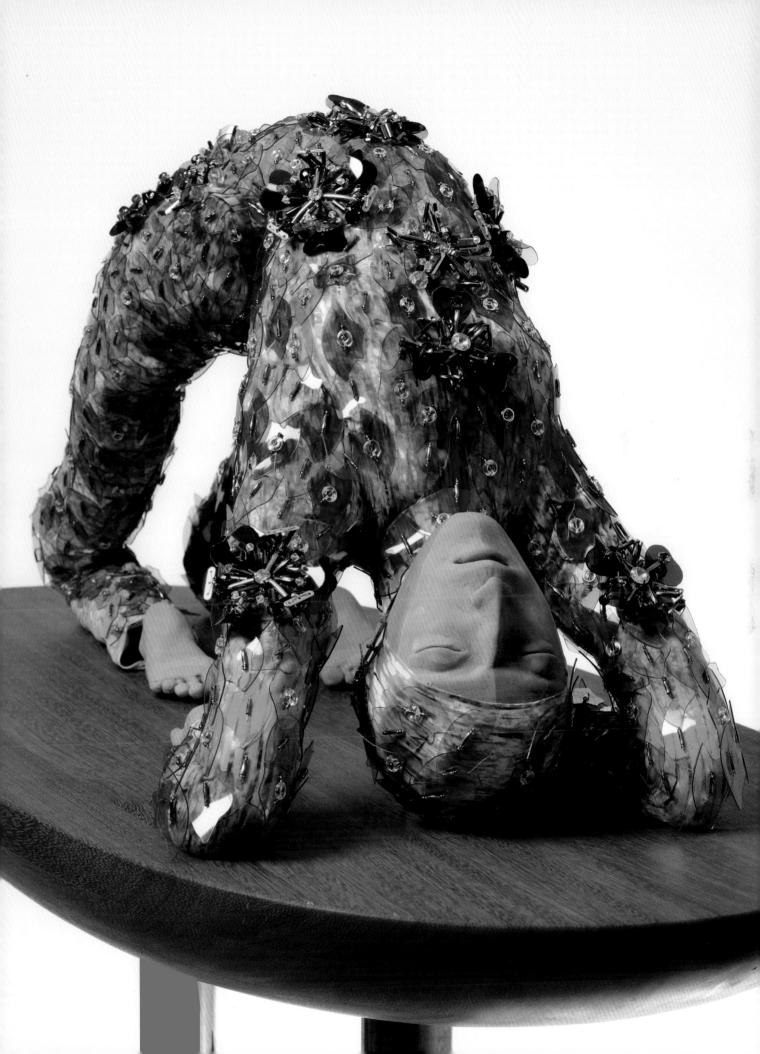

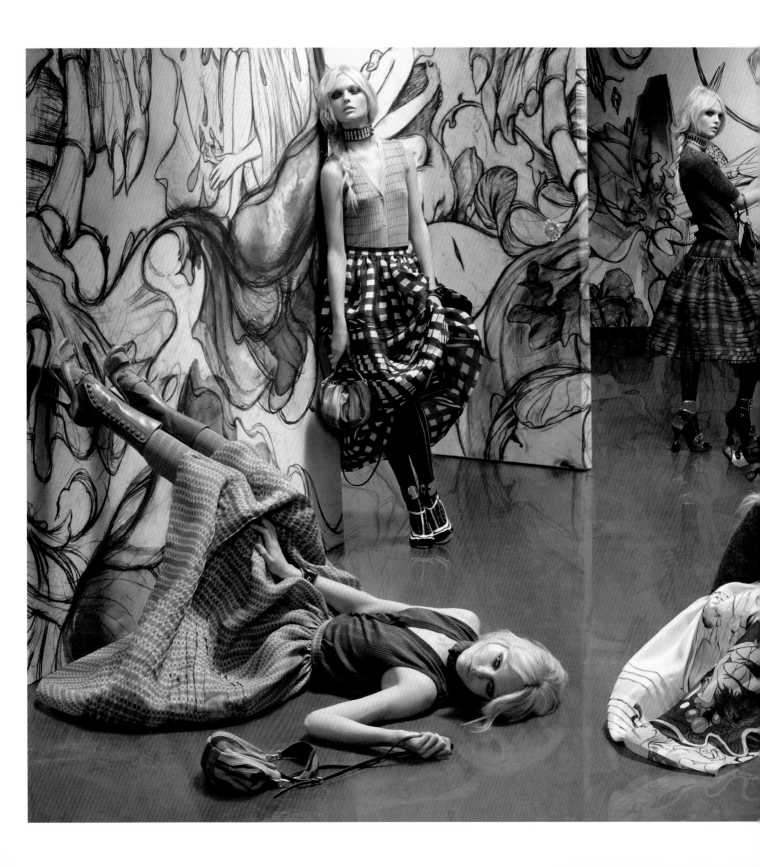

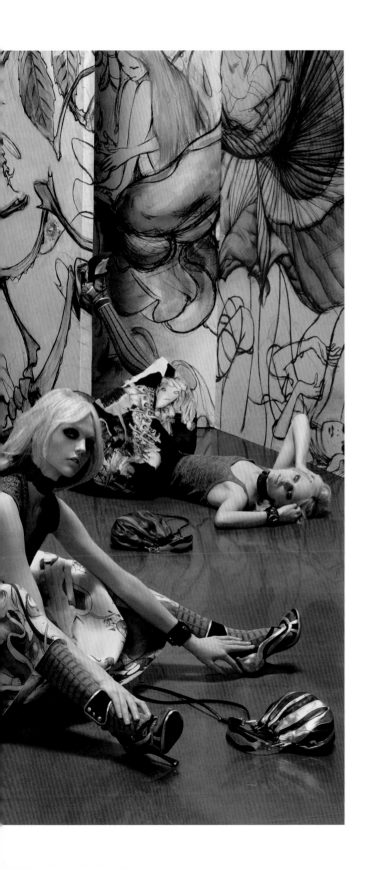

Prada & James Jean

In 2008 the Italian luxury house Prada engaged illustrator and comic artist James Jean to collaborate on its Spring/Summer 2008 collection, in what represented the first such partnership in the label's history. The project, which resulted in over one hundred pieces, including dresses, shoes and bags, was not confined to clothing and accessories, however. Jean was invited to create a mural for Prada's Rem Koolhaas-designed Epicenter store in New York as well as a backdrop for the collection's runway presentation in Milan (shown to the press in 2007) and his artwork was integrated into the seasonal advertising campaign, photographed by Steven Meisel, that promoted the Spring/Summer 2008 collection.

Jean also wrote and developed an animated short film, *Trembled Blossoms* (2008), which he made with the assistance of Los Angeles-based director James Lima and a team of animators who used motion-capture technology. The film, a dark fairytale in which creatures turn into fashion products, brought to life the characters in the watercolour prints Jean had created for Prada. The film was screened in Prada's Epicenter stores in New York, Los Angeles and Tokyo, where the windows of the building in the city's Aoyama district were covered in coloured film printed with a giant image of the lead character reaching for a peach from a tree.

The choice of Jean as a collaborator for Prada was surprising. Jean is best known as a cover artist for DC Comics, work that has garnered multiple Eisner and Harvey awards. His style of hand-painted watercolour designs, with their organic modernism, would at first seem at odds with Prada's more streamlined, industrial aesthetic, yet the collaborative project has largely been regarded as a successful one.

Prada campaign featuring clothing reproducing artwork by James Jean and photographed on a set designed by the artist, Spring/Summer 2008.

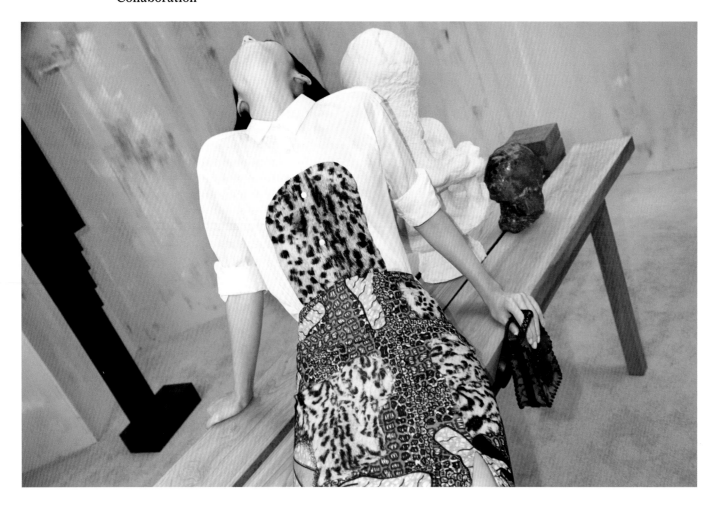

In conversation:
Jonny Johansson, Acne

Launched in Stockholm in 1996, Acne was conceived as a creative collective to work across the borders of fashion, film and advertising. Its co-founder, Jonny Johansson, sees this cross-disciplinary practice as a natural characteristic of Swedish culture. In addition to its seasonal ready-to-wear collections featuring denim, the house's core product line, Acne has worked on projects in film, furniture and industrial design, engaging with filmmaker Daniel Askill, artist Katerina Jebb and Italian bicycle manufacturer Bianchi, among others. The company also launched its own biannual magazine, *Acne Paper,* in 2005, with contributions from stylist Carine Roitfeld and photographers David Lynch, Lord Snowdon and Sarah Moon, as well as actor and fashion muse Tilda Swinton. One of Acne's most important artistic crossovers was its Spring/Summer 2012 collection, the result of a collaboration with London-based artist Daniel Silver, who made cut-and-paste collages that were then applied to the pieces.

Above, opposite and overleaf: Acne, collection reproducing artwork by Daniel Silver, Spring/Summer 2012.

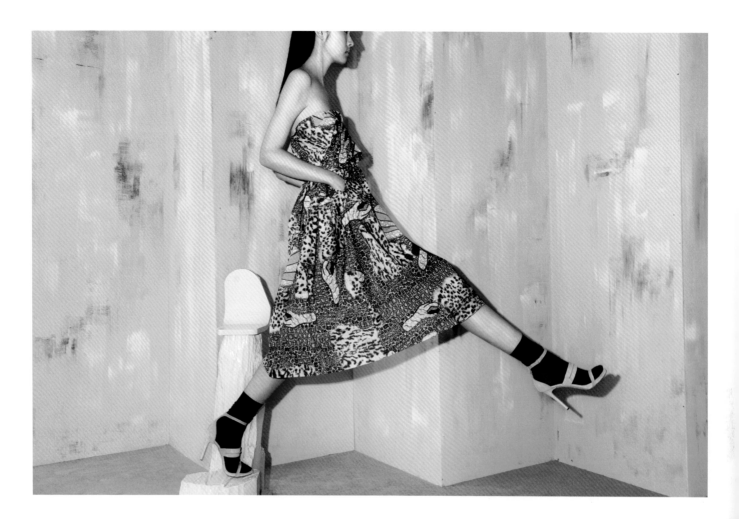

MITCHELL OAKLEY SMITH *Acne has collaborated with countless artists and creatives, from Michelle Jank to Daniel Silver and all of the people involved in Acne Paper. Did you always intend for the house to be so collaborative?*

JONNY JOHANSSON Absolutely, yes. To me, Swedish culture is very social and democratic, so it's a natural feeling that our work should be about sharing in a group, about bringing different people from different disciplines together to create something new.

MOS *Do you find that working across various disciplines – furniture, film – influences what you do as a designer?*

JJ I think that you should explore any medium or form of creativity you are interested in, no matter if it's fashion or architecture or art. To work with people who really have something to say is inspiring but also challenging because you must step outside of your comfort zone. It's important for me to try different disciplines, but I can't say I'm a connoisseur. I'm just a playful, happy kid in the art world.

MOS *What is the process of integrating art into fashion, as you have done with Daniel Silver and the* **WHITE ART / T-SHIRT PROJECT** *(2010).*

JJ Well, firstly, I believe there is a line between fashion and art. They are two different disciplines.

Nothing I do is art, but I draw inspiration from it and admire the way it allows my mind to think in new ways. I make it clear that I'm not an artist and that we don't make art. We can then step into these projects with mutual acceptance.

MOS *But does working with an artist add artistic value to your clothing? If you work with an artist on a collection, do those clothes become art?*

JJ It's not an easy question. To be successful today, artists need to be able to work with different mediums, but I can't answer that question. It comes back to me: art opens boxes in my mind that I can't open myself, and that's why I do it.

MOS *Tell me about the* **WHITE ART / T-SHIRT PROJECT.**

JJ It's such a simple idea but, I think, very smart and democratic: to offer art to a fashion consumer is a good way of raising the profile of both the artist and art as a field.

MOS *Is the thinking behind working in film the same?*

JJ We have always worked with film as a format at Acne, and then all of a sudden everyone was doing fashion films. I felt like we had to do something contemporary that would reach beyond the house, which is when we looked to Michelle Jank and Daniel Askill (page 218). I never wanted to create films just because it's fashionable. Whatever we do has to feel really natural to Acne.

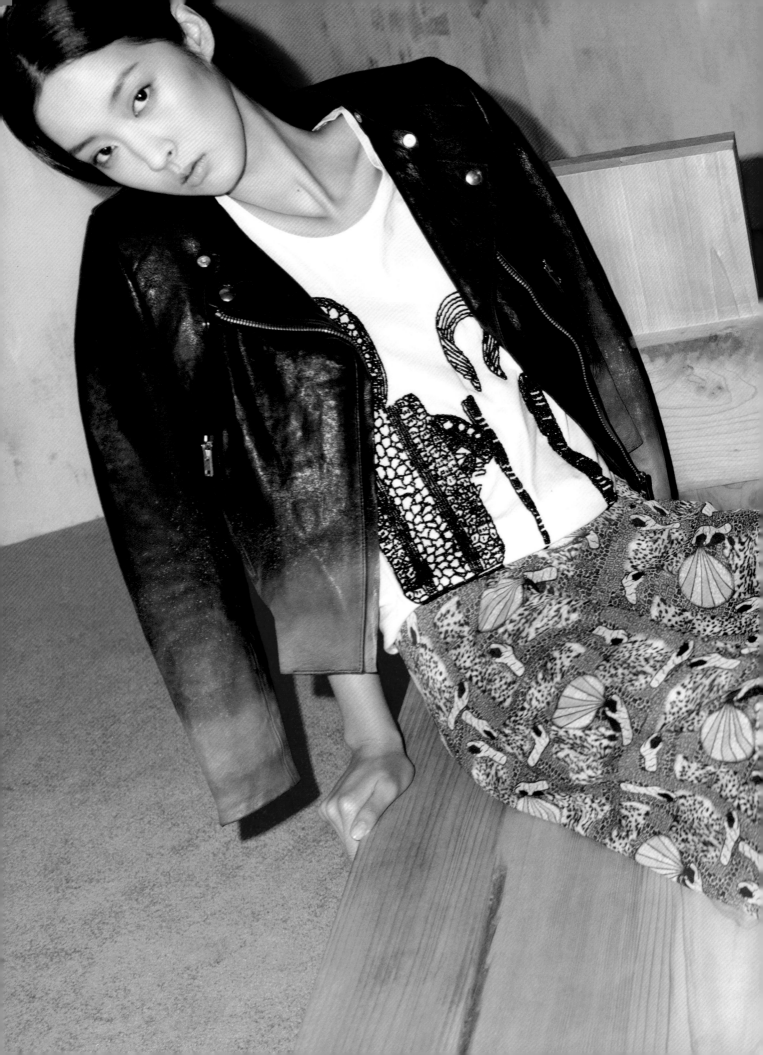

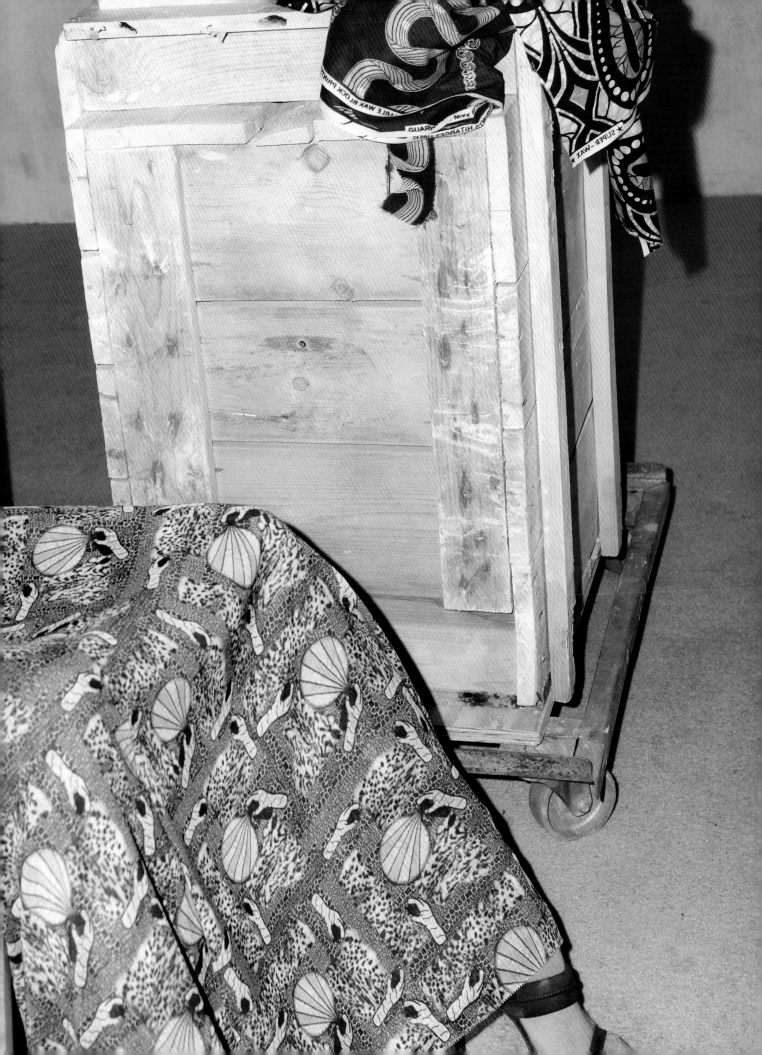

Christian Dior & Anselm Reyle

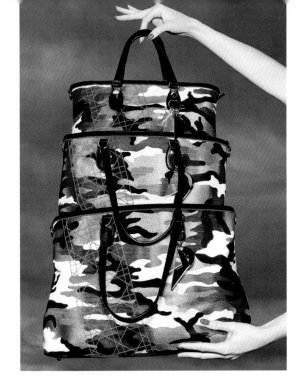

In 2012 Christian Dior presented a product-based collaboration with German artist Anselm Reyle, the first such project undertaken by Dior. Reyle was given free rein to re-envision the house's famous Lady Dior and Miss Dior handbags, and also produced a series of accessories and shoes, utilizing his signature fluorescent camouflage and coloured triangle motifs as a means of reinventing the classic pieces. For a house so venerated for its history of exquisite couture, Reyle's incorporation of street-art

> 'I loved working on the Lady Dior handbag. Most of my work builds on objects that already exist, which I then transform. [Here] I applied the same philosophy.'
>
> *Anselm Reyle*[3]

elements was an irreverent gesture that appealed to a younger audience well versed in the contemporary language of appropriation. The idea for the collaboration, which marked a new direction for the brand in the wake of the departure of creative director John Galliano in 2011, followed the success of two major museum exhibitions that celebrated Christian Dior in an artistic context: 'Christian Dior & Chinese Artists' (2008), at the Ullens Center for Contemporary Art, Beijing, which asked contemporary Chinese artists to comment on what Dior stands for; and 'InspirationDior' (2011), a retrospective at the Pushkin Museum, Moscow, which explored Dior's oeuvre alongside major artworks from the 19th and 20th centuries.

Above and opposite: Shopping totes (above) and wedges (opposite) designed by Anselm Reyle for Christian Dior, 2012.

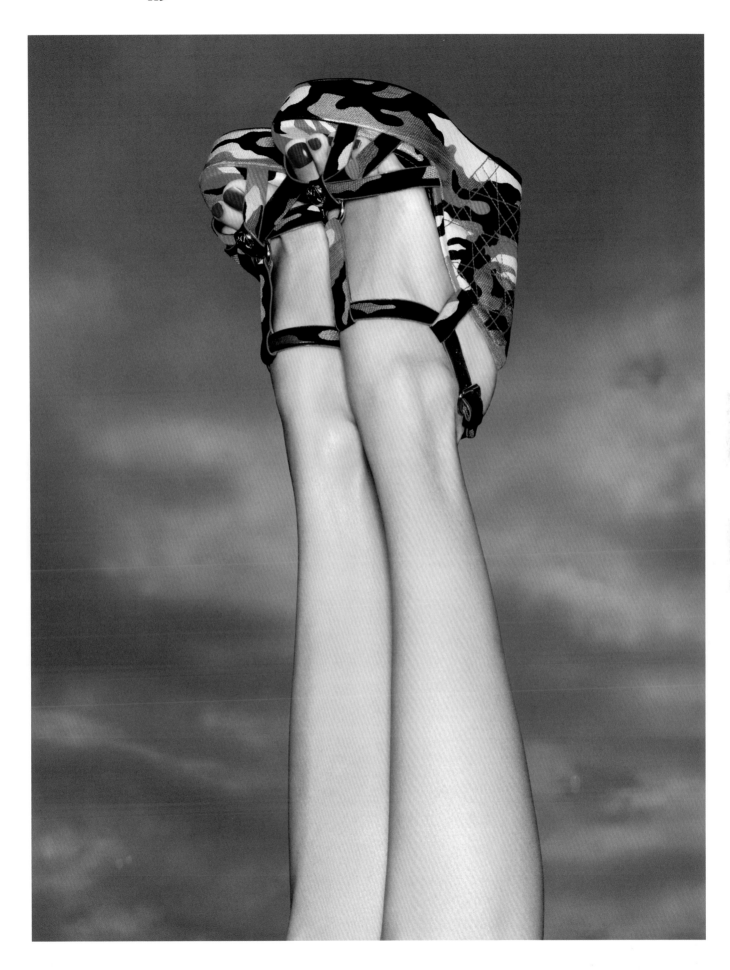

Bally Love:
Olaf Breuning
& Philippe Decrauzat

Swiss leathergoods, shoes and accessories company Bally is arguably the only major Swiss brand in the fashion industry, with the exception of several well-known watch manufacturers. Founded by Carl Franz Bally in 1851 in the Swiss hamlet of Schoenewerd, the company's long history and Swiss heritage have always been a source of pride for the brand. It is still headquartered in Switzerland, and maintains its own in-house craftsmen and designers, headed by Graeme Fidler and Michael Herz at the company's design office in London. Despite Bally's identity as a historic brand, it is also a house that prominently embraces and supports contemporary art and design. The brand has a strong history of working with artists, and is well known for its iconic, historic 20th-century posters in collaboration with graphic illustrators.

Since Bally, as a specialist leathergoods house, produces a smaller collection of ready-to-wear than other fashion houses, it does not show its wares via traditional runway shows, with their attendant publicity; instead, it increasingly uses contemporary art projects as a vehicle to raise awareness of the brand. In 2010 the company began sponsorship of the globally recognized contemporary art fair Art Basel and its American counterpart Art Basel Miami Beach. In the same year it also founded Bally Love, an annual project in which the house teams with a contemporary artist to create a capsule collection. Philippe Decrauzat, known for his geometric Op art, was the project's inaugural artist, followed by Olaf Breuning in 2012

The boundaries and specific product aims of Bally Love are flexible but its underlying intention is to produce covetable, well-made items with a contemporary flair. The project also gives Bally's in-house designers a welcome resptite from the commercially orientated fashion industry. 'We spend so much of our time

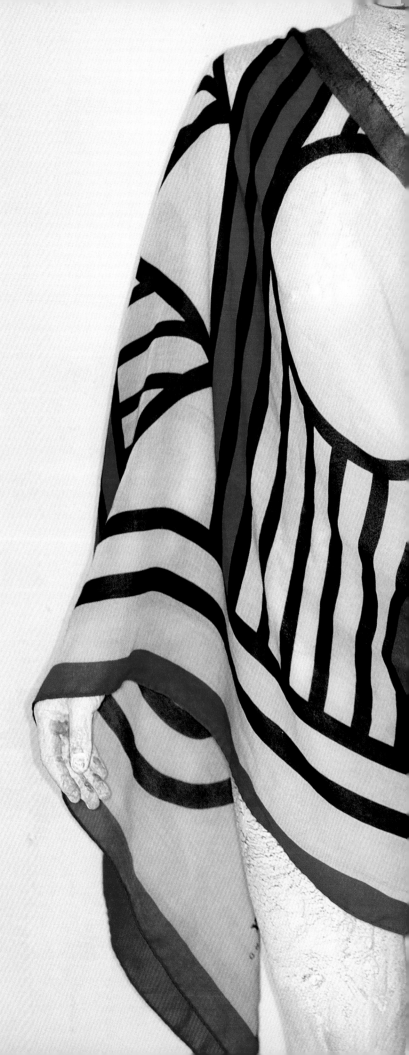

Scarf designed by Olaf Breuning in collaboration with Graeme Fidler and Michael Herz for Bally Love #2, 2012.

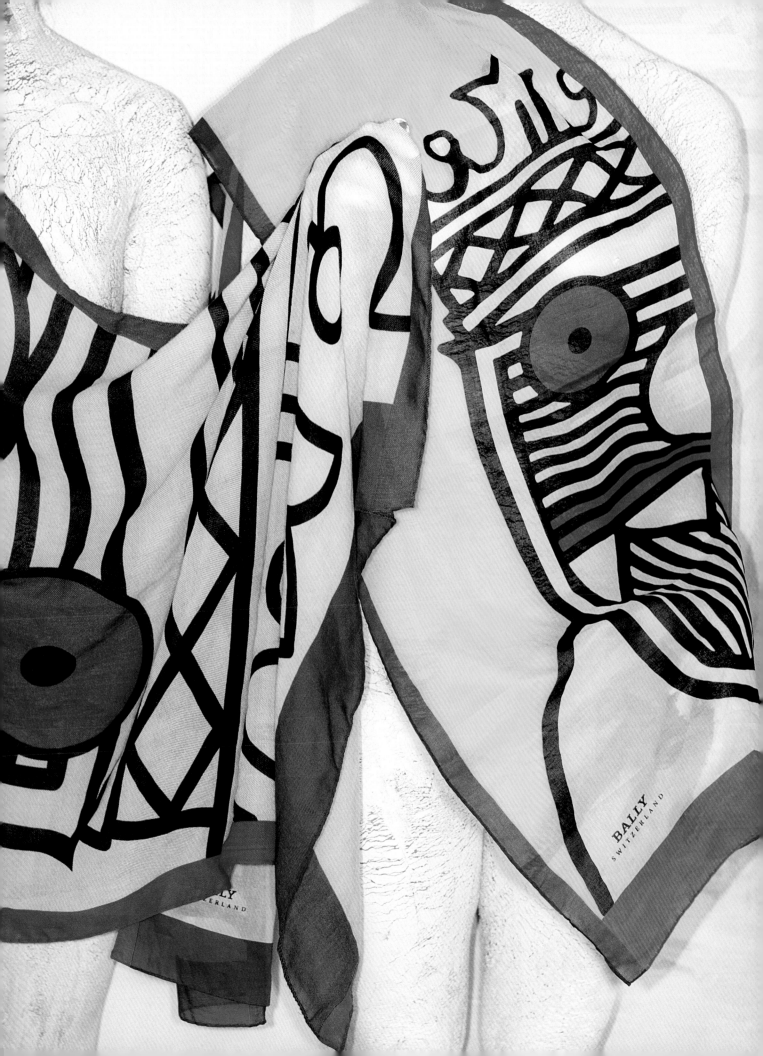

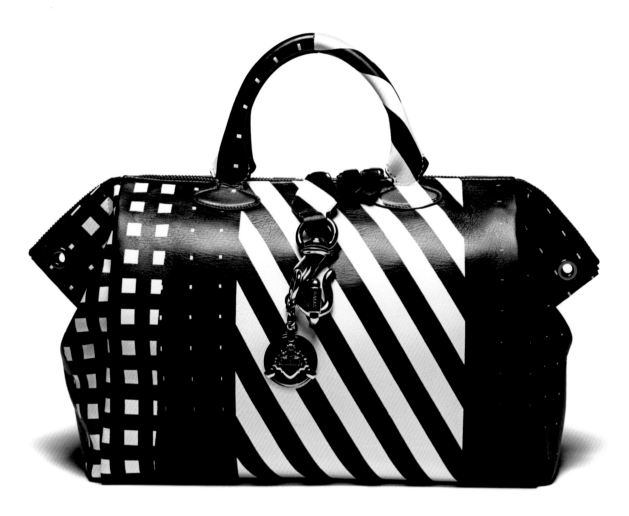

Above: Bag designed by Philippe Decrauzat for Bally Love #1, 2010.
Opposite: Shoes designed by Philippe Decrauzat for Bally Love #1, 2010.

looking at the needs of our market, on planning and production, and so many other things, which is the framework you work within as a designer, [but Bally Love] is a moment of collaboration [that is] about the creation of a special piece and not so much about sales figures,'⁴ explains Fidler. Although the project was initiated prior to Fidler and Herz's appointment, they enthusiastically embraced the concept. 'I think it's important for all brands to contribute in areas that are related to them, like art, which very much relates to us as designers,' explains Herz. While the inaugural project had simply reproduced Decrauzat's graphic prints on leathers and fabrics, Fidler and Herz took a more collaborative approach. 'We find it much more interesting to have a conversation and to create something *with* an artist,' says Fidler. 'When we worked with Olaf, he produced imagery – the papier-mâché shapes, the big painted people – and was really interested in creating fashion product, so we as a design team worked on the proportions and the technical requirements. It was a proper, very inspiring collaboration, and I think we created a collection that was much more than simply an artist's image on product.'

'It's like visiting a gallery; you might see something you may not have expected to see in our store, which helps to keep everybody's mind a little bit more open.'

Michael Herz

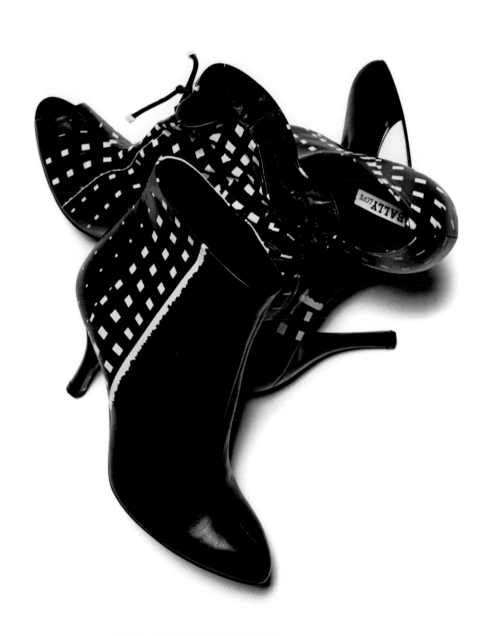

Stella McCartney & Jeff Koons

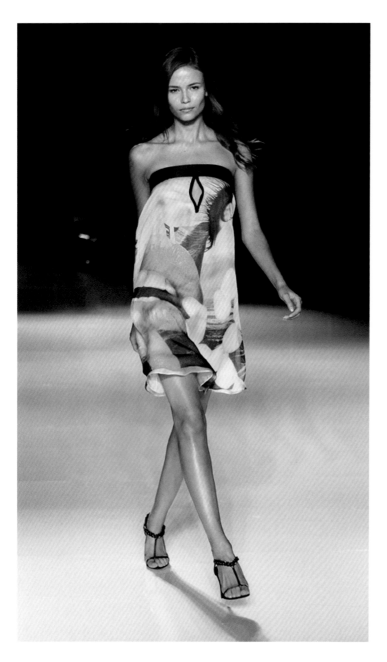

The Spring/Summer 2006 collaboration between Stella McCartney and American post-pop artist Jeff Koons was doubly a celebrity event. Koons is one of the most collectable and successful artists of the 21st century, famous not only for his iconoclastic statues, which have included subjects such as Michael Jackson and his chimp Bubbles, but also for his marriage to Hungarian-born Italian porn star Cicciolina that produced *Made in Heaven* (1989–1991), a controversial series of paintings, photographs, billboards and scuptures that showed Koons and his wife in explicit poses. Stella McCartney, daughter of the Beatles' Paul McCartney, has earned a critical reputation for her ecologically and ethically sound clothing – the designer eschews all animal products – designed for the forward-thinking contemporary woman with an aesthetic of easy luxury. Her collections include lingerie, sportswear for Adidas and a range for children for mass retailer Target. In a short time McCartney's recognition that there is a connection between fashion and personal lifestyle has transformed the contemporary definition of a 'brand'.

McCartney's collaboration with Koons involved a series of prints of his pop paintings reproduced on diaphanous dresses, as well as a jewelry collection that included small-scale reproductions of Koons's now-iconic *Rabbit* (1986), a huge stainless steel rabbit that mimicked a balloon animal, which was cast in miniature for charms on necklaces and bracelets. An advertising campaign featuring supermodel Kate Moss, a friend of the designer, further elevated the collaboration to iconic status. Although the collaboration seems incongruous given the contrast between Koons's obsession with kitsch and excess and McCartney's preference for a more restrained aesthetic, it was an extraordinarily successful project for both participants.

Above and opposite: Stella McCartney, dresses reproducing artwork by Jeff Koons, Spring/Summer 2006.

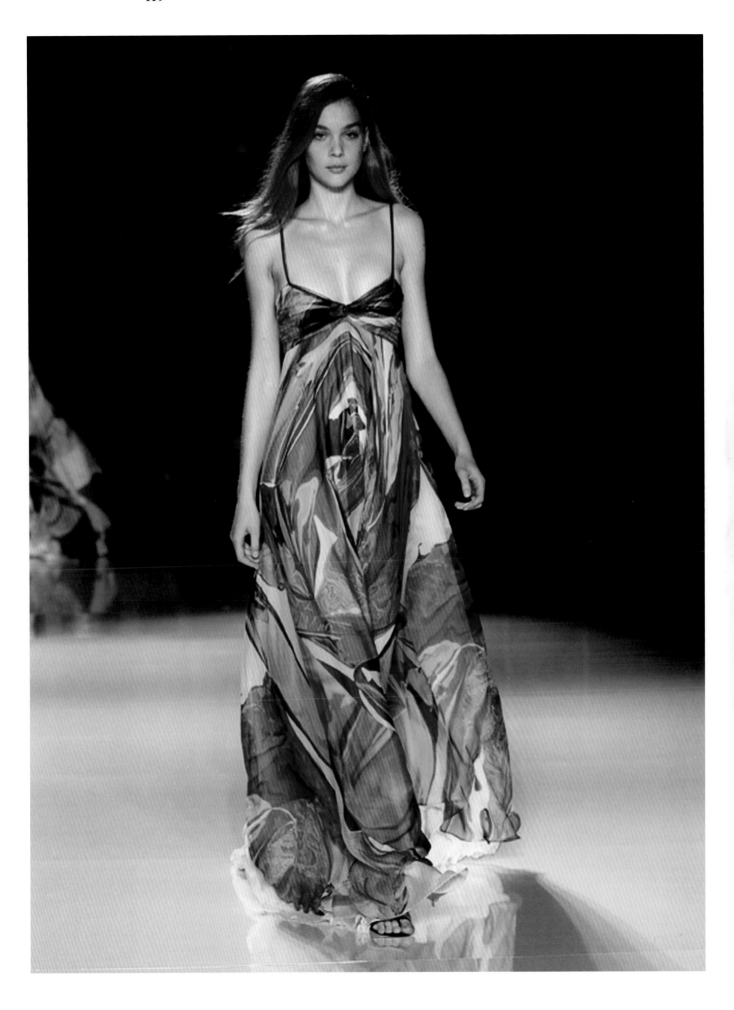

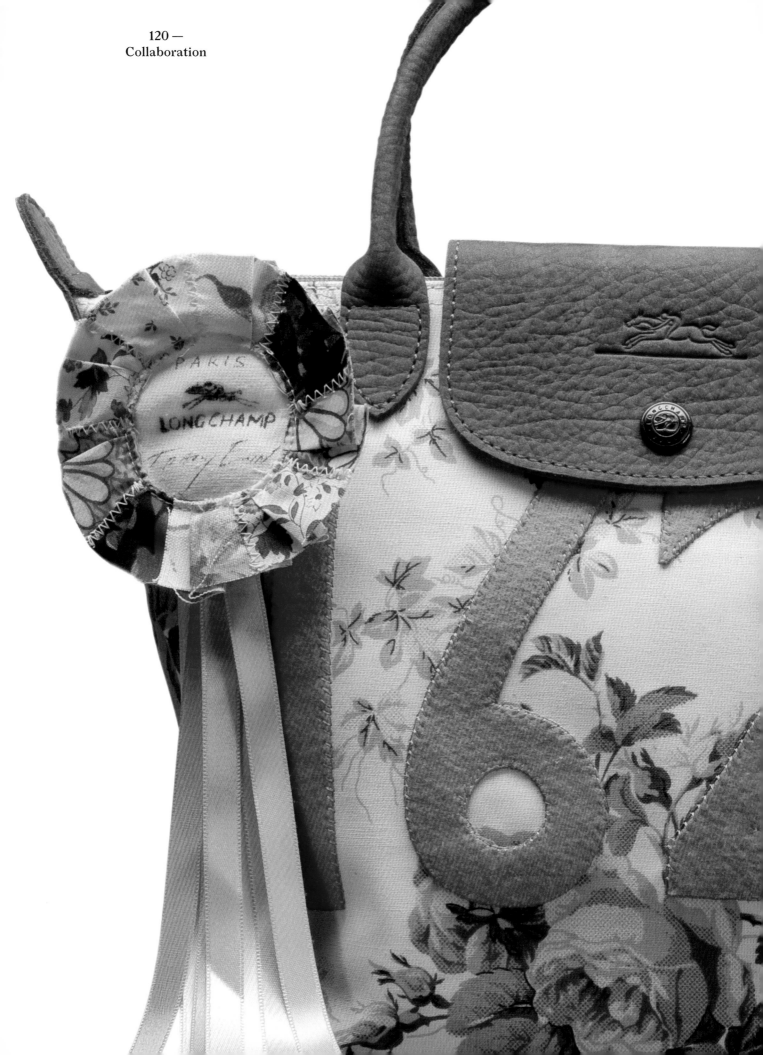

Longchamp
& Tracey Emin

British conceptual artist Tracey Emin enjoys an international reputation as a provocateur. Her practice is frequently described as confessional, featuring autobiographical and emotionally complex installations, etchings, drawings and needlepoints. She quickly rose to prominence in the 1990s as one of the group of Young British Artists, or YBAs, achieving household-name status in Britain. As a finalist in the Turner Prize in 1999, she courted controversy with *My Bed,* her unmade bed replete with condoms. Emin has engaged with the fashion world on several occasions: she appears on Nick Knight's SHOWStudio website as a contributor, and has modelled in photographic advertisements for Vivienne Westwood, with whom she shares an irreverent post-feminist spirit and post-punk aesthetic.

Emin's collaboration in 2004 with the gentrified French leathergoods label Longchamp, however, seemed at first to be an odd fit. The house invited Emin to collaborate on its bestselling line

Emin's collaboration cleverly turned on her playful assessment of her personal 'baggage'.

of foldable travel bags, 'Le Pliage', as well as producing a suitcase. Emin's response was, like her work, distinctively handmade and hands-on: incorporating embroidery, the bags were made in a limited edition of two hundred, individually signed by the artist to give them the authenticity of artworks. Emin's collaboration cleverly turned on her playful assessment of her personal 'baggage'. Each bag was embroidered with the name of a place – a hotel, city, or street – where the artist had fallen in love, transforming it into a souvenir of her own romantic adventures.

Opposite: 'Le Pliage' bag redesigned by
Tracey Emin for Longchamp, 2004.

Louis Vuitton:
Takashi Murakami, Richard Prince, Yayoi Kusama & Stephen Sprouse

As the distinguished fashion curator Olivier Saillard so saliently expressed, 'No other fashion house has wielded as much influence on the work and reputation of an artist in the way Louis Vuitton cultivated its highly visible relationships'.[5] Its founder, Gaston-Louis Vuitton, collaborated with decorative artists such as Pierre-Émile Legrain, Jean Puiforcat and René Lalique. In the 21st century the house has worked with visual artists to create ready-to-wear or accessories capsule collections on an almost annual basis. Its artistic collaborators have included Julie Verhoeven (2002), Takashi Murakami (2003), Richard Prince (2008), Yayoi Kusama (2012) and Stephen Sprouse, who was responsible for the label's successful 'Graffiti' (2001) and 'Leopard' (2006) patterns.

One especially important area of collaboration for Louis Vuitton has been the regular updating of its signature prints – most prominently the 'LV' monogram – by contemporary artists. Georges Vuitton, the founder's son, created the company's current monogram, which represented a break from the house's traditional geometric patterns. Incorporating floral motifs, Georges's pattern, based on Japonisme and Art Nouveau designs, not only served to modernize the brand at the turn of the century but also to distinguish the house's wares from its counterfeits, of which there were as many then as there are today. This practice of updating the monogram was

Below and opposite: Works by Takashi Murakami for Louis Vuitton, including his many reinterpretations of the house's monogram print (below and opposite, on the walls) and anime-style scuptures (opposite), displayed in the exhibition 'Louis Vuitton: A Passion for Creation', at Hong Kong Museum of Art, 2009.

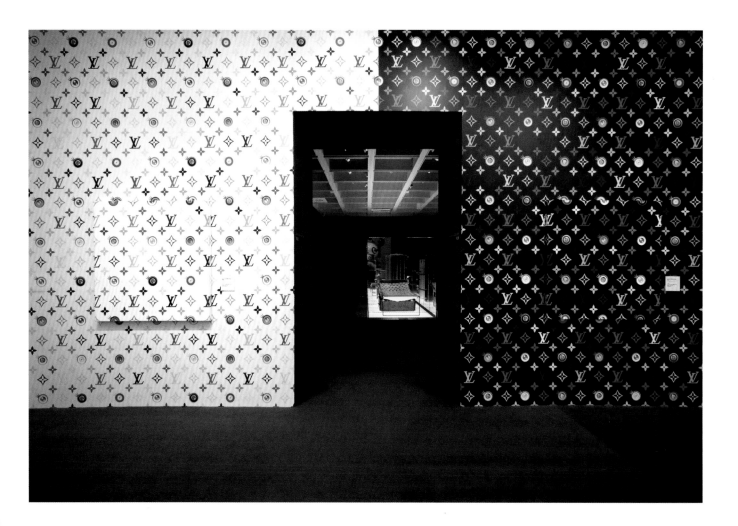

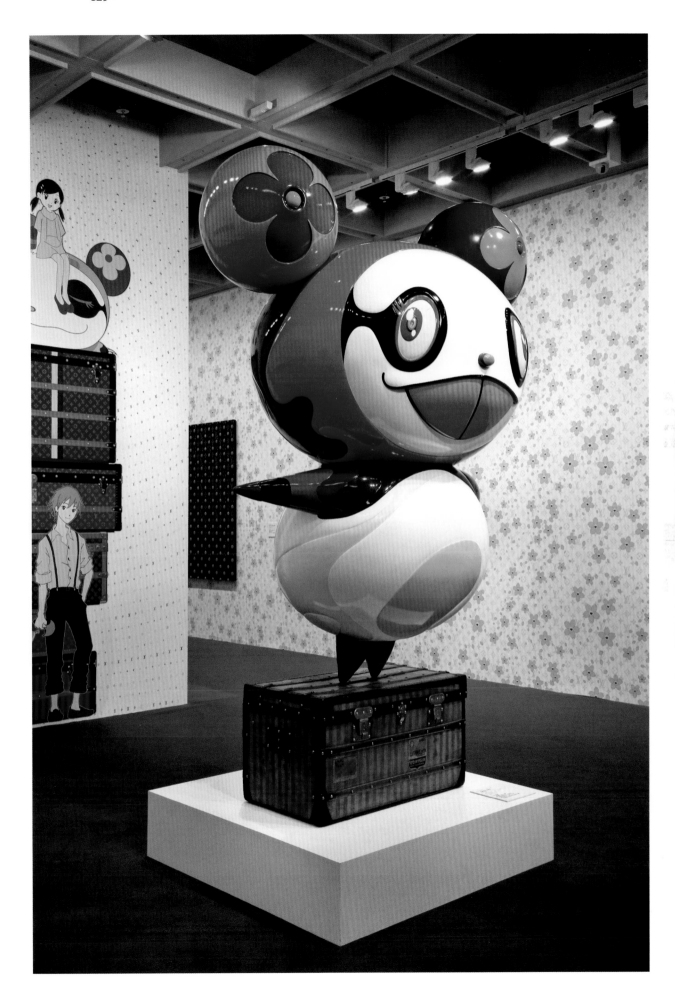

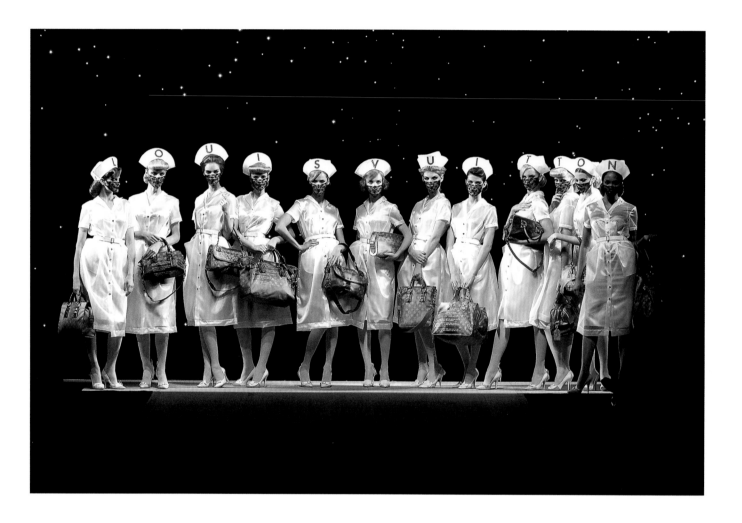

Above: Finale of the Marc Jacobs for Louis Vuitton
Spring/Summer 2008 presentation, which included
bags and other pieces customized by Richard Prince
and worn by models dressed to resemble his notorious
Nurses series of paintings.

'These projects represent more than a mere contract for services, as is the case with other collaborations in the fashion industry between a designer and an artist that may produce a particular pattern or dress. Louis Vuitton, however, invited artists as full participants in the creative process, and with every partnership, codifying the process.'

Olivier Saillard[6]

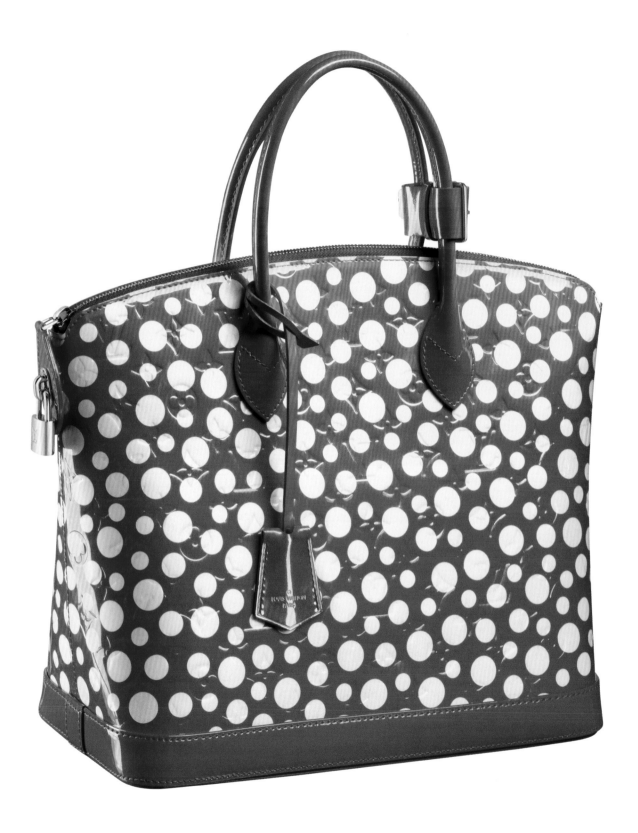

Above and opposite: Marc Jacobs for Louis Vuitton,
Lockit MM bag (above) and Lockit Vertical MM bag,
dress and jewelry (opposite), reproducing *Dots Infinity*
artwork by Yayoi Kusama, 2012.

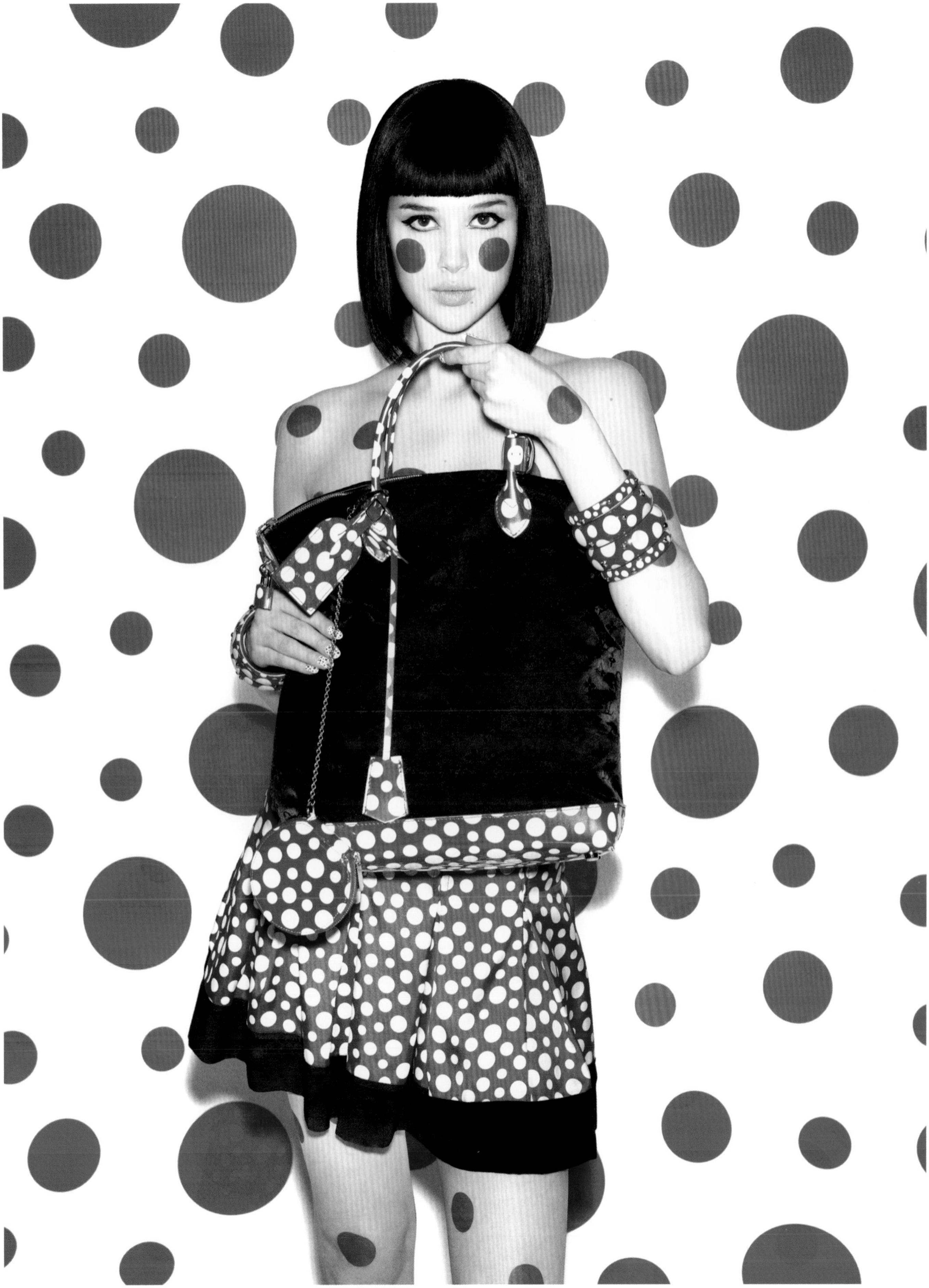

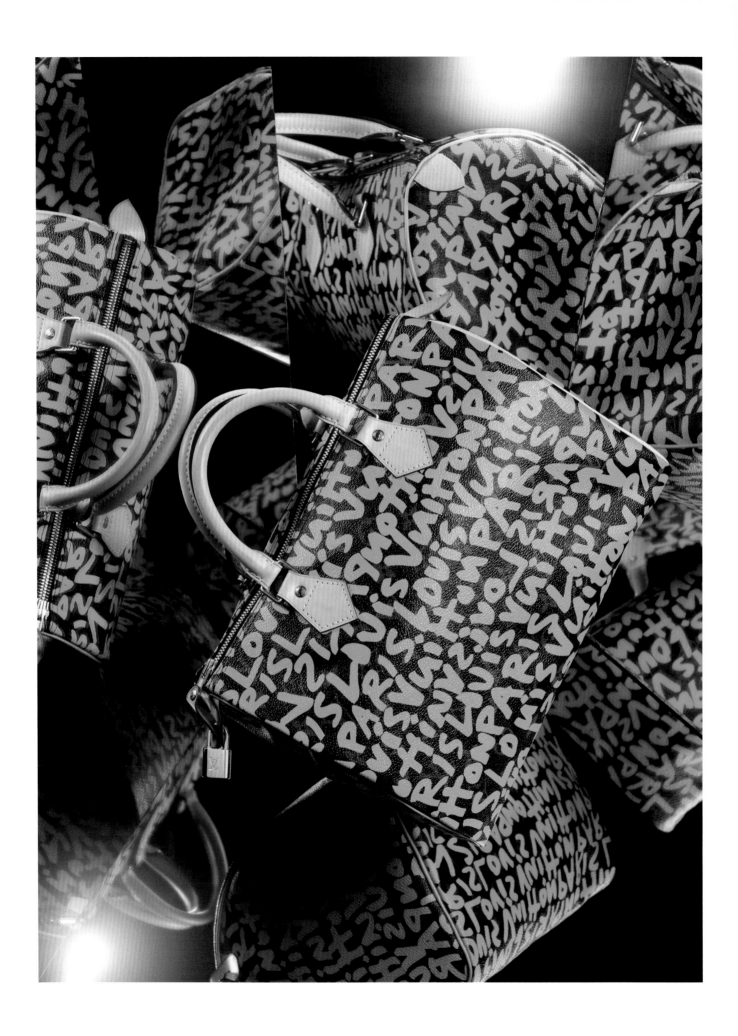

continued by the company's current owner, Bernard Arnault of luxury conglomerate LVMH, which assumed a controlling interest in 1990, with a centennial re-release of the house's signature monogram products in 1996. The celebratory collection featured bags personalized by some of the world's leading fashion designers including Azzedine Alaïa, Helmut Lang, Sybilla, Manolo Blahnik, Isaac Mizrahi, Romeo Gigli and Vivienne Westwood.

In 2003 creative director Marc Jacobs invited Japanese anime artist Takashi Murakami to redesign the house's iconic monogram, resulting in one of its greatest commercial successes to date. Murakami first reinterpreted the monogram in acid colours on black and white backgrounds, and later diversified in a number of versions, some incorporating anime-style images of cherry blossoms, cartoon characters and toy animals. This radical melding of high and low culture is typical of Murakami, who founded the Japanese postmodern art movement Superflat that conflates Japanese graphic design with the hyper-consumerism of Japanese society. He also designed in-store installations to house the products, as well as sculptures to accompany them. The artist later reappropriated the paintings and sculptures he had produced for Louis Vuitton, showing them in his solo exhibitions, thereby further collapsing the distinction between commercial and high art.

Throughout his tenure at Louis Vuitton, Jacobs has attempted to honour its founder's vision that the house should straddle both the fashion and art worlds. Jacobs himself is an avid collector of contemporary art, but equally understands the intimidating nature of a sparse gallery space. 'I had in my mind that only incredibly grand, extremely wealthy people lived with art of any sort,'[7] he explained of his early career. In an attempt to break down this barrier, Jacobs uses Louis Vuitton's collaborative projects to communicate the work of an artist to the wider public in an accessible medium: fashion. Speaking of his collaboration with Japanese avant-garde artist Yayoi Kusama, he reflects that 'it's a wonderful thing, the way contemporary art sort of permeates...and changes the environment, and for many people who don't look at art or go to galleries, there will be a new venue, a new place to see [the] work and to come to appreciate it through the eyes of Vuitton.'[8]

Opposite: Louis Vuitton, Speedy bag reproducing artwork by Stephen Sprouse overlaying the house's own signature monogram, 'Stephen Sprouse Tribute Collection', 2009.

Versace & Tim Roeloffs

As creative director and vice president of Versace since the death of her brother Gianni in 1997, Donatella Versace has restored the house he founded in 1978 to its former glory by imbuing its seasonal ready-to-wear collections with what can only be described as an Italian sexiness. One of her greatest commercial and critical successes has been her one-off collaboration with Dutch-born, Berlin-based collage artist Tim Roeloffs, whom she commissioned to create twelve prints, which appeared on four dresses for the house's Autumn/Winter 2008 womenswear collection. Roeloffs employed his trademark aesthetic of bricolage, physically cutting and pasting his own photographs of Berlin as part of a collage of archive imagery from past Versace campaigns. Roeloffs was given complete artistic freedom to create the prints, and was also provided access to details of Gianni Versace's personal interests, which included a love of 1960s wallpaper. The gritty imagery of Berlin marked a departure from the house's typically luxurious, sexy style and love of classical Roman imagery (its logo is the head of Medusa), but, as Roeloffs explained, 'Donatella wanted to do something about Berlin because Gianni loved Berlin.'[9] The resulting images, a mélange of a fragmented skyline and neo-classical furnishings digitally printed on neon pink, purple and yellow silk dresses were, however, ebullient and baroque in the very spirit of Versace. As a collaboration it embraced the conceptual ambitions of both artist and brand, creating new audiences for both.

'I was very impressed with the result as I didn't know how they planned to put photo-montages onto clothing. They did it very well and still maintained the dimensionality that's in my work.'

Tim Roeloffs[10]

Opposite: Versace, dress reproducing artwork
by Tim Roeloffs, Autumn/Winter 2008.

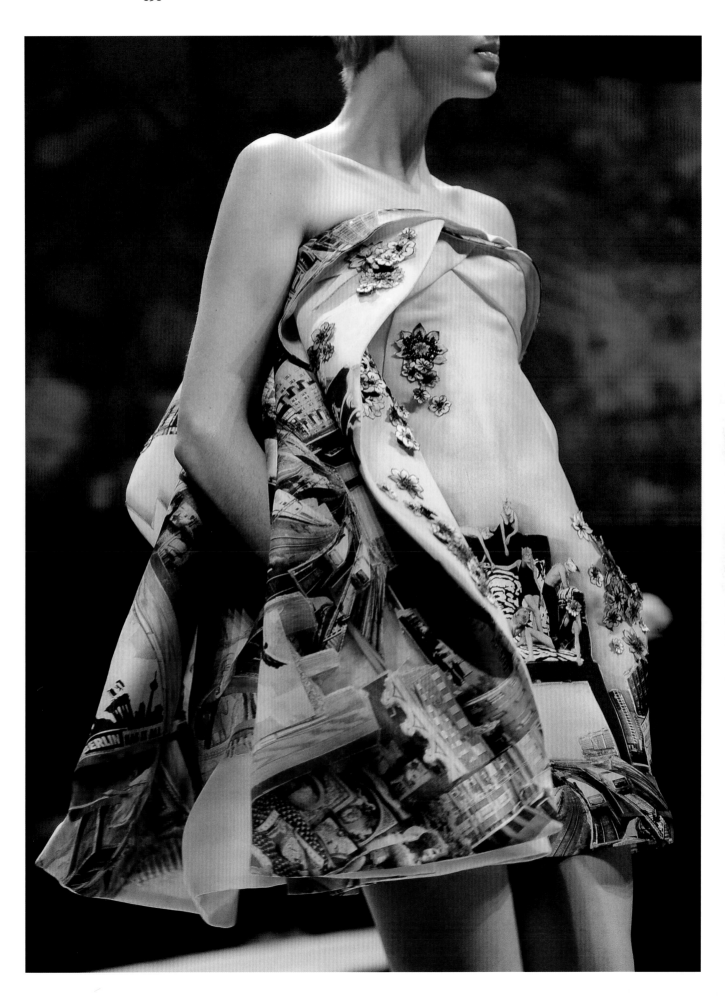

Pringle of Scotland & Liam Gillick

Established in 1815, Pringle of Scotland is one of the world's oldest luxury brands, best known for its 'Argyle' pattern and signature twinset made famous by celebrities such as Grace Kelly and Brigitte Bardot in the mid-20th century. Both were the work of Otto Weisz, who was the company's head designer from 1934. This long history has been both a boon and a challenge for the house. In a gesture designed to infuse its history with a contemporary vision, the company invited Turner Prize-nominated British artist Liam Gillick, known for his colourful Plexiglas sculptures, to collaborate with design director Alistair Carr on a capsule collection of accessories and knitwear. 'LIAMGILLICKFORPRINGLEOFSCOTLAND' was unveiled in May 2012 at Art Basel Miami Beach. The capsule collection took its cue from a series of the artist's abstract colour-block permutations, offset by a black-and-grey palette, and comprised clutch bags, weekenders, tote bags, an iPad holder and a wallet, as well as two cashmere pieces. For a preview of the capsule collection, Gillick created an intervention at the Pringle womenswear runway show at London Fashion Week in 2011. The vast length of the stark, white audience benches was monogrammed with black-vinyl text fragments from Gillick's then unpublished book *Construction of One*. In addition, the artist created a retail installation of bold, colour-blocked benches for the presentation of the 'LIAMGILLICKFORPRINGLEOFSCOTLAND' products in stores. The project successfully reinvigorated a venerated, traditional brand and brought it back into contemporary dialogue.

Pringle has also collaborated no less than three times with actress Tilda Swinton, who embodies both the edgy sensibility to which the brand aspires and the traditional Scottish values it mythologizes (Swinton, though born in London, is of prominent Scottish descent and has made her home in the Highlands for many years). In 2011 she starred alongside Scottish artist Jim Lambie in a Pringle advertising campaign shot by Swiss photographer Walter Pfeiffer against the backdrop of the Glasgow School of Art, further expanding the brand's consumer demographic and exploding clichés about its cardigan-wearing clients.

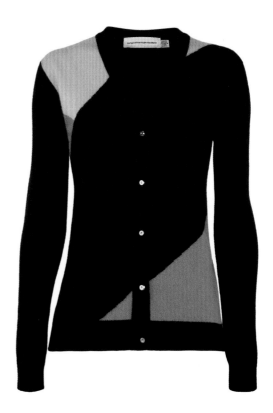

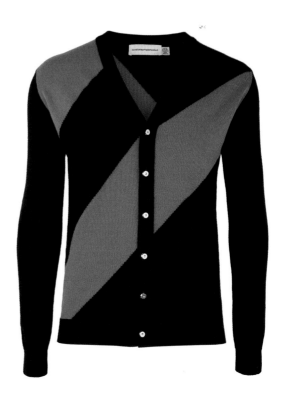

Top and above: Cardigans from the capsule collection 'LIAMGILLICKFORPRINGLEOFSCOTLAND' by artist Liam Gillick and designer Alistair Carr, 2012.

'Pringle of Scotland is closely associated with contemporary art; we partnered with the Serpentine Gallery for our 195th birthday and worked extensively with leading Scottish artists such as Richard Wright and Douglas Gordon to get their take on our heritage. Our project with Liam Gillick is a natural progression. We pride ourselves on creating truly authentic collaborations with the art world.'

Benoit Duverger,
Managing Director, Pringle of Scotland[11]

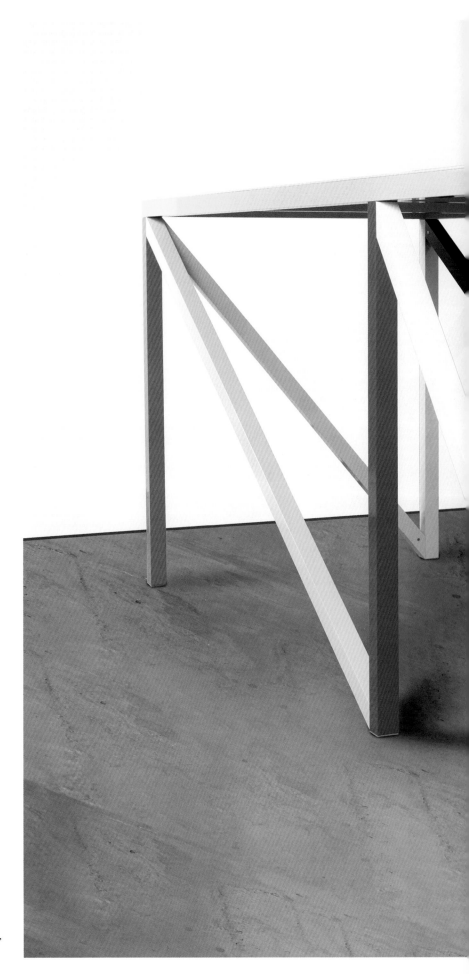

A retail installation created by Liam Gillick
to display the 'LIAMGILLICKFORPRINGLEOFSCOTLAND'
capsule collection in stores, 2012.

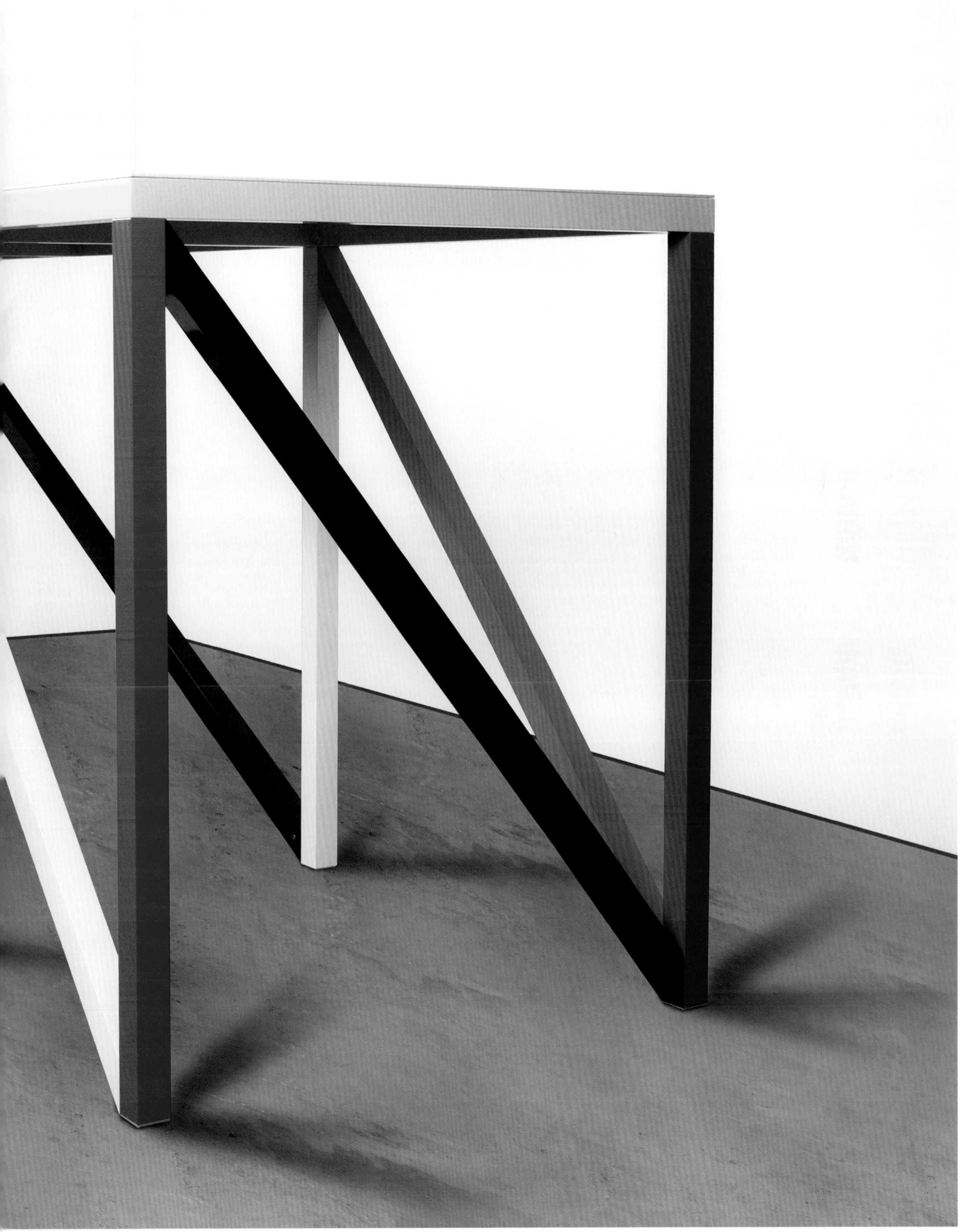

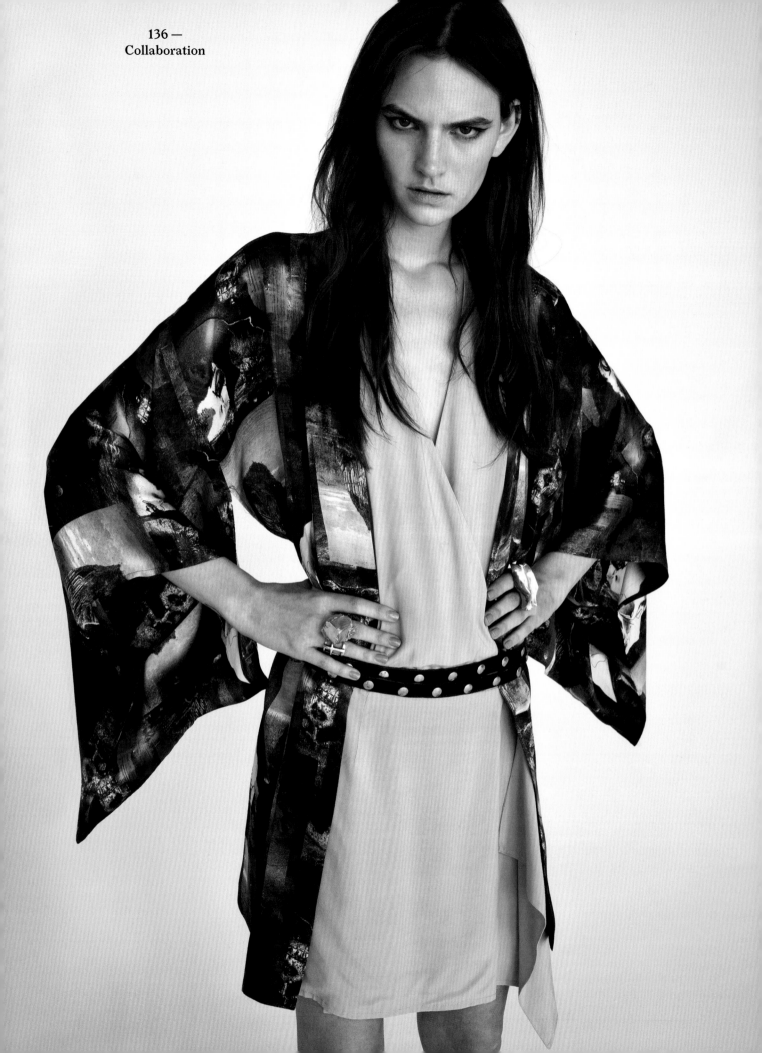

Something Else
& Julie Verhoeven

For Australian label Something Else's Spring/ Summer 2012 collection, British artist and illustrator Julie Verhoeven was engaged to create a series of unique artworks that were digitally printed onto clothing. Verhoeven, recognized as one of the most prolific collaborators in the fashion world, had previously worked with Louis Vuitton, Mulberry, Peter Jensen and Loewe, among others. The collaboration with Something Else was unusual, however, in that it offered Verhoeven wide-ranging freedom of interpretation. 'I like to merely inspire an idea and let the artist shape it from there,'[12] explained Natalie Wood, the label's founder and designer, of the process. Wood first came up with a loose theme – travelling across a desert, with a free-spirited woman in mind – which was first interpreted by Australian-born, New York-based writer Indigo Clarke in a series of short stories that were to accompany the collection. These stories were then sent to Verhoeven as possible inspiration. 'I didn't set a brief for her, just [asked her] to illustrate what came to mind. I had full trust in her creative process,' says Wood.

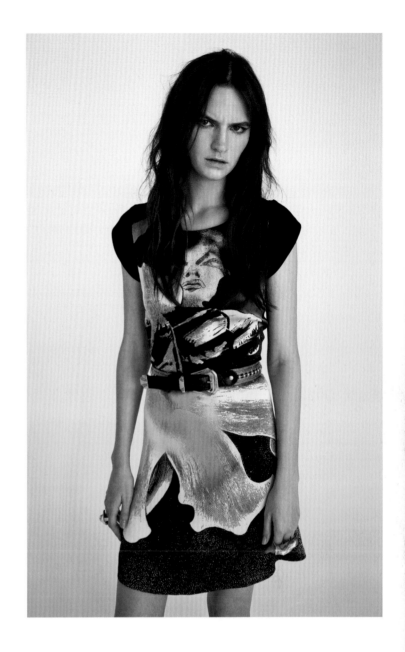

'I like to merely inspire an idea and let the artist shape it from there.'

Natalie Wood

Above and opposite: Something Else, dress (above)
and overshirt (opposite) reproducing artwork
by Julie Verhoeven, Spring/Summer 2012.

In conversation:
Pamela Easton & Lydia Pearson,
Easton Pearson

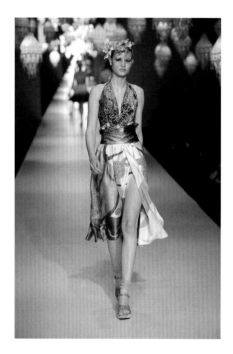

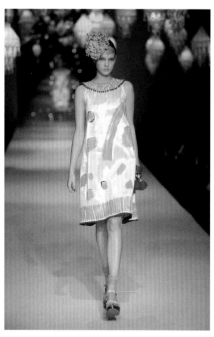

Australian label Easton Pearson is known for its mélange of Asian and Pacific influences, manifested via the hand-craft techniques and fabrics encountered in founding designers Pamela Easton and Lydia Pearson's extensive travels. Another important element has been their collaboration with Australian artists, including Stephen Mok, Graham Davis and Fukutoshi Ueno. In 2009 a retrospective of the label's more than twenty-year history at the Gallery of Modern Art, Brisbane, highlighted the mesh of cultures, ideas and techniques that underpin the label's collections, and explored how its artistic aesthetic has evolved, matured and mutated over the course of two decades.

ALISON KUBLER *What has prompted you to look outside of your own artistic ability and engage in collaborations?*

EASTON PEARSON Visual art isn't fashion, and fashion isn't visual art – they require different skills. We can do surface decoration to a certain extent, but we're not painters. We've had to look to artisans in India to achieve the painted look we desired. For our collaboration with Stephen Mok, his aesthetic was very much what we wanted for the collection: a celebration of the imperfect and naïve nature of our style. His painting incorporates loose, fluid strokes and lots of bold colour and line – witty and irreverent, which we love. In our collaborations with Indian artisans, we give them the shapes and colour palettes, but don't direct them – they have an enormous amount of freedom.

AK *What do you think a good collaboration brings to fashion?*

EP Collaborating means introducing a different perspective and extending your design. We have a vision, but to have someone else make their mark and express themselves is very special.

AK *Would you say that the hardest part of collaborating is the risk of injecting someone else's style into yours?*

EP We're very lucky in the sense that we've had really good relationships with the artists we've worked with. With Stephen, communicating was easy as he's not a precious type of artist. We were taking his drawings that were very witty and humorous and applying painstaking hand-beading and other very expensive processes to the final product.

AK *Is the result of collaboration with an artist then art?*

EP Fashion isn't really art, but then you have to ask yourself what the definition of art is. The lines have become blurred. Art used to be a creation from an individual's mind, body and soul, but today it's not like that in many ways, so I think it really depends on the intent of the designer.

AK *Well there's the commercial element to fashion that has historically precluded it from being considered art. Do commercial objectives play a part in the planning of a collaborative project?*

EP We don't approach any of our work with the view that a certain number of garments must sell; it's really the last thing we think of. It's our folly but also our luxury because we are in control of our business.

AK *But, needless to say, collaborations are hugely popular.*

EP Definitely, and they're happening in film, dance and music as well as fashion. Maybe it is because we all have more access to people via the internet, or because people constantly need more stimulation and it's a case that two minds are better than one.

Above, top and opposite: Easton Pearson,
dresses reproducing artworks by Stephen Mok,
Spring/Summer 2008.

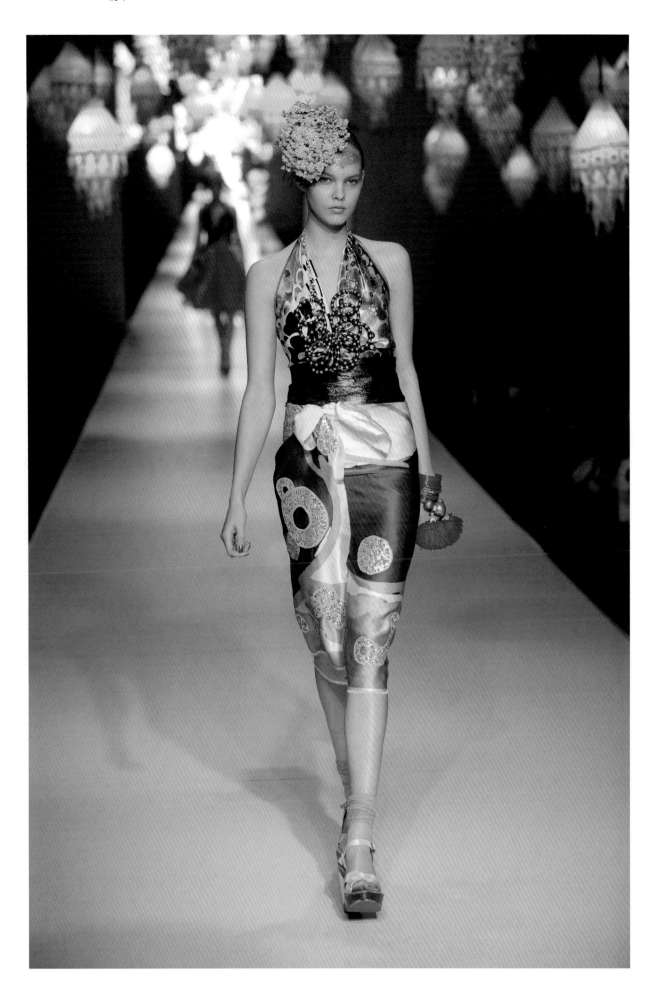

Coach: Hugo Guinness & James Nares

Founded in 1941 and still headquartered in New York, American luxury leather goods company Coach, best known for its women's handbags, luggage and accessories, has long been viewed as a relatively conservative brand, associated with its loyal uptown New York clientele. To help dispel this notion, in early 2012 Coach teamed with London-born, New York-based artist Hugo Guinness, known for his woodblock and linoleum prints. Guinness created four exclusive design motifs for the label – a coffee cup, sunglasses, a key ring and a tire pattern. 'Coach is a New York institution, so I created what I see every day on the streets of the city,' explained the artist.[13] The block prints were applied to a seventeen-piece collection of bags and accessories to appeal to a more youthful audience.

Following the success of the collection with Guinness, Coach teamed with British-born, New York-based artist, filmmaker and musician James Nares on a limited-edition capsule collection. The house employed five of Nares's single-brushstroke paintings, which it then applied to its classic canvas tote bag. Although the prints Coach employed were existing pieces from Nares's archive, the house significantly altered the construction of the bag, using a single heavy-duty seam so as to not interrupt the flow of the artwork. The collection was limited to 175 bags produced in each of the five different designs; all were individually numbered and stamped with Nares's signature, offering a witty take on the idea of the artist's mark: the brushstroke.

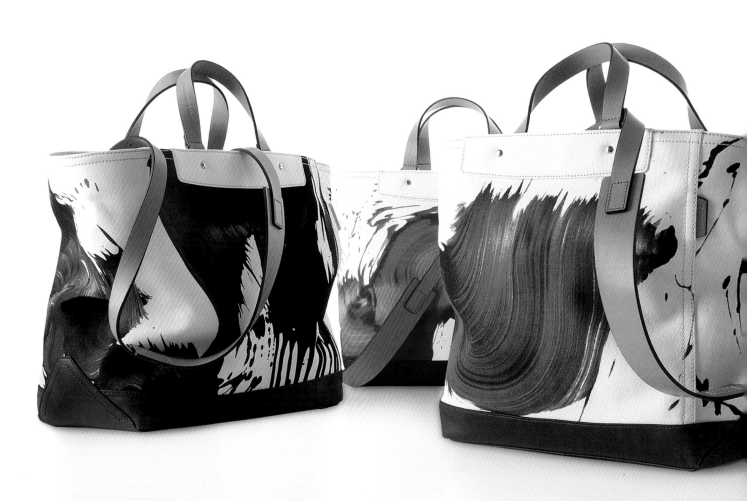

'When one of these bags is carried past you, you have the impression of a painting set in motion. They really are works of art.'

Jason Weisenfeld, Senior Vice President of Global Brand Communications and Collaborations, Coach

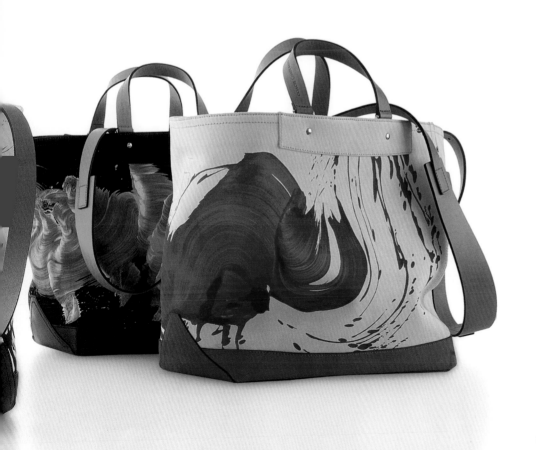

Coach tote bags, each colourway made in limited editions of 175, reproducing artworks by James Nares, 2012.

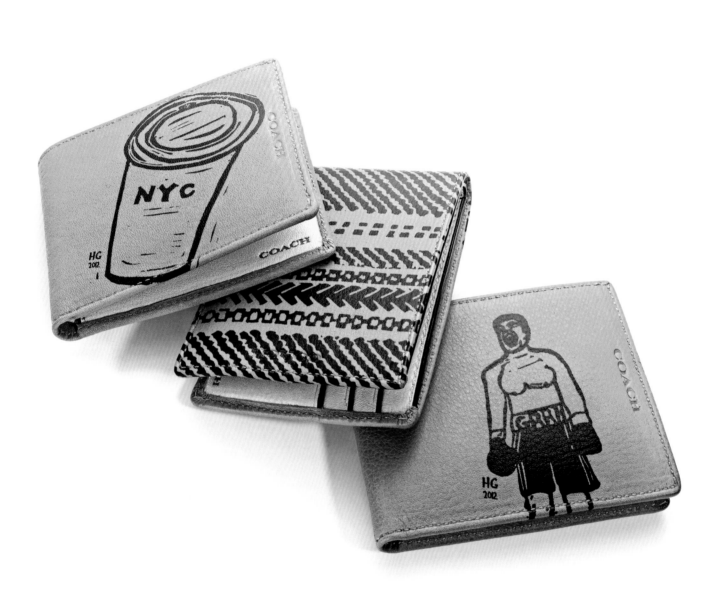

Above and opposite: Coach, leather wallets
(above) and tote bags (opposite) reproducing
artworks by Hugo Guinness, 2012.

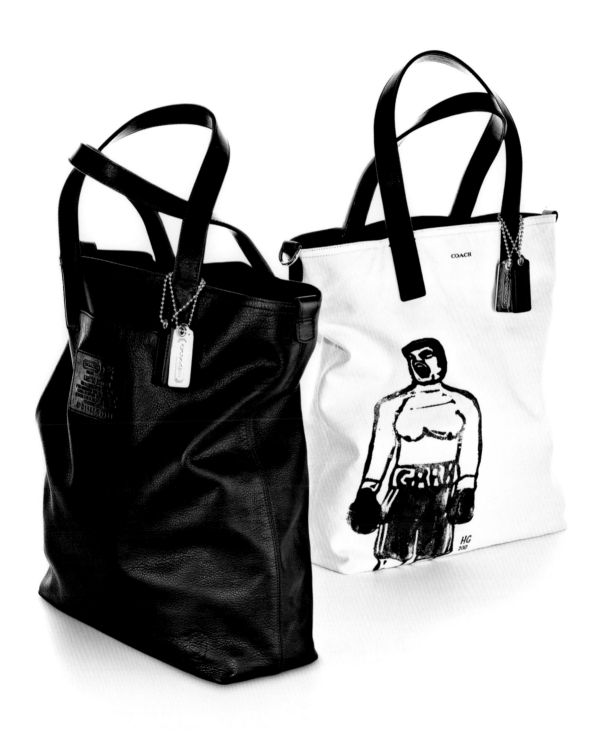

Marni: Richard Prince,
Gary Hume
& Claude Caillol

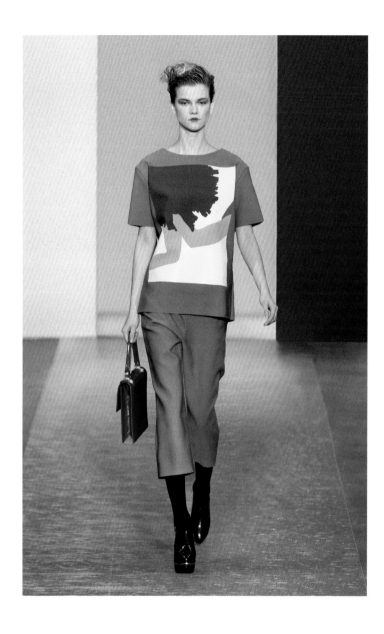

Above and opposite: Marni, shirts reproducing artworks
by Gary Hume, Autumn/Winter 2010.
Pages 146–47: Marni, sleeveless shirts reproducing artwork
by Peter Blake, Spring/Summer 2009.

Established in 1994, Italian label Marni produces seasonal ready-to-wear collections and accessories such as handbags, eyewear and jewelry that are characterized by a bold use of print and colour, displaying a casual and understated, yet often eccentric, elegance. This aesthetic has been developed further over the years via collaborations with carefully selected artists, musicians and illustrators who reflect head designer Consuelo Castiglioni's own interests. The Marni website prominently displays a catalogue of such art projects, demonstrating the importance of these collaborations to the brand's identity.

In 2007 Marni worked with American painter and photographer Richard Prince, borrowing a suite of watercolours that were reproduced on T-shirts (Spring/Summer 2007 and Autumn/Winter 2007). This low-key approach to working with such a highly collectable artist displayed the confidence and cultural cachet of the brand. In 2010 the label collaborated with British painter Gary Hume on a series of printed cotton shirts for its Autumn/Winter 2010 collection. Hume, a past Turner Prize finalist, takes the subjects of his figurative paintings from popular culture, reducing them to simplified colour abstractions. The collaboration with Marni had conceptual significance in that it eventually resulted in the returning of Hume's source images (many of which had been taken from fashion magazines) to their original context when the collection was reported in the press.

French artist and furniture designer Claude Caillol collaborated with Marni to produce 'The Plastic Collection' for Autumn/Winter 2010. In a clever extension of his own practice, which involves drawing on recycled shopping bags, Caillol translated his free-hand drawings onto Marni-branded ephemeral plastic shopping bags that were then applied to more permanent PVC tote bags with leather handles. In creating an object that would become collectable as opposed to recyclable or disposable, Marni made a playful, knowing comment on the nature of consumer culture, of which it is a complicit part.

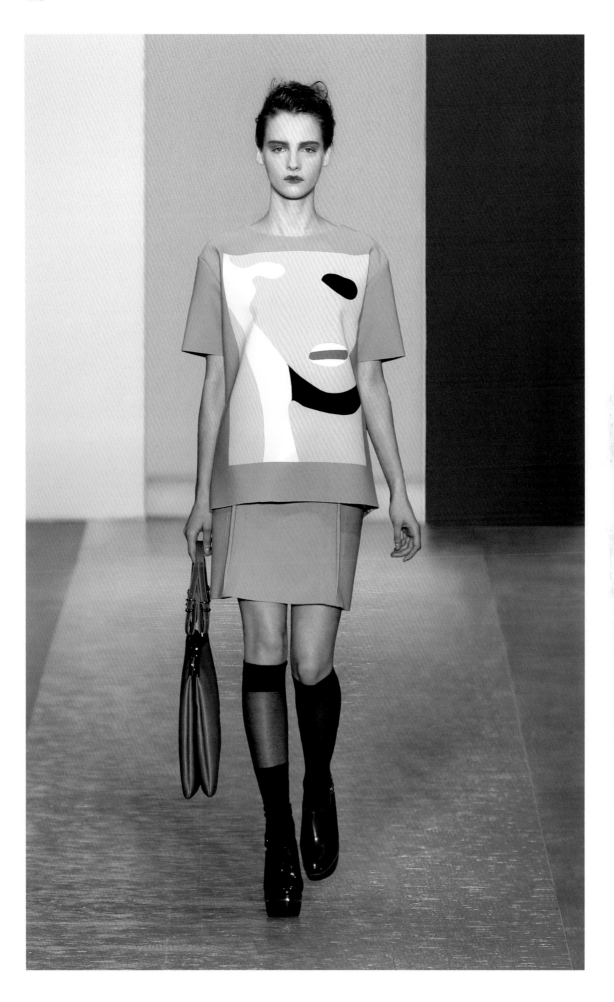

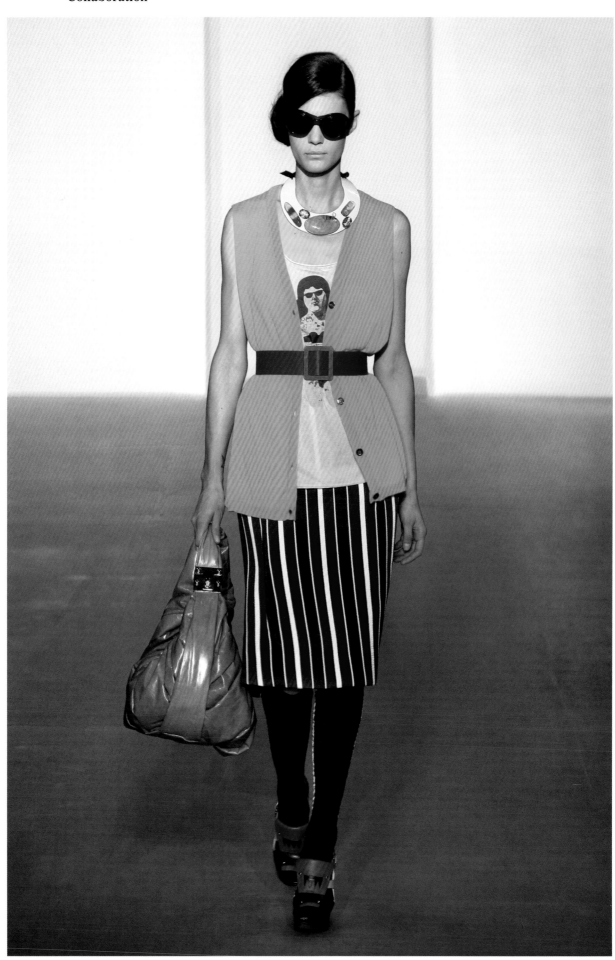

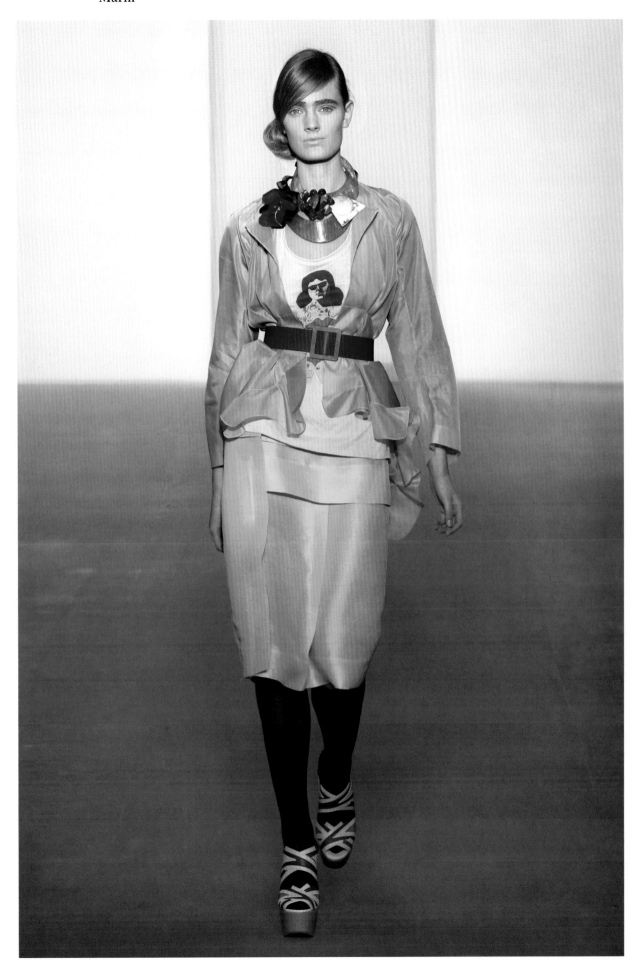

Hermès & Erwin Wurm

Austrian artist Erwin Wurm's approach to sculpture is distinctly non-traditional. He is best known for his *One Minute Sculptures*, an ongoing series of body-based works in which random everyday objects are used to create three-dimensional assemblages that are then documented photographically. The series offers a humorous riposte to the monumental sculptural tradition. Wurm's collaboration with the venerable French luxury accessories house Hermès, renowned for its silk scarves and leathergoods, is as surprising as the juxtapositions in his work – and therein lies its strength.

In contrast with other historic fashion brands, such as Louis Vuitton, which maintain their contemporary relevance by periodically inviting artists to reinterpret their classic designs, Hermès favours purely artistic collaborative projects in which its products and the artist's presentation of them engage in a dialogue, although the label does also have a long tradition of product-based artist collaborations on its silk scarves. In 2008, at the invitation of Véronique Nichanian, Hermès's artistic director for menswear, Wurm created a series of incongruous and witty photographs, entitled *Monde Hermès*, depicting people engaging with Hermès products in the style of his *One Minute Sculptures*. In one image, a man stands upon a horse's back in a subversive take on the typical triumphal pose of an equestrian statue, carrying a Hermès Birkin bag; in another, a man sits in an elegant salon balancing a Hermès vase precariously on his head. These photographs were exhibited in Hermès stores alongside surreal sculptures such as a mirrored leg dressed in clothing and shoes, and a boxy jacket and legs that distorted the traditional shapes of mannequins,

and, by extension, the human form. In accord with Hermès's preferred mode of collaboration, these photographs and sculptures were conceived purely as artistic works, and not as eventual promotional material. 'I did not do any advertising for Hermès,' explains Wurm, 'and not a single photograph or image may be used for advertising purposes; they are only permitted to display the works [in-store] and reproduce them in a company magazine.'[14]

Wurm feels that the close 21st-century relationship between art and fashion justified his decision to work with Hermès. 'The fashion world has gained a much greater affinity with art, and the world of art is steeped in fashion. In my eyes, fashion designers like Alexander McQueen are brilliant artists.' Moreover, he found the experience of working with a top luxury brand so wholly alien to him that it became a source of artistic inspiration in its own right. 'I was intrigued by the firm's position in the absolute luxury segment. At the outset I couldn't even imagine how bizarre and unfathomable it all is. I was totally fascinated by one example in their product line: hooded sweat jackets, so-called "hoodies" – which of course are a synonym for the youth movement and rebellion – are made of Nile crocodile skin and sold for an outrageous 80,000 euro apiece. I found that extremely interesting, since you don't even need to say anything about a jacket like that, you can just display it – and that's what I did.'

Opposite: Erwin Wurm, *The Anarchist*, from his *Monde Hermès* series, 2008.
Pages 149–50: Erwin Wurm, sculptures from his *Untitled* series commissioned for display in Hermès stores, 2008.

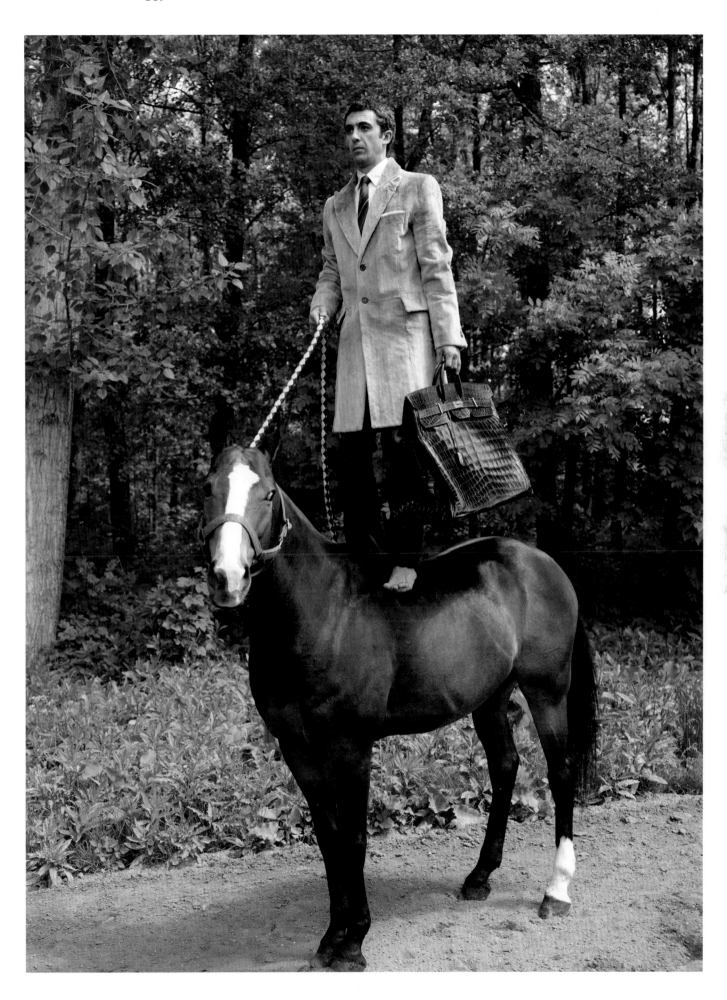

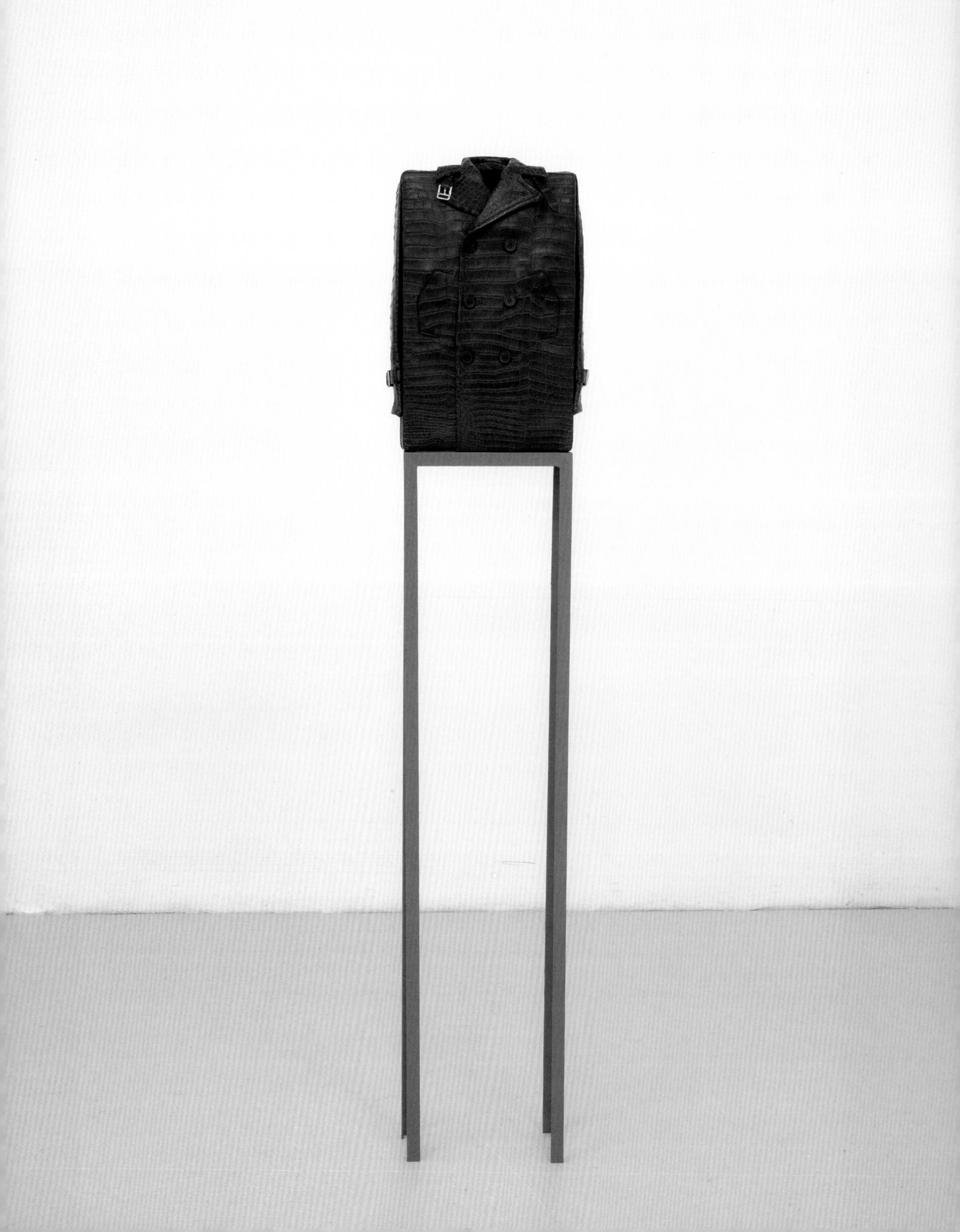

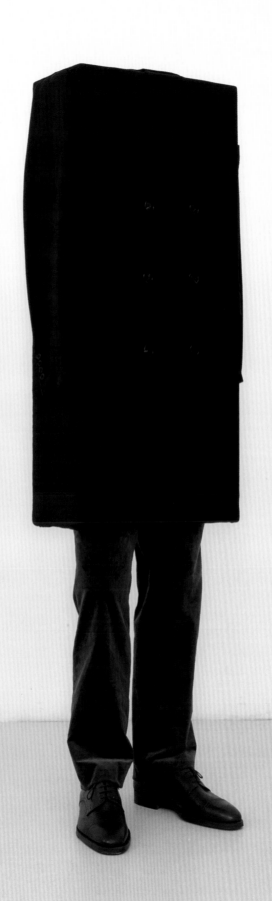

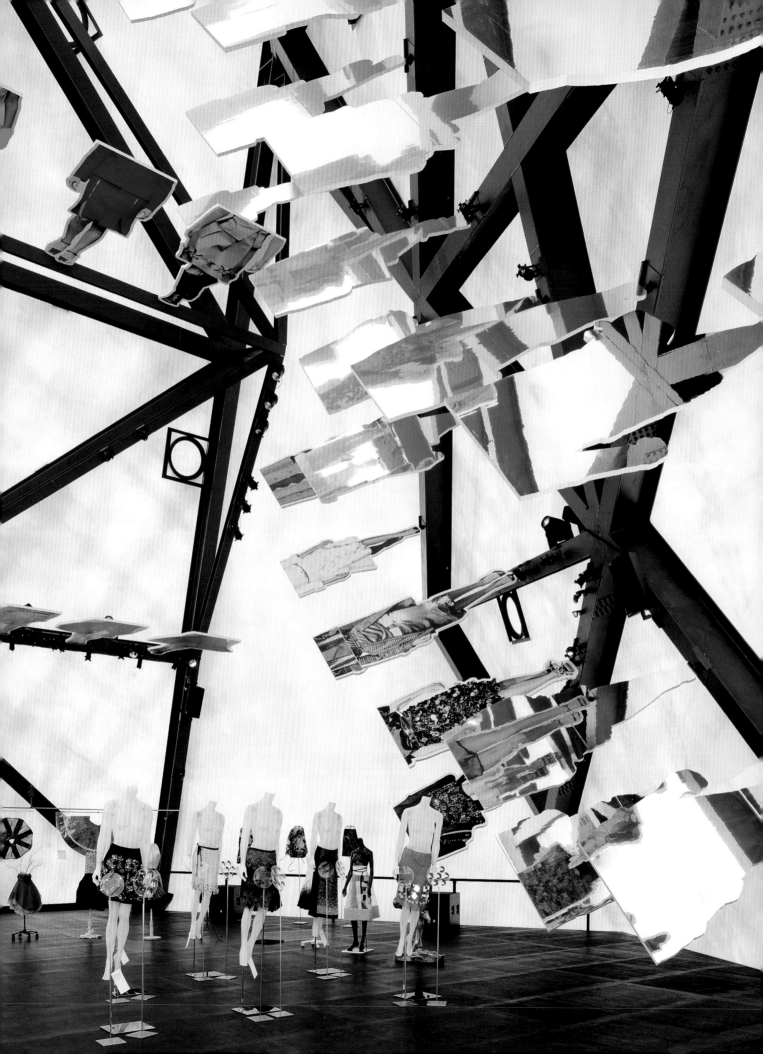

Eye candy and ideas: Fashion as exhibition

Introduction:
Eye candy and ideas

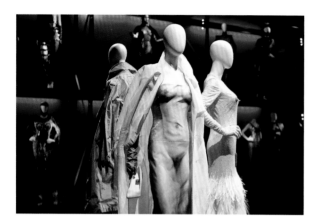

'The Fashion World of Jean Paul Gaultier:
From the Sidewalk to the Catwalk' exhibition at
the Montreal Museum of Fine Arts, 2011.

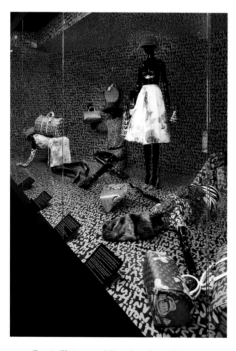

'Louis Vuitton – Marc Jacobs' exhibition
at the Musée de la Mode et du Textile,
Les Arts Décoratifs, Paris, 2012.

Put simply, a fashion exhibition is eye candy and ideas rolled into one. Fashion has a unique ability to connect with viewers on multiple levels of meaning. Its theatricality and grand gestures attract fashion and non-fashion audiences alike to museum exhibitions in order to experience an extraordinary visual spectacle. On a deeper level, fashion is also an art form that speaks to a universal understanding of the body. Audience demand for both aesthetic and intellectual content has been increasing steadily since the turn of the millennium, resulting in a plethora of fashion exhibitions in traditional art venues.

When the Metropolitan Museum of Art, New York, staged the retrospective exhibition 'Alexander McQueen: Savage Beauty' in 2011, the response was overwhelming; the show attracted more than 650,000 visitors, an unprecedented number for any previous exhibition in any artistic genre. Public interest in the label was already at an all-time high due to its founder's recent suicide and Kate Middleton's patriotic decision to wear a dress by Alexander McQueen designer Sarah Burton when she married Prince William in April 2011, but 'Savage Beauty' nonetheless proved a litmus test of fashion's cultural worth and established the bankable appeal of fashion exhibitions in a fine art context. Since 2009 there have been a number of other successful museum retrospectives focused on a single designer or label, including Jean Paul Gaultier, Cristóbal Balenciaga, Christian Louboutin, Yves Saint Laurent, Madame Grès, Hussein Chalayan, Rodarte, Comme des Garçons and Chloé. These exhibitions have focused on designers whose practice is defined by a rigorous attention to detail and a high level of craftsmanship, as opposed to fast or high street fashion – an important distinction in terms of fashion's new standing in the art world.

A key exhibition that directly addressed the question of fashion's new credibility within the art world was 'The Art of Fashion: Installing Allusions', at the Museum Boijmans van Beuningen, Rotterdam, in 2009. Curated by eminent fashion historians Judith Clark and José Teunissen, 'The Art of Fashion' presented the work of some twenty-five international artists and avant-garde designers, and included pieces by Viktor & Rolf, Chalayan and Walter Van Beirendonck, who (together with Anna Nicole Zeische and Naomi Filmer) were among the five designers invited to make new work for the exhibition. The exhibition resembled a series of installations, which largely eschewed the traditional mannequin/garment approach to presentation, and, by exhibiting both fashion

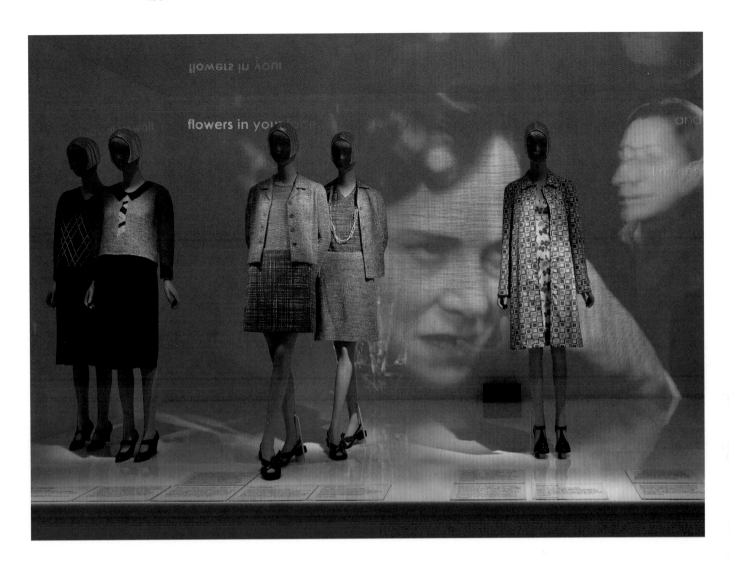

Above: 'Schiaparelli and Prada: Impossible Conversations'
exhibition at the Costume Institute at the Metropolitan
Museum of Art, New York, 2012.

and contemporary art in a shared platform, successfully
bridged the perceived cultural divide between the two.

Just as the discipline of architecture boasts its
cast of 'starchitects', this critical re-presentation of
fashion has been led by a roll call of 'It' curators that
includes Andrew Bolton of the Costume Institute at the
Metropolitan Museum of Art, New York; Valerie Steele
of the Museum at the Fashion of Institute of Technology,
New York; and Pamela Golbin of the Musée de la Mode
et du Textile, Paris. Their new breed of fashion exhibition typically focuses on a designer's cross-disciplinary
practice and features dynamic and innovative means of
presentation, often the result of the designer's creative
engagement with artists, filmmakers, stylists and architects. For instance, 'Hats: An Anthology', a travelling
exhibition curated by milliner Stephen Jones for the
Victoria & Albert Museum, London, in 2009, displayed
both Jones's own work and other famous hats in vitrines
like exotic hothouse flowers, presenting them both as
works of art and as important artefacts of social history.

As fashion exhibitions increasingly move outside the
remit of leading fashion institutions and into mainstream
art museums and galleries, they challenge the ways in

'Clothes are never a frivolity; they always mean something.'

James Laver, fashion historian[1]

Opposite: 'Alaïa: Azzedine Alaïa in the 21st century' exhibition
at the Groninger Museum, the Netherlands, 2011.

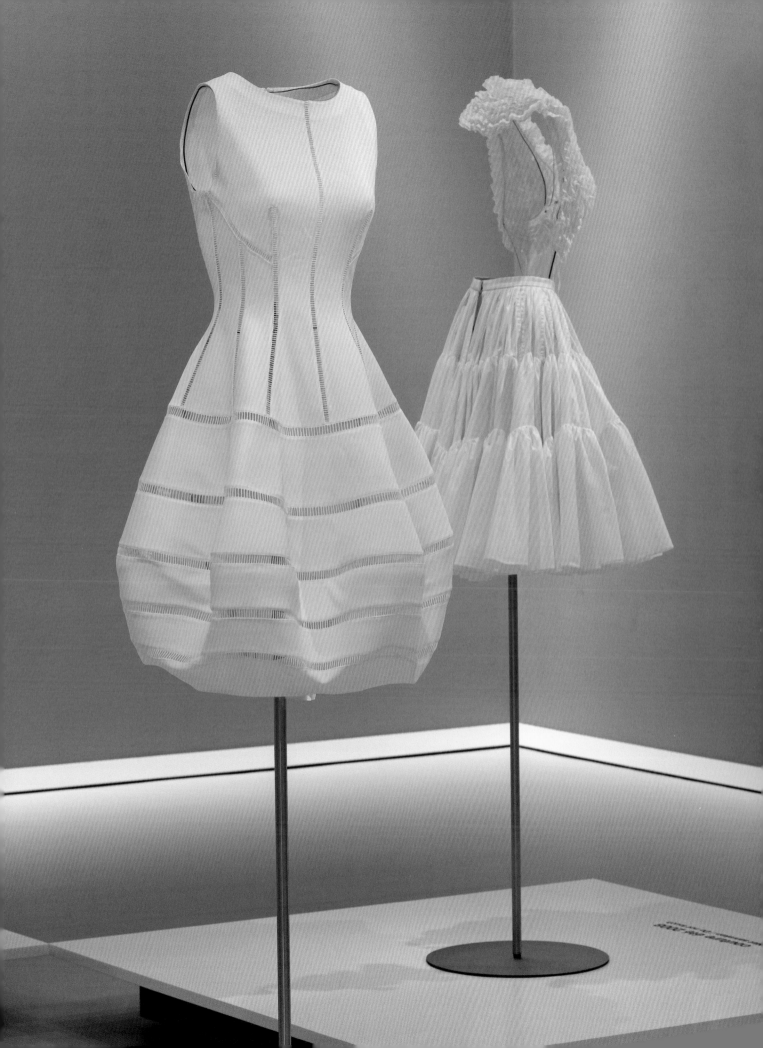

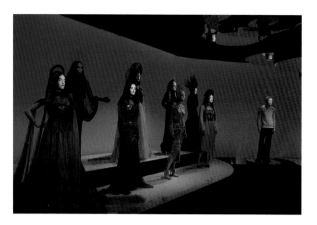

'The Fashion World of Jean Paul Gaultier:
From the Sidewalk to the Catwalk' exhibition at
the Montreal Museum of Fine Arts, 2011.

which fashion has traditionally been presented to the public. The mannequin, for instance, with its allusion to the human form, is difficult to do away with, both a physical support for clothing and a vehicle for its expression. Clark observes that the sight of a garment displayed on a mannequin triggers an automatic appraisal of the work as a potential purchase, a reaction unlike that normally elicited by other types of fine art: 'We usually have an immediate identification with the garment – Do we like it? Would we wear it? How far does it differ from our taste, style, period, assumptions, etc.? We may not identify with actually wearing the garment but we know how it works. We use our own dictionary of style to judge the designer's project – is it daring, sexually exciting, glamorous, etc. by our own moral code? – And we do this in a way that we cannot do with any other applied art.'[2] The dilemma for curators, then, is how to use the mannequin, with its prosaic references to the high street shopping experience, within the design of a fine-art exhibition. The major retrospective 'The House of Viktor & Rolf' at the Barbican Art Gallery, London, in 2008 offered an unconventional solution to this problem, eschewing conventional mannequins in favour of 1/3-life-size dolls dressed in miniature bespoke versions of the Dutch duo's most famous designs, displayed in a large dollhouse. This conscious thwarting of scale disrupted familiar elements of fashion presentation while highlighting the absurdity of haute couture and mocking its pretensions to artistry.

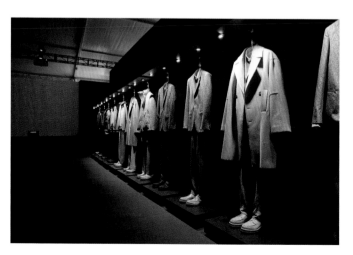

'Infinite Loop' temporary exhibition for the Calvin Klein
Autumn/Winter 2012 presentation, Seoul.

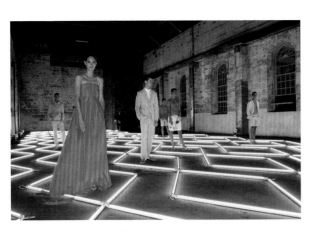

Light installation by Jonathan Jones for
Calvin Klein Spring/Summer 2009 collection presentation,
Cockatoo Island, Sydney, 2008.

Inspired by the popularity of such high-profile exhibitions, fashion brands are at the same time increasingly styling their stores to resemble art galleries or miniature museums, blurring the line that once existed between art and fashion, or, in the view of some critics, between creativity and commerce. Products are displayed on plinths, in Perspex cases or artfully arranged on a wall in the manner of a salon hang, mimicking art curation as they offer democratic entry to its rarefied world. This similarity in appearance between art galleries and fashion boutiques also reflects the reality that shopping and visiting exhibitions are both forms of contemporary entertainment in which one can consume ideas and products – via the all-important museum shop in the case of art museums.

Another important aspect of the increasingly close relationship between fashion and art exhibition in the 21st century is that fashion houses have emerged as influential patrons of both contemporary and traditional fine art. In 2012 Salvatore Ferragamo sponsored a major exhibition of the work of Leonardo da Vinci at the Louvre in Paris, setting a new precedent for the revival of traditional patronage. In return for its significant financial support, the Louvre granted permission for Ferragamo to stage a runway show on a 120-metre (394-foot) catwalk in the hallowed halls of the Denon Wing, the first time such a prominent fashion event had been hosted by a leading art museum. Also in 2012, Louis Vuitton sponsored Yayoi Kusama's touring survey exhibition that was organized by Tate Modern in London, increasing Kusama's public profile as the brand embarked upon its own collaborative projects with the Japanese avant-garde artist. Italian fashion house Prada also enjoys a reputation as a major supporter of the arts through its Fondazione Prada, which maintains exhibition spaces in Milan and Venice, and its extensive financial sponsorship of art projects. Unlike Louis Vuitton, Prada has traditionally eschewed collaboration in favour of high-profile projects as part of an artist's ongoing work, such as Francesco Vezzoli's *24Hr Museum* (2012), a temporary installation in the Palais d'Iéna, Paris, described by the artist as a 'self-parodying fake retrospective/introspective'.[3]

This chapter looks at the growing place of fashion within the art gallery, in creative, curatorial and patronage roles. As some of the world's leading fashion curators explain in the interviews that follow, the 21st century is a pivotal moment for fashion, which – by right of its considerable financial resources, gift for dynamic presentation and ability to attract enormous new audiences to art museums – now finds itself both scrutinized and admired as an influential force in the shifting hierarchy of the art world.

In conversation: Andrew Bolton, The Costume Institute at The Metropolitan Museum of Art, New York

The Costume Institute at the Metropolitan Museum of Art, New York, houses what is arguably the greatest costume collection in the world, made famous by *Vogue* editor Diana Vreeland, who served as a special consultant from 1972 until her death in 1989, and who in many ways made popular the concept of fashion as exhibition. Under the direction of curators Harold Koda and Andrew Bolton, the Costume Institute continues to set a global standard for fashion exhibitions ('Alexander McQueen: Savage Beauty', which opened in 2011, attracted a total of 661,509 visitors, placing it among the museum's top ten most visited exhibitions). They range in theme from monographs on a single designer, such as the McQueen show, to conceptual pairings such as 'Schiaparelli and Prada: Impossible Conversations' (2012), a study of the parallels between Italian designers Miuccia Prada and Elsa Schiaparelli.

ALISON KUBLER *I wanted to start by asking, rather broadly, if you think fashion sits comfortably within an art museum?*

ANDREW BOLTON I think it can. Fashion isn't just about wearability or about the pragmatics of clothing, but also about ideas and concepts. Designers like Hussein Chalayan and Alexander McQueen, for example, use fashion to talk about ideas of gender, identity, politics, religion; fashion is a vehicle to express ideas about the subject. And that, too, is what art is all about. So, yes, fashion does have a place within the art gallery. I think fashion is an art form. You just need to think of haute couture in terms of craftsmanship – there's extraordinary talent in technical expertise; it is the art of fashion. So this, coupled with the ideas and concepts [behind it], makes it hard for me to see a distinction between art and fashion. I also think fashion is a really important art form because it's accessible and it's democratic: people aren't afraid of fashion and can relate to it more than other art forms. People don't need to have a prior knowledge of fashion to appreciate it because they wear clothes everyday.

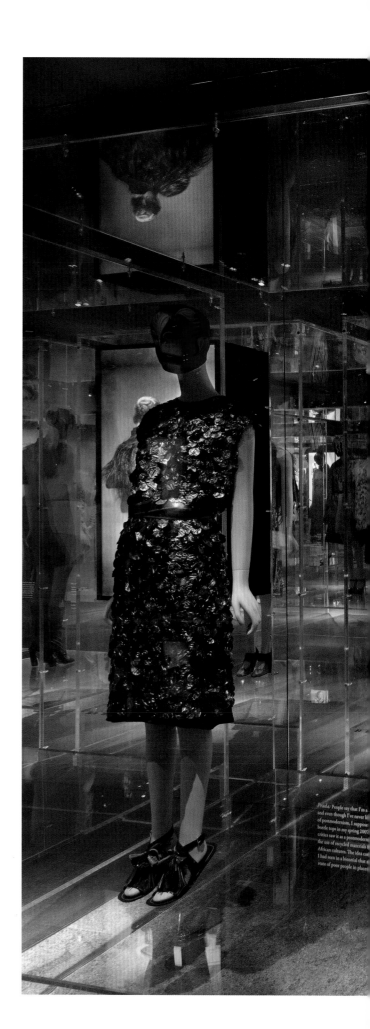

'Schiaparelli and Prada: Impossible Conversations' exhibition at the Costume Institute at the Metropolitan Museum of Art, New York, 2012.

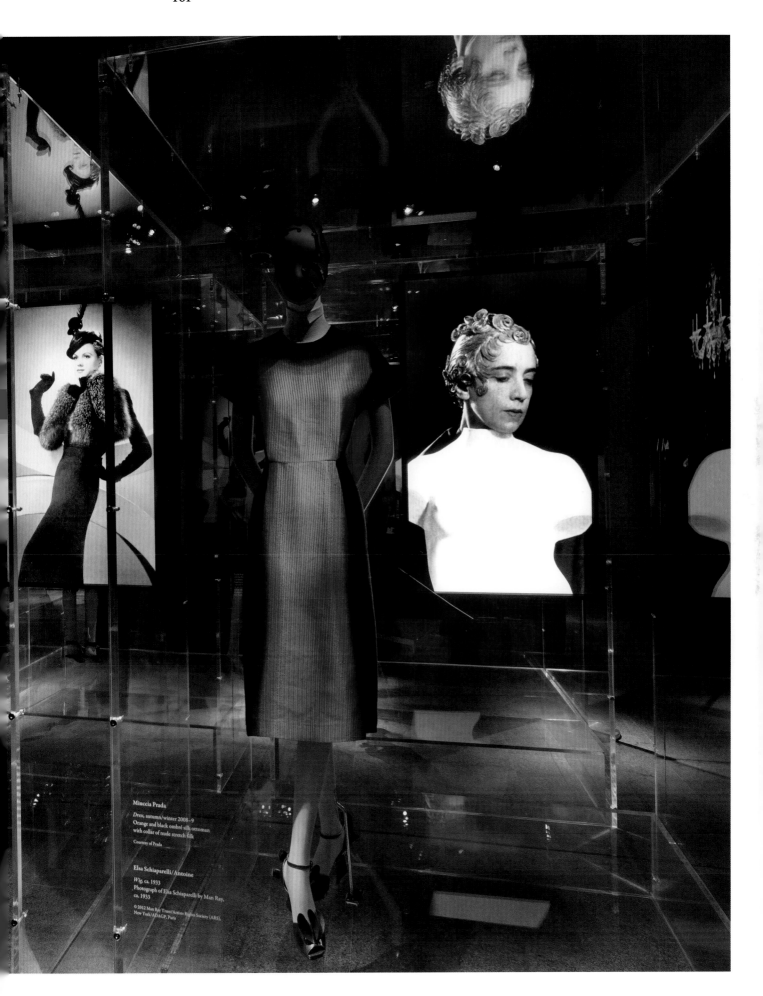

Miuccia Prada

Dress, autumn/winter 2008–9
Orange and black ombré silk ottoman
with collar of nude stretch silk
Courtesy of Prada

Elsa Schiaparelli/Antoine

Wig, ca. 1933
Photograph of Elsa Schiaparelli by Man Ray,
ca. 1933

© 2012 Man Ray Trust/Artists Rights Society (ARS),
New York/ADAGP, Paris

Below and overleaf: 'Alexander McQueen: Savage Beauty'
exhibition at the Costume Institute at the Metropolitan
Museum of Art, New York, 2011.

AK *How do you view collaborations between artists and designers? There have been
an enormous number in recent years.*

AB The majority of collaborations are banal; they're not thought out, they
don't expand the argument of art and fashion, and they're too simplistic.
I don't think that fashion designers need to work with artists to elevate
fashion because I really do think that fashion is an art form. There have,
however, been interesting collaborations, like that between Marc Jacobs's
Louis Vuitton and [Takashi] Murakami, where there was a focus on the
argument of [both] fashion and art as commerce.

AK *Were you surprised by the response to the McQueen show?*

AB Yes, absolutely. The whole experience was extraordinary. To show it so
soon after his death was very emotional for me. I was working directly
with the McQueen house, which I wanted to do very much, I really wanted
to speak with Sarah [Burton, creative director of Alexander McQueen]
about the McQueen design process, and it was extraordinary to learn
how McQueen worked. Sam Gainsbury, who is responsible for producing

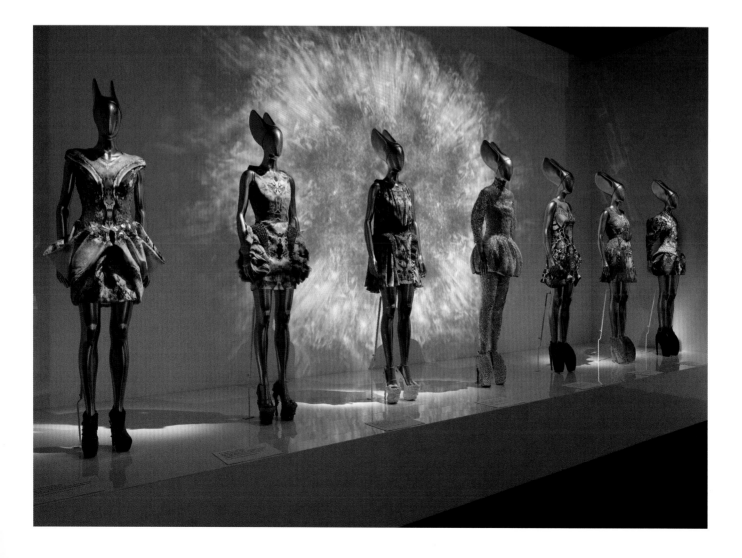

the McQueen shows, talked about the ideas McQueen had for the runway and Trino Verkade, who was his first employee, would talk about the commercial side. Having access to those people was extraordinary. What was unique about McQueen was that he used fashion to channel, convey and evoke emotions in the viewer. He didn't care if you liked or hated his work, he just wanted you to have a reaction. He was shamanistic about his work; the materials he'd use were outside of fashion, like shells and enormous feathers, which had a fetishistic quality about them. What was amazing was how people responded to it emotionally. I think if he hadn't died people wouldn't be quite so emotional about it, as emotions were enhanced

AK   *What is it that defines a designer worthy of selection for an exhibition?*

AB   A lot of what we focus on is designers who really have advanced fashion in one way or another, whether through techniques and construction, or conceptually. The consideration is focusing on designers who have made a contribution to fashion history, such as [Coco] Chanel, [Cristóbal] Balenciaga, [Gianni] Versace, [Alexander] McQueen, [Hussein] Chalayan and [John] Galliano; designers who have engaged with the boundaries of fashion in one form or another. Chalayan was more about concepts, where McQueen is about construction. All of the designers have advanced fashion through one form or another. The Prada and Schiaparelli

'Fashion responds to current events quickly, acting as a mirror of our time.'

Andrew Bolton

by the circumstances of his death, but people were responding to his pure vision expressed through fashion.

AK   *Do you think the impact of a show like that helps to shift attitudes towards fashion in a traditional museum context? Is it less of an uphill battle to get fashion into those spaces?*

AB   The uphill battle is with art critics rather than the museum itself, particularly in America where there's a bias against fashion, because they see it very low down on the ladder when it comes to art – the bottom rung. I find it frustrating to constantly argue with critics that fashion is art, that it very deservedly has a place in a museum context because it taps into all of the other artistic references that other designers have used, particularly postmodern artists. I love the fact that it has contextualized fashion within a broader design environment.

show took on a different strategy, creating a dialogue between two different designers, using less formal but more conceptual similarities – designers that use fashion to convey notions of beauty or style. We wanted to create a fictional conversation between these women who share similarities. It's also a conversation between the past and present that worked on different levels.

AK   *On a rudimentary level, why do you think art and fashion have collided so much in the past decade?*

AB   I think that people are very much aware of the power of fashion to express ideas of gender, politics and the body. The commonality and themes between artists and fashion designers represents the breakdown of boundaries of the disciplines. A lot of it is realizing how integral fashion is to contemporary culture. Fashion responds to current events quickly, acting as a mirror of our time.

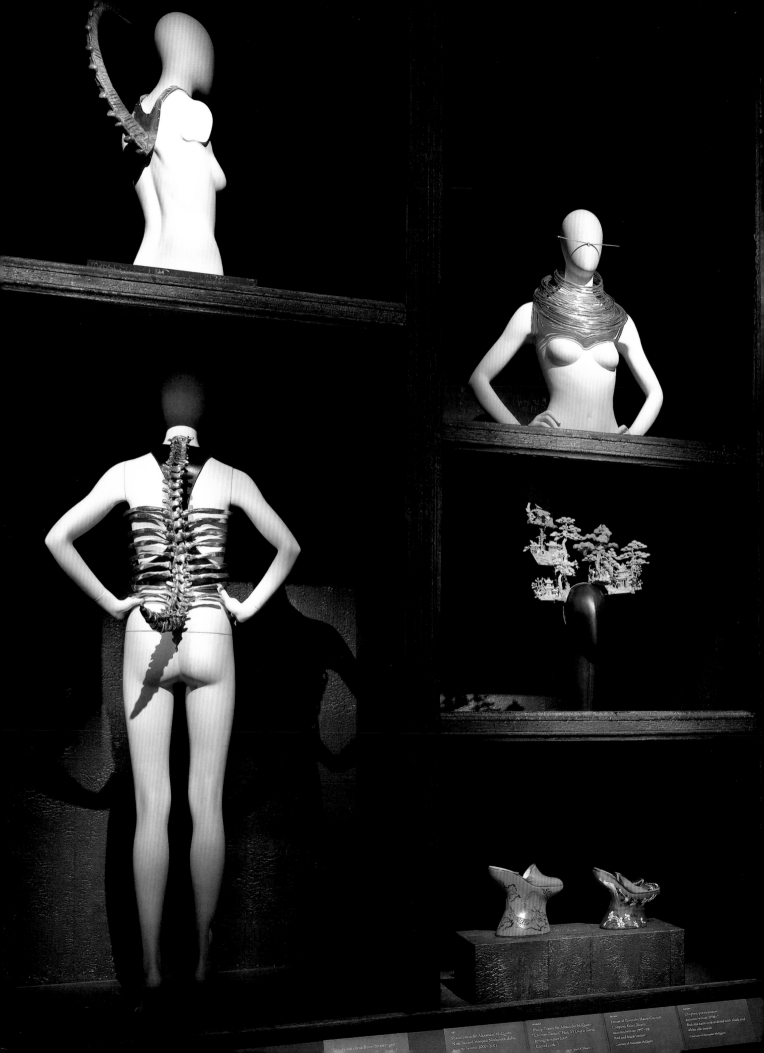

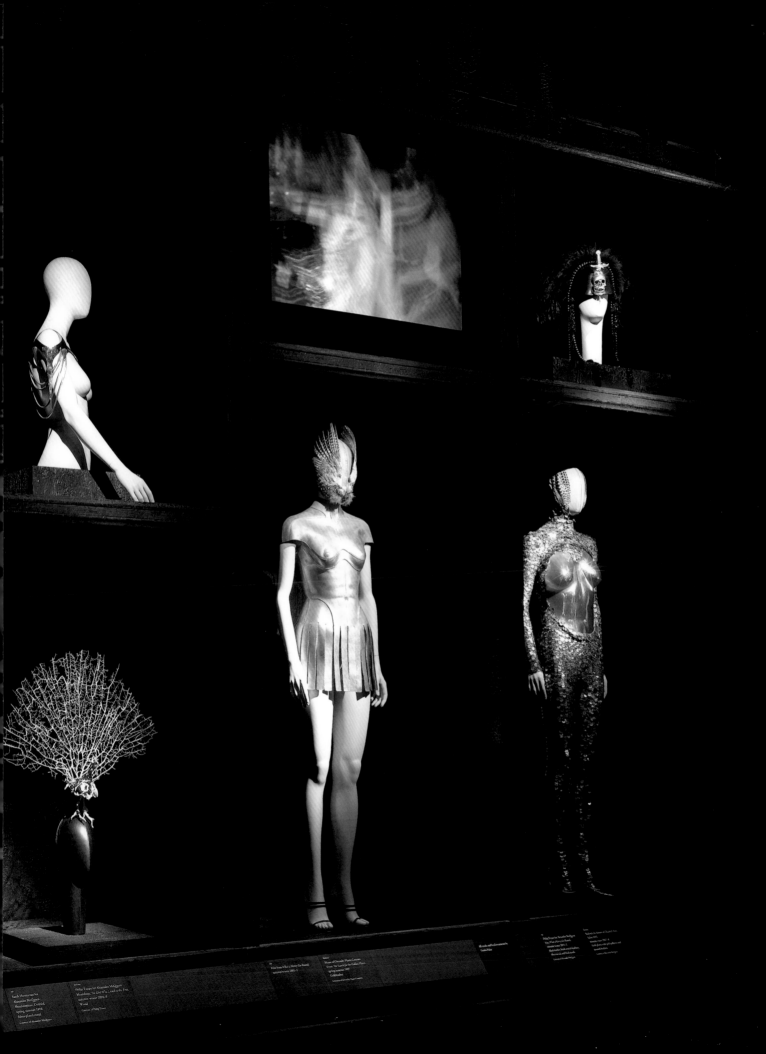

'Waist Down – Skirts by Miuccia Prada'

'Waist Down – Skirts by Miuccia Prada' was a travelling exhibition consisting of more than two hundred skirts, including pieces drawn from the designer's first collection for the house in 1988. Conceived by curator Kayoko Ota of AMO – the research arm of OMA (Office for Metropolitan Architecture), the firm of longtime Prada collaborator Rem Koolhaas – the exhibition was initially presented within Koolhaas's Prada Transformer in Seoul (see page 280) in 2008, before travelling to the brand's Epicenter stores in Tokyo, Shanghai, New York and Los Angeles. As the pieces shown were no longer available for purchase, the intention of these in-store exhibitions was not to encourage sales but to celebrate the artistic heritage of the brand and offer an unexpected view of fashion more generally. To this end AMO created site-specific installations in which some skirts twirled on rods suspended from the ceiling, demonstrating the dynamic movement that occurs from the waist down on the human body. Others were shown like tapestries, splayed open, conceptually 'dissecting' the garment that has formed the basis of Miuccia Prada's international reputation for more than twenty years. In 2012, the exhibition concept was loosely adapted for part of the Metropolitan Museum of Art, New York's 'Schiaparelli and Prada: Impossible Conversations'. The section 'Waist Up/Waist Down' highlighted Schiaparelli's use of decorative detailing and Prada's focus on the skirt as a tool to express femininity.

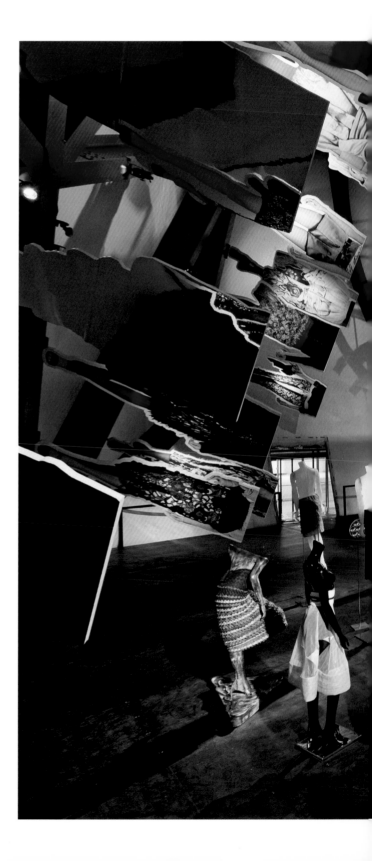

'Waist Down – Skirts by Miuccia Prada' exhibition inside the Prada Transformer in Seoul, 2008.

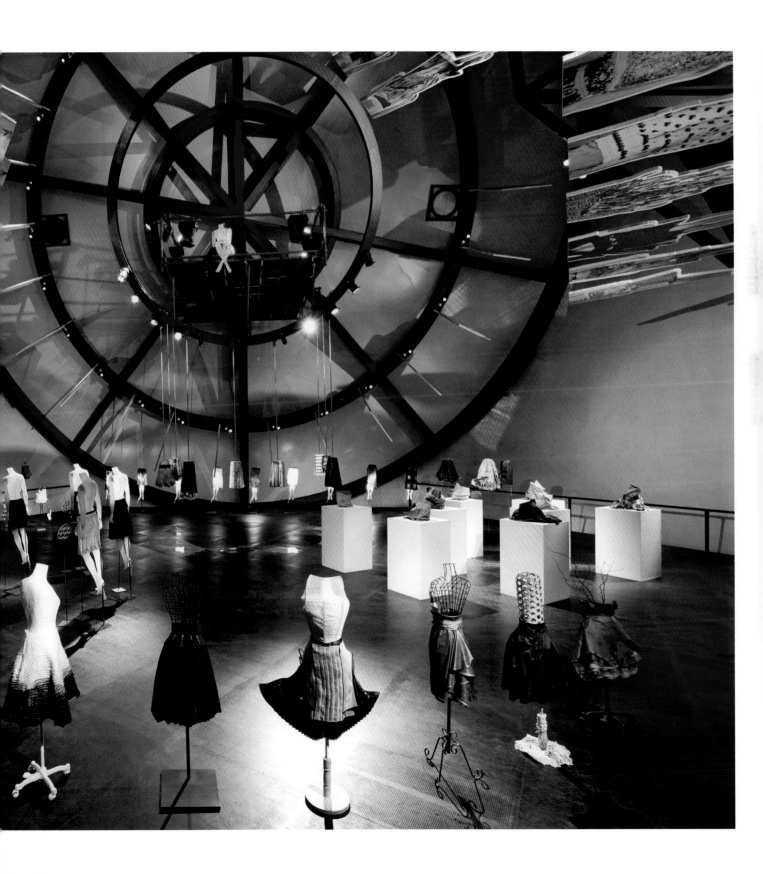

Christian Louboutin
at the Design Museum, London

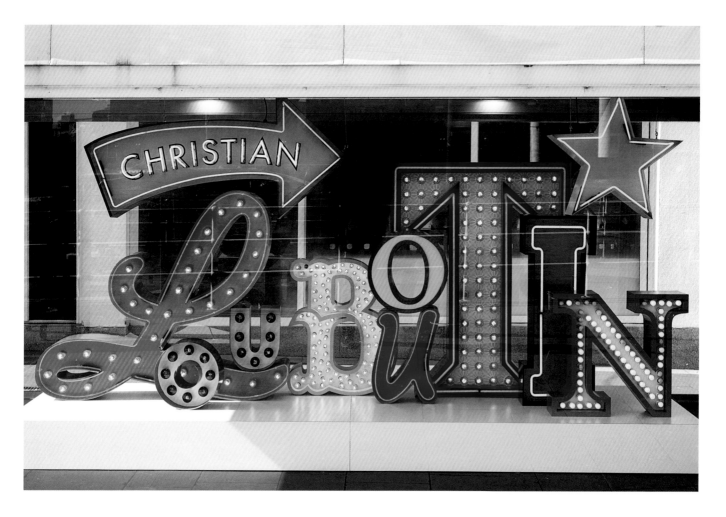

Since 1989, the Design Museum in London has presented exhibitions of architecture, fashion and industrial design, including the work of Paul Smith, Zaha Hadid and Jonathan Ive, with the aim of placing design at the centre of contemporary culture and demonstrating the richness of its creativity. In 2012, the museum presented the first British retrospective of iconic French shoe designer Christian Louboutin, celebrating a twenty-year career that has pushed the boundaries of shoe design and spawned a celebrity following. The exhibition was housed in a specially designed environment that evoked Louboutin's sources of inspiration, including art, film and travel. The sparse, white interior of the Design Museum was painted black and decorated with neon signs, red-velvet sofas and a wall of cobblers' moulds in Louboutin's signature red, as well as a holographic performance by burlesque artist Dita Von Teese. The works, drawn from Louboutin's personal archive, ranged from his most celebrated early designs – including the original sketches of his iconic red soles – to his latest collection, which for the first time included a range for men. The inclusion of Louboutin's then-current line in the exhibition created a link between retail and gallery space and highlighted the commercial considerations at the heart of contemporary design.

This page and opposite: 'Christian Louboutin' exhibition at the Design Museum, London, in 2012, including neon and light installations (right and opposite), a wall of red cobblers' moulds (below) and a holographic performance by Dita Von Teese (bottom).

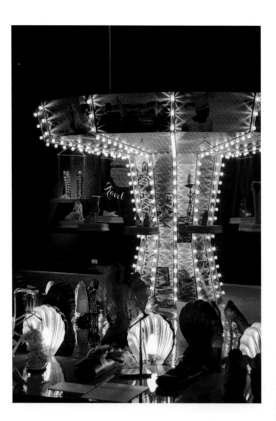

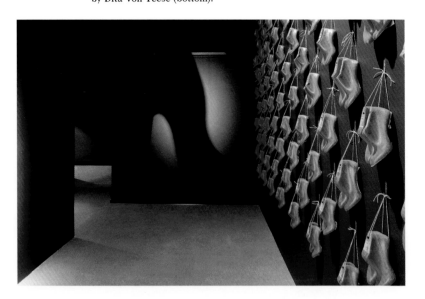

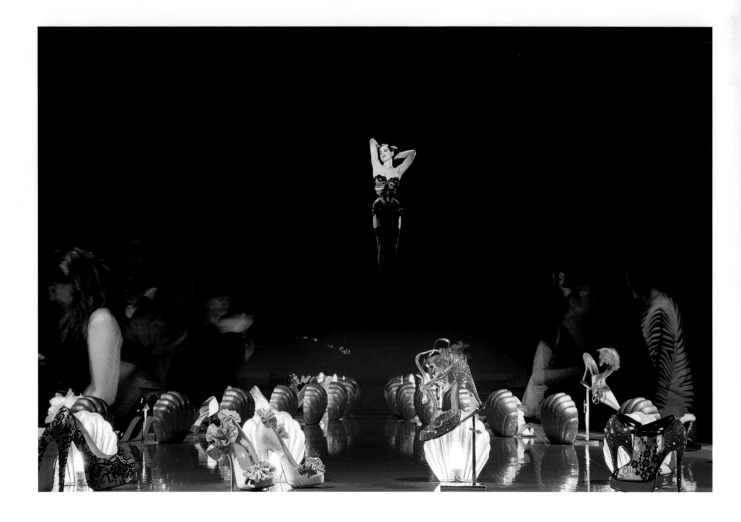

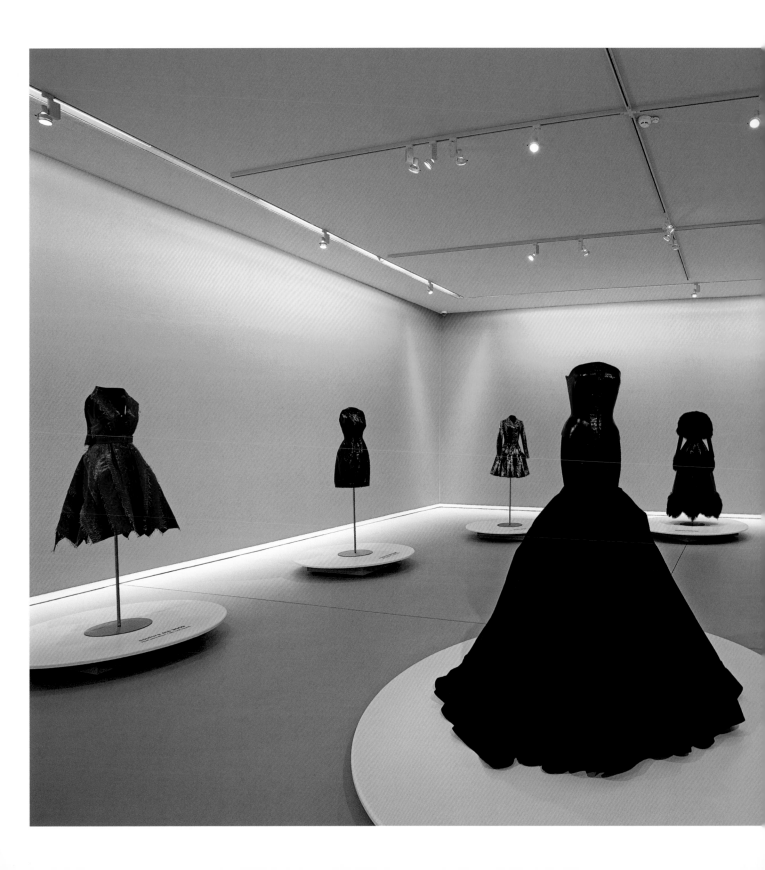

Azzedine Alaïa at the Groninger Museum

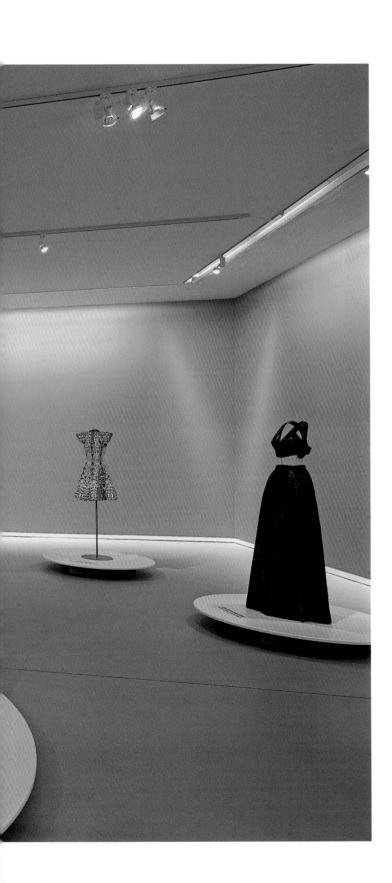

Tunisian-born designer Azzedine Alaïa, considered one of the last great traditional couturiers, has been the subject of several survey exhibitions throughout his career. 'Alaïa: Azzedine Alaïa in the 21st Century' at the Groninger Museum, the Netherlands, in 2011 was the sequel to another show of his work at the museum in 1998 that also travelled in 2000 to the Guggenheim in New York, where Alaïa's designs were displayed alongside complementary artworks from the Guggenheim's Brant collection: a bandage dress from 1990, for example, was paired with a number of Andy Warhol's *The Last Supper* screenprints, with the implication that both works represent artistic masterpieces. The existence of no fewer than three separate curatorial iterations of Alaïa's work is demonstrative of both his prolific output and the critical respect his work commands across the art–fashion divide.

'Alaïa: Azzedine Alaïa in the 21st Century', curated by Mark Wilson, brought together work from the beginning of the millennium, organized with a taxonomic as opposed to a thematic approach. Each room in the exhibition was devoted to a different material that the designer had used in the past decade: velvet, fur, wool, leather, cotton, animal skins, chiffon and knitwear. By focusing on the physical medium rather than abstract collection themes, the exhibition was able to showcase Alaïa's celebrated cutting and tailoring skills and his signature body-conscious aesthetic in a manner in keeping with his refutation of the seasonal fashion cycle.

Left and overleaf: 'Alaïa: Azzedine Alaïa in the 21st Century' exhibition at the Groninger Museum, the Netherlands, 2011.

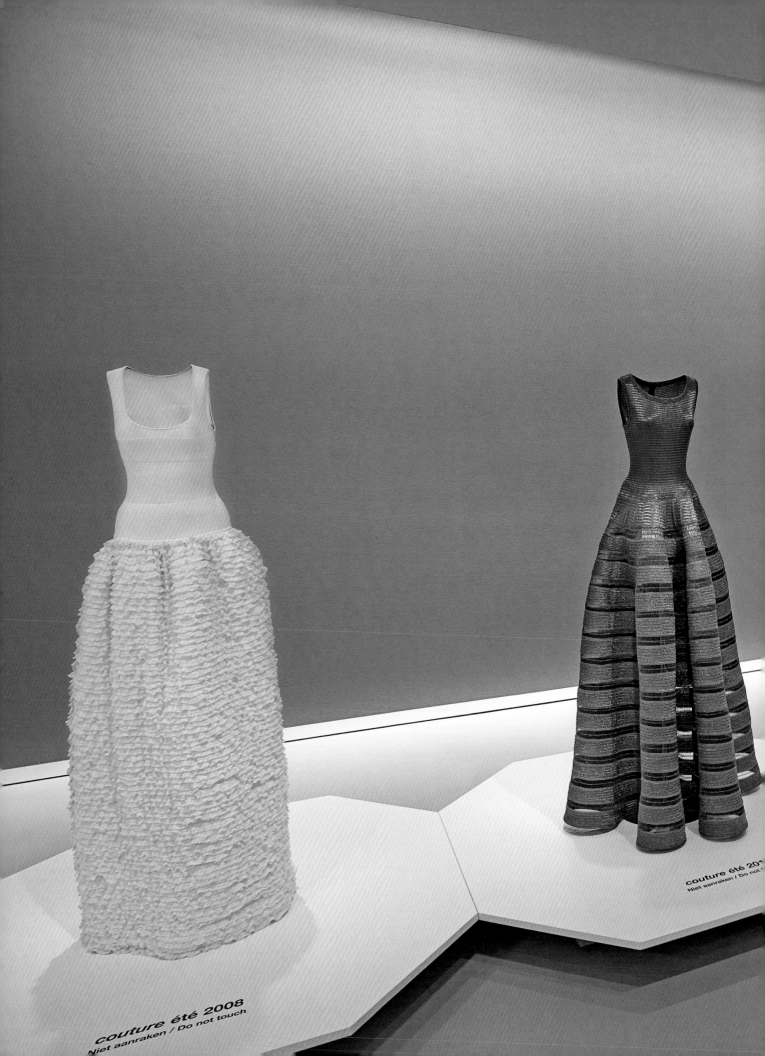

couture été 2008
Niet aanraken / Do not touch

couture été 20•
Niet aanraken / Do not •

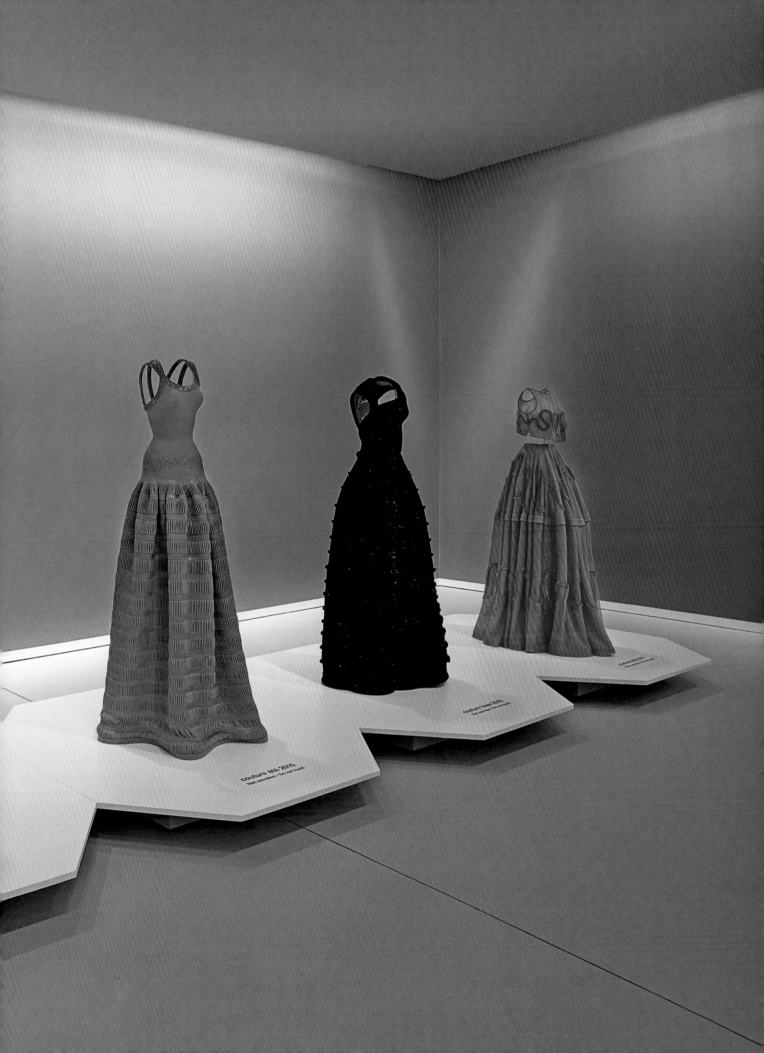

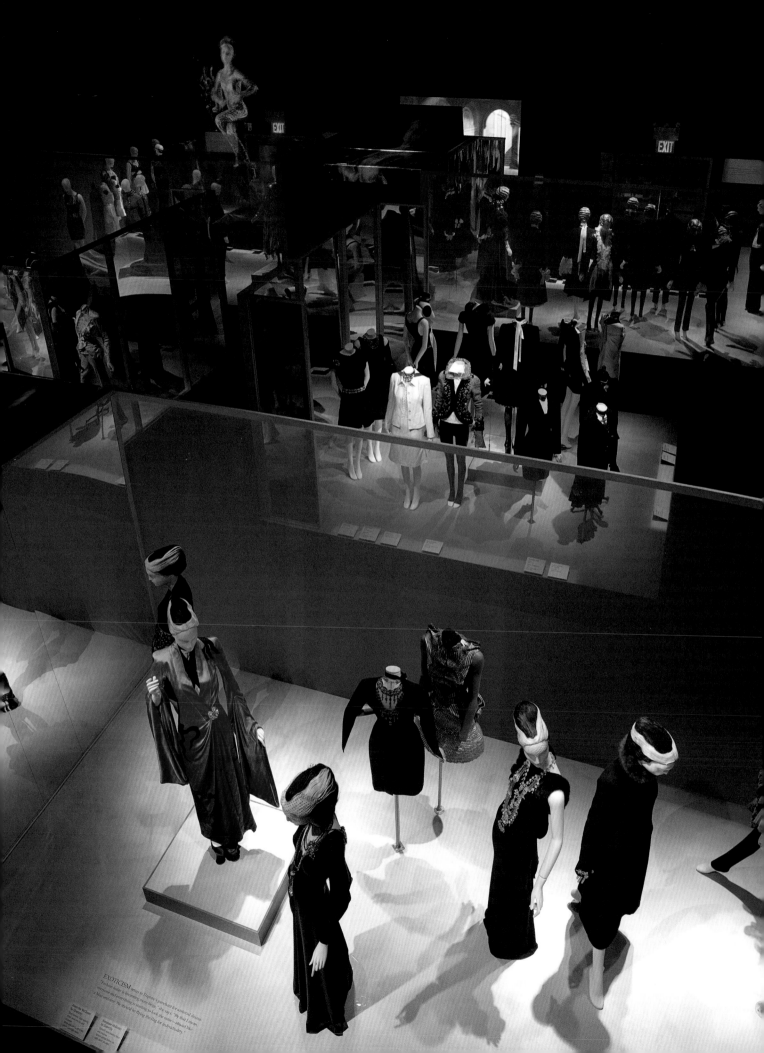

EXOTICISM refers to Diaghilev's penchant for sartorial drama
— overseas and everything is starting to look the same.—Alfred Stieglitz
«Just notice, he should be flying the flag for individuality.

Daphne Guinness at The Museum at The Fashion Institute of Technology, New York

The history of fashion has included a long line of designers' muses and champions of couture; among the most famous have been Anna Piaggi, Marchesa Luisa Casati, Iris Apfel and Isabella Blow. Daphne Guinness, a close friend of Blow, is considered one of the most daring and creative living contemporary fashion supporters, known not only for her devotion to designers such as Alexander McQueen and Gareth Pugh but also for her unique way of wearing their clothes, which has made her an international style icon in her own right. Heiress to the Guinness brewery fortune and granddaughter of Diana Mitford, one of the original It-girls, Daphne Guinness is more than an actress wearing clothing as endorsement: she personally supports fashion designers and purchases their pieces, particularly from emerging talent. Her keen curatorial eye is legendary, as is her respect for fashion as an art form; she famously halted the posthumous auction of Blow's wardrobe in 2007, purchasing the collection in its entirety to ensure that it would be kept together, and establishing the Isabella Blow Foundation to raise funds to exhibit it for posterity.

In 2011, the Museum at the Fashion Institute of Technology (FIT) in New York staged an exhibition of Guinness's own impressive fashion collection entitled 'Daphne Guinness', co-curated by Guinness herself and Valerie Steele, the museum's director. The exhibition featured some hundred garments from Nina Ricci, Azzedine Alaïa, Gareth Pugh, Rick Owens, Christian Lacroix, Chanel and Valentino, shown alongside accessories such as millinery by Philip Treacy, and footage and images of Guinness wearing the pieces on display. Guinness's loyal patronage of McQueen was demonstrated by her large collection of his work, both from his time at Givenchy and also from his own house, including more than twenty-four garments that had never been exhibited previously. The works on display also included some of Guinness's own designs, reflecting her interest in uniforms, and her films, such as her *Tribute to Alexander McQueen*. In presenting one living woman's wardrobe as equivalent to a collection of fine art, the exhibition demonstrated how patronage from a leading personality and celebrity can make a fashion designer's career in a manner analogous to that of an art collector or museum curator, and highlighted the creative significance of this role.

Opposite: The 'Daphne Guinness' exhibition at the Museum at the Fashion Institute of Technology, New York, 2011.

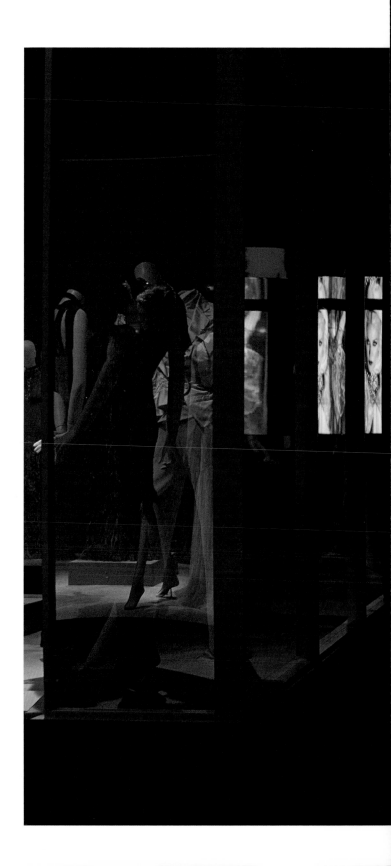

Daphne Guinness's film *Tribute to Alexander McQueen*
in the 'Daphne Guinness' exhibition at the Museum
at the Fashion Institute of Technology, New York, 2011.

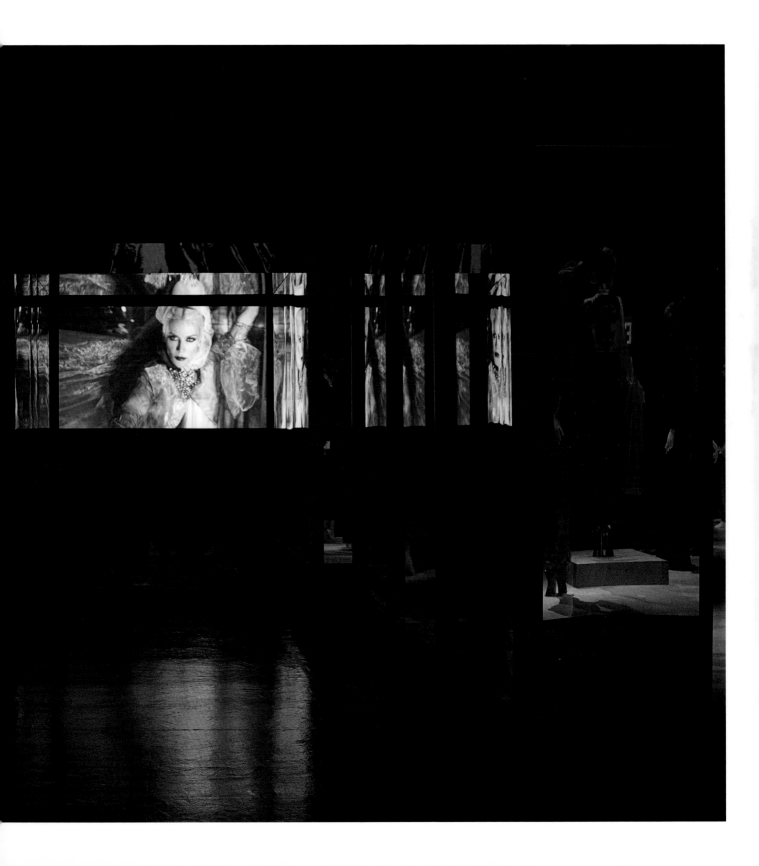

In conversation:
Katie Somerville, National Gallery
of Victoria, Melbourne

The National Gallery of Victoria is Australia's largest visual arts museum and the only one with a significant permanent fashion collection. Its fashion department – headed by Katie Somerville, curator for Australian Fashion and Textiles, and Roger Leong, for International Fashion and Textiles – is made up of a team of five curators who typically produce two or three exhibitions on an annual basis, including 'Together Alone' (2009), which exhibited the work of leading Australian fashion designers alongside that of their New Zealand counterparts to explore the dynamic relationship that exists between the two geographically close yet culturally divergent countries.

MITCHELL OAKLEY SMITH *How has the perception of fashion within an art museum changed in recent years?*

KATIE SOMERVILLE We find ourselves in a pivotal position. I have been at the gallery for seventeen years so inevitably have seen some significant shifts, perhaps most noticeably that there's now an expectation among the public that they'll see fashion within their visit to the gallery. We've gone from a position when the collection was called Costume and Textiles and contained within the Decorative Arts department, tucked away in a small corridor, to having dedicated staff and a series of major seasonal exhibitions within dedicated fashion gallery spaces and beyond.

MOS *The retrospective exhibition is probably the most popular today.*

KS Certainly in terms of attendance, which partly explains why the retrospective has become the predominant model for fashion exhibitions internationally: it's accessible; the fashion designer as artistic hero, whose body of work warrants that [level of] display and scrutiny where you can look at [both] the patterns in and [the] evolution of their practice.

MOS *It's evident that there's been a significant shift in the way fashion is viewed, in that it's now appreciated in the same way art is. Why do you think that has occurred?*

KS On a rudimentary level, people come to an art gallery to be fed creatively, nourished and informed, but also for the wonder factor: finding a particular thing that you think is marvellous and are drawn to. At the end of the day it doesn't matter if that's a painting or a dress; they're both aesthetic objects and both have the ability to connect with an audience on that level. Fashion and textiles do remain on the outer [fringe] when it comes to the hierarchy of the art world, as photography has done in the past. That's partly because there's a notion that fashion is frivolous or transient, but of course so much of contemporary art practice could be construed to be like that, too. In truth, there's room for both, and in all respects there's a hunger among audiences to access objects, whether fashion or prints or graffiti, through the lens of a curated space.

MOS *Do you think the growing presence of fashion in the gallery space changes what a gallery stands for?*

KS There is a cynical, but perhaps not incorrect, perception that fashion is also a means of making accessible a space like an art gallery to an audience that wouldn't ordinarily come through [the doors]. Fashion plays a powerful role in popularizing the traditional art space. Of course, it doesn't do this exclusively – we're also challenging our own ideas and values.

MOS *Is it challenging then to have the gallery dedicate resources or space to the fashion department?*

KS The most common questioning or resisting of the presence of fashion exhibitions within the gallery comes from journalists, actually. Fashion journalists, at least in Australia, are traditionally experienced in talking about fashion in a seasonal, trend-driven way rather than from a reflective cultural perspective. At the same time art writers seem to shy away from the discussion of fashion exhibitions. That remains one of the more interesting challenges we are yet to overcome, because audiences [themselves] are well and truly up to speed.

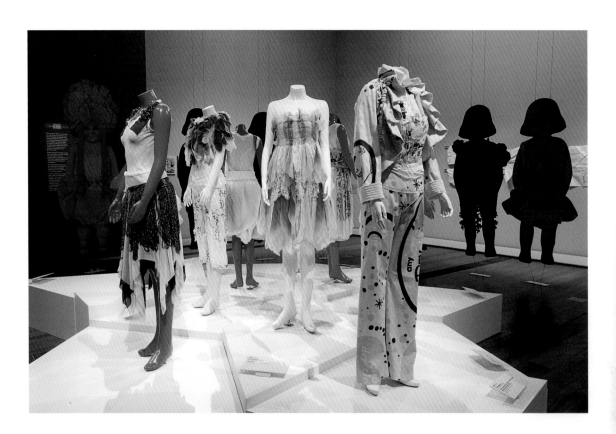

'Fashion plays a powerful role in popularizing the traditional art space.'

Katie Somerville

MOS *Do you acquire fashion works in much the same way as do your colleagues in other departments of the gallery?*

KS Absolutely – the general principals are the same. The approach varies depending on what era you're looking at. In the contemporary realm we usually watch someone over a few seasons, and if it's the first representation of their work [for the gallery], we typically look for a suite of work that foregrounds their signature approach to design. Subsequent acquisitions are about deepening or following on from a particular thread of that designer's work. There's not a very large secondary market for Australian fashion, so it's really about what you can track down and what private individuals can offer from their collections, making it much more case-by-case. We have certain criteria, which continually evolve and can change with forthcoming programming, with exhibitions planned for four to five years in advance. But the principals are ultimately about asking whether it will make sense in years to come as to why we collected this work.

Above: 'Together Alone' exhibition at the National Gallery of Victoria, Melbourne, 2009.
Overleaf: 'ManStyle' exhibition at the National Gallery of Victoria, Melbourne, 2011.

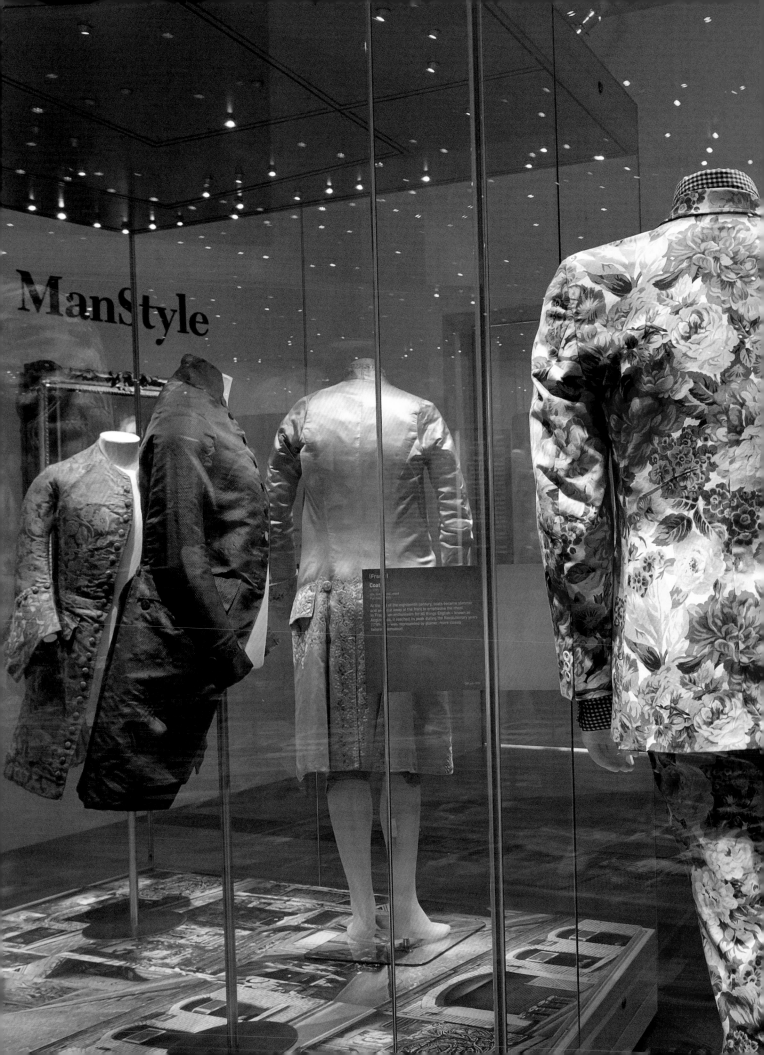

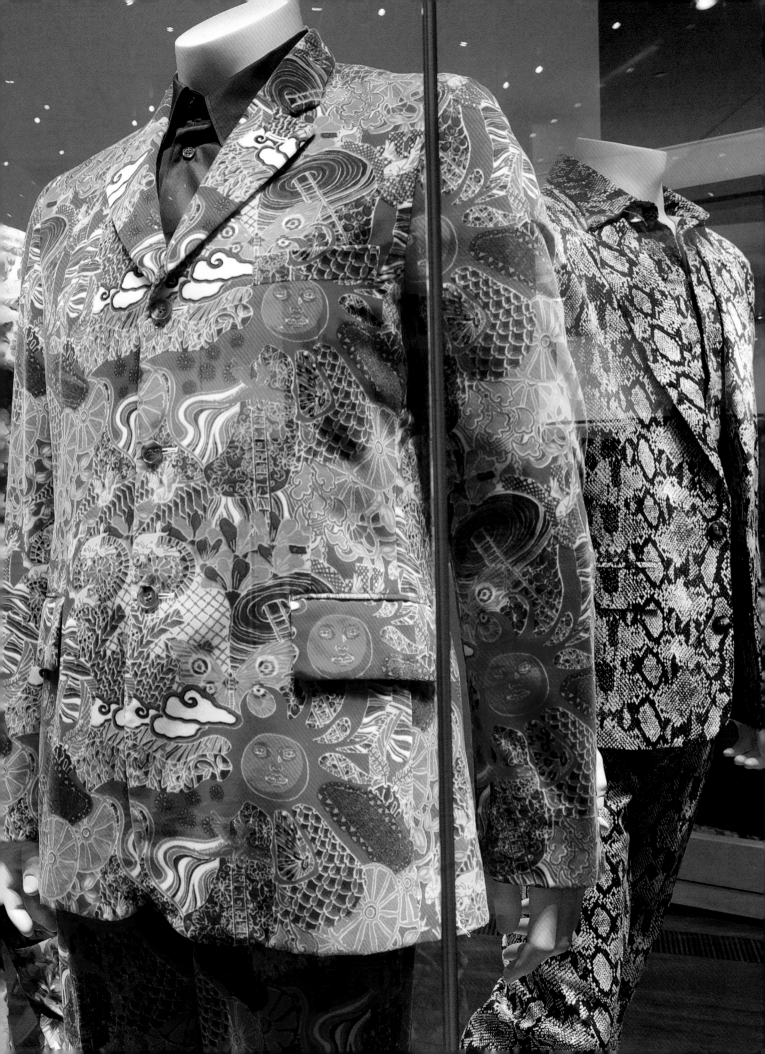

Calvin Klein event installations: Jonathan Jones & Geoff Ang

For the past few years, Calvin Klein has been collaborating with emerging and mid-career artists on experiential exhibitions of its clothing, with the aim of presenting these artists' work to a broader audience within the framework of a global fashion business. In celebrating the brand's fortieth anniversary in 2008, Calvin Klein engaged light sculptor James Turrell and renowned minimalist architect John Pawson, who designed several of the brand's flagship stores, to create an event on the High Line, the former elevated railway that extends twenty-two blocks along the west side of Manhattan. Although Calvin Klein is headquartered in New York, the brand selects artists local to the region of each event, inviting, for instance, Japanese minimalist architect Shinichi Ogawa to collaborate on a temporary, open-plan glass house on the grounds of the Meiji Jingu Gaien Museum in Tokyo in 2007. These high-profile collaborative exhibitions are another public medium through which Calvin Klein – famed since the 1980s for its edgy and hugely influential advertising campaigns, most recently those produced by French art director Fabien Baron – remains an innovator of communication in the fashion world.

In 2008 Australian light artist Jonathan Jones created a spectacular installation for a Calvin Klein event on Cockatoo Island, a former penal colony and shipyard in Sydney Harbour that is now home to the Biennale of Sydney. Jones created lightscapes of fluorescent lighting mounted on scaffolding; on and around them stood models wearing clothing from Calvin Klein's Spring/Summer 2009 collections, which were unveiled at the event. The bright colours of the collections – pink, yellow, red – appeared even more vivid and sharp under the lighting, providing a new perspective on both the designs and Jones's work, which is more typically white and industrial. For the Sydney-based artist, the change of context was a welcome one: 'Most of the time artwork exists within a sterile environment, the white box, but this engagement gave the work a whole new life.'[4]

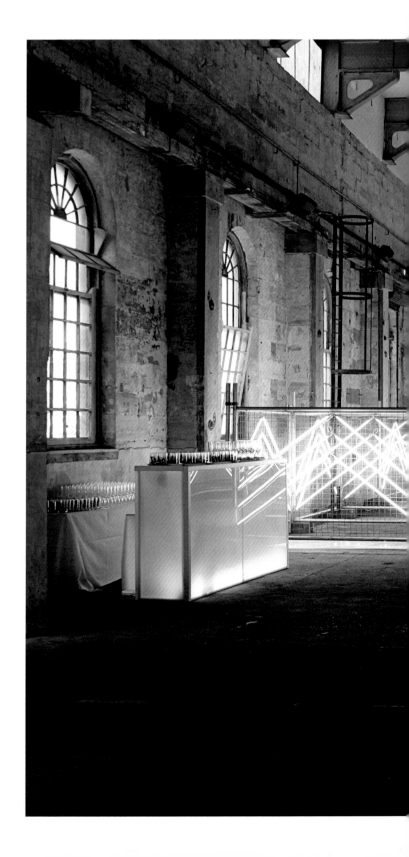

Light installation by Jonathan Jones for Calvin Klein
Spring/Summer 2009 collection presentation,
Cockatoo Island, Sydney, 2008.

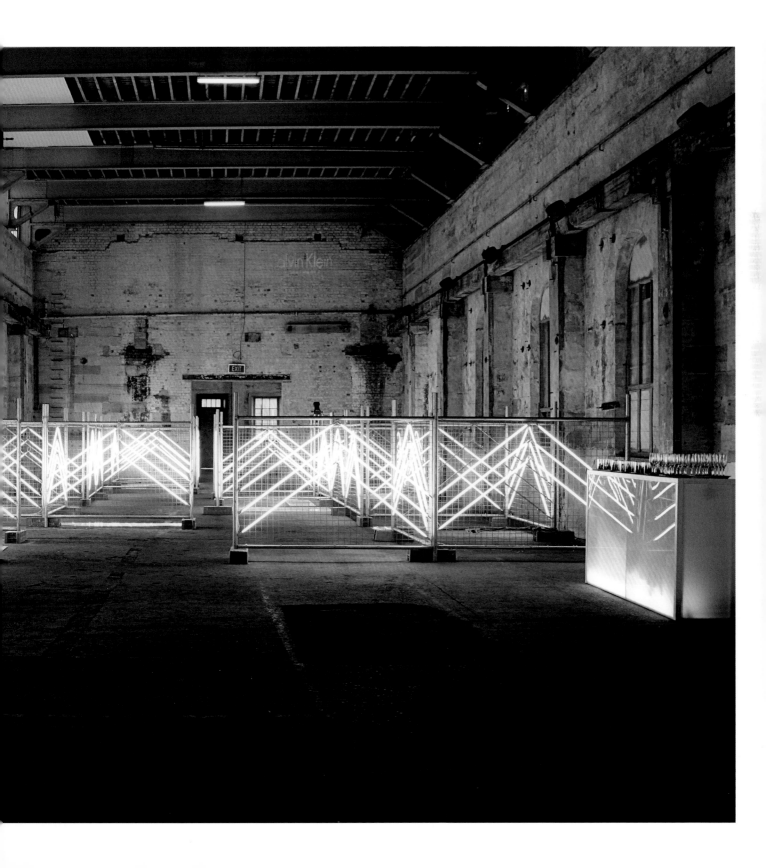

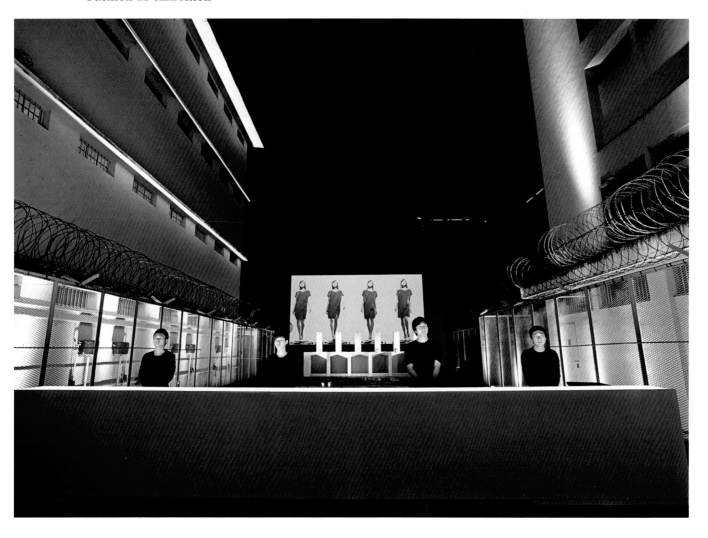

Above: A film by Geoff Ang screened as part of his installation
for a ck Calvin Klein Spring/Summer 2010 collection event,
Queenstown Remand Prison, Singapore, 2010.

In 2010, the brand's mid-priced line, ck Calvin Klein, headed by Kevin Carrigan, collaborated with video artist Geoff Ang to create a large event in the decommissioned Queenstown Remand Prison in Singapore. Since ck Calvin Klein does not show its collections on a runway in the manner of Calvin Klein Collection, the event provided an alternative means of presenting the designs. The event, which took place just weeks before the prison's scheduled demolition, included a line-up of models showcasing the range in front of large-scale video installations by Ang. He created a two-minute film in which motionless models, wearing the colour-block designs featured in the collection, were slowly rotated in a vacant, wind-swept space, while other models moved quickly across the screen in a blur, leaving a trail of digital pixels in their wake. They appeared and then disappeared into the ether, much like the prisoners who once had inhabited Queenstown's tiny 2×4-metre (6×12-foot) cells. Ang also installed a raised white platform – similar to a fashion catwalk – running the length of the cellblock, so that the models stood in the same place where the prison's inmates had once reported for the daily headcount. The statuesque symmetry of the models' straight, sharply cut clothing mirrored the regimented architecture of the building. The installation was inspired, said Ang, by the theme of freedom and liberty, evident in his emphasis on movement and strong colour. His work fittingly evoked the Calvin Klein aesthetic – the brand is known for its clean, minimalist, easy-to-wear clothes. At the same time, Ang made a powerful artistic statement that could be interpreted as a comment on Singapore's notoriously tough justice system.

In May 2012, Calvin Klein hosted a one-night event in Seoul organized in conjunction with the New Museum of Contemporary Art, New York. Lauren Cornell, the museum's adjunct curator, organized the exhibition, 'Infinite Loop', which integrated fashion-based installation works with the video art of Rafaël Rozendaal, Scott Snibbe and collective Flightphase in a tribute to the video art pioneer Nam June Paik. Their specially commissioned interactive video installations accompanied groups of models wearing Calvin Klein's Autumn/Winter 2012 designs from its various lines – the upper-tier Collection and mid-priced ck Calvin Klein as well as its Underwear collection – some of which had already been presented in traditional runway shows earlier in the year. As such, the exhibition was not conceived as a replacement for the seasonal runway presentation, but as a unique opportunity to show the garments in a different light.

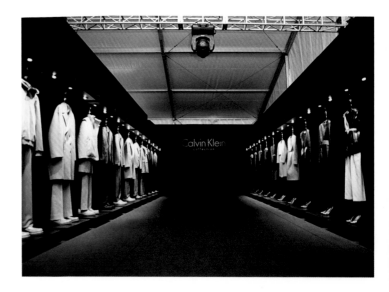

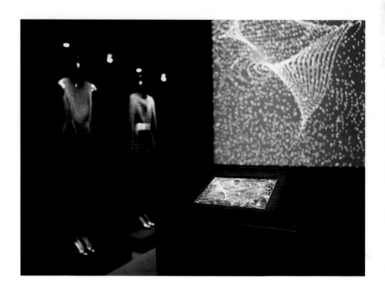

Above and top: Installations in the 'Infinite Loop' temporary exhibition for the Calvin Klein Autumn/Winter 2012 presentation in Seoul.

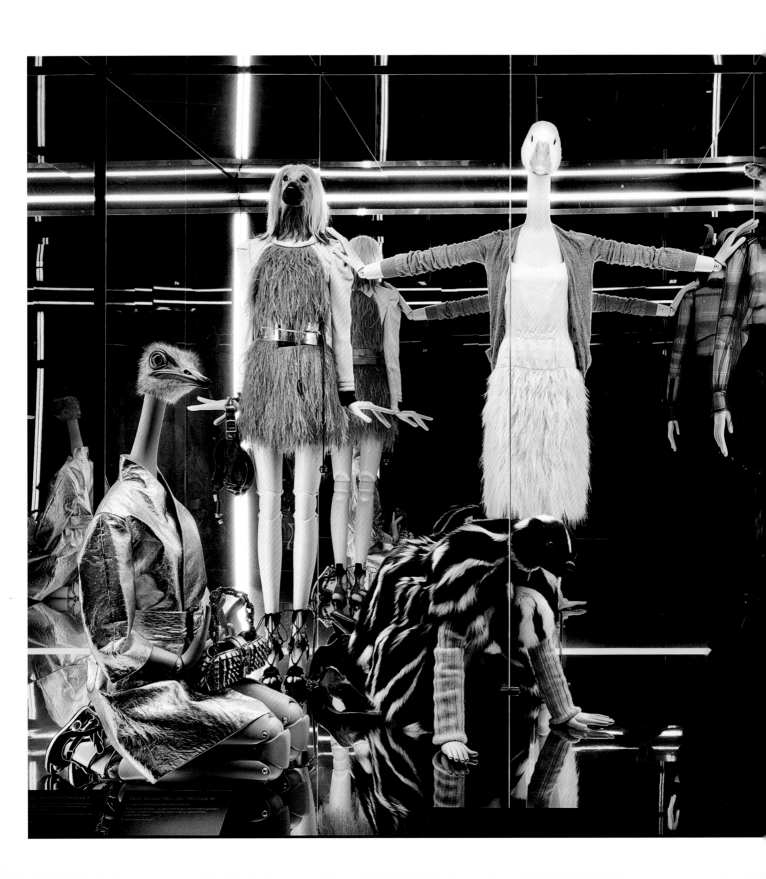

In conversation: Pamela Golbin, Musée de la Mode et du Textile, Les Arts Décoratifs, Paris

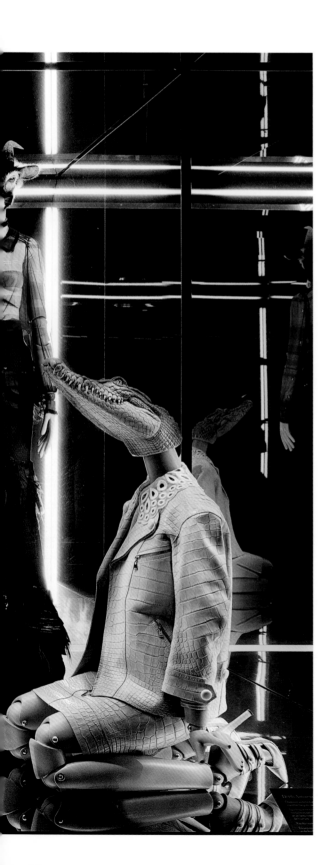

Les Arts Décoratifs is a private, non-profit museum of decorative arts dating back to 1882, and occupies three sites in Paris. The Musée de la Mode et du Textile, its gallery dedicated to fashion and textiles, occupies 1,500 square metres (16,146 feet) over two levels. Its archives, from which part of its seasonal fashion exhibitions are drawn, contain some 16,000 costumes, 35,000 fashion accessories and 30,000 pieces of textiles acquired through private donations or directly from designers and manufacturers. Pamela Golbin, its chief curator of 20th century and contemporary fashion, has been responsible for a number of blockbuster fashion exhibitions that have travelled the globe and generated important catalogues; among the most successful have been retrospectives of fashion greats including Madeleine Vionnet, Christian Lacroix, Yves Saint Laurent, Valentino, Balenciaga, and most recently 'Louis Vuitton – Marc Jacobs'.

ALISON KUBLER *What makes fashion worthy of discussion and appreciation within a museum framework?*

PAMELA GOLBIN Haute couture has always been exhibited in museums because of its value and the level of skill involved. Creativity remained in the hands of couturiers until the 1970s when ready-to-wear was introduced by designers such as Jean Paul Gaultier, Kenzo and Comme des Garçons...It took a long time for museums to express this shift in the creative process. Fashion is an industry, and what makes it so dynamic and important is the fact that it's relevant to the cultural phenomena of today. We have no problem embracing designers who are industrially focused, hence why ready-to-wear is adaptable for exhibition, because we believe in the creative process behind the fashion. We have always worked closely with fashion designers and collected prototypes from archives. So it's never off the rack, but focused on the raw elements of the creative process. The creative output is the priority; whether [the collected piece] is haute couture or ready-to-wear, it doesn't matter.

AK *So ready-to-wear, like haute couture, can be considered art?*

PG I've always had a problem with this question. Fashion and art are two distinct domains that sometimes have a dialogue and sometimes don't. I think pairing them together as a single entity is a disadvantage to all of the incredible industrial

Left and overleaf: 'Louis Vuitton – Marc Jacobs' exhibition at the Musée de la Mode et du Textile, Les Arts Décoratifs, Paris, 2012.

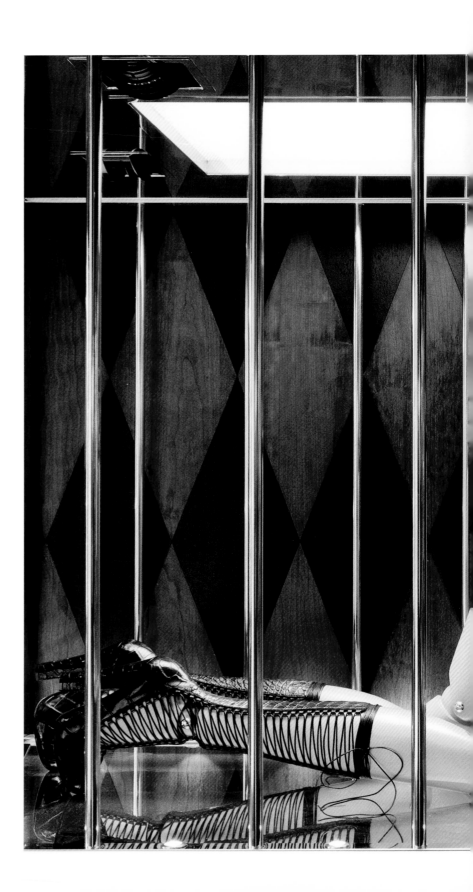

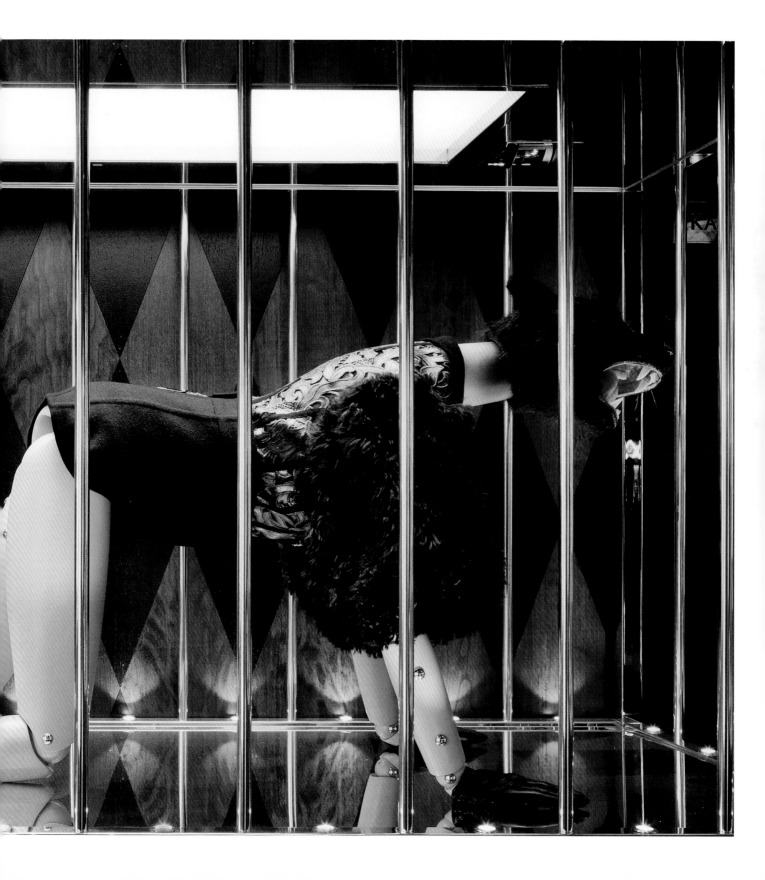

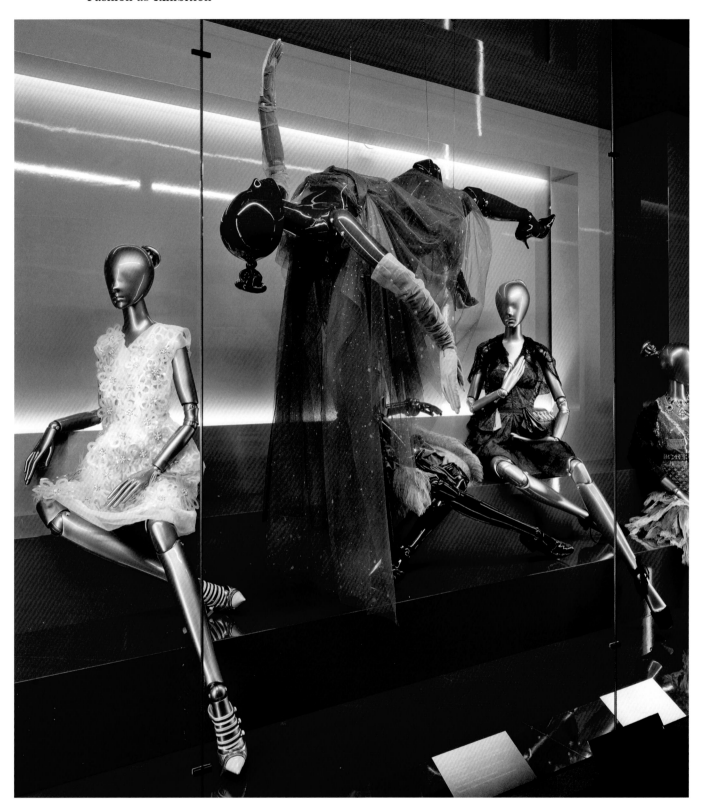

Above: 'Louis Vuitton – Marc Jacobs' exhibition at the Musée
de la Mode et du Textile, Les Arts Décoratifs, Paris, 2012.

'People often talk about what fashion sees in art, but what's really interesting is what art sees in fashion. Art is looking for an edge and fashion delivers it, as it is highly transient and based on a lot of money. Maybe fashion doesn't need art as it's already moving on to the next thing, but art might not be ready to give up on fashion so easily.'

Pamela Golbin

aspects of fashion. Fashion will never attain the prices that art does, and yet people push fashion aside because of its associations with commerce. Fashion and art have gone through major paradigm shifts in globalization and commerce. The level of sophistication in both sectors has increased dramatically and museums have played a major role in raising the profile of each, but I don't think one can become the other. While both speak to the same audience, fashion has always been viewed with a little 'f' and art with a big 'A', but I think fashion is more important now. People don't often comment on the fact that the art world has changed just as much as the fashion world.

AK *How do you make an exhibition different in the case of 'Louis Vuitton – Marc Jacobs', given that Louis Vuitton has mounted its own exhibitions in the past?*

PG We have one of the largest permanent [fashion] gallery spaces and because of its structure we decided quite early on that for every exhibition we would form an artistic team with individual roles. This allowed us to work directly with the designer and rethink the spaces each time. For the Vuitton–Jacobs exhibition we worked directly with Marc [Jacobs] and stylist Katie Grand, who is part of the Louis Vuitton team. I believe it's imperative for the designer and their team to be part of the process. Collaborating with designers always pushes our limits and creates an incredible dialogue between a creative and commercial culture. This dialogue makes us and the designers rethink the way we work on many levels.

AK *How do you identify designers to work with when it comes to programming?*

PG We have collections at the museum that range from 16th-century costume to contemporary pieces...and one of the most important factors is the balance between the contemporary and the historical. We must ask ourselves, how can contemporary designs play into our collections for the public? Fashion is an extremely

sophisticated language with an incredible syntax and vocabulary, and we must find a way of bringing the world of each individual designer to the exhibitions. Hussein Chalayan and Marc Jacobs have completely contrasting points of view, for example, but each brings a different facet of fashion to our visitors and offers them a more objective view of the spectrum of fashion today. This variety and independent perspective is extremely important.

AK *What do you think prompts the art and fashion worlds to look at each other?*

PG The final consumer of art and fashion is the same. For artists, the creative process has the advantage of time while fashion designers have to concentrate on producing at least four collections a year. And yet time is waning for artists today and they must be constantly producing work or another artist will take their place. Both art and fashion are now global entities – each one has exploded in terms of scale. People often talk about what fashion sees in art, but what's really interesting is what art sees in fashion. Art is looking for an edge and fashion delivers it, as it is highly transient and based on a lot of money. Fashion also has an incredible way of appropriating art, but it chews it up and spits it out. Maybe fashion doesn't need art as it's already moving on to the next thing, but art might not be ready to give up on fashion so easily.

Opposite: Original Louis Vuitton luggage trunks displayed alongside images of historical garments, 'Louis Vuitton – Marc Jacobs' exhibition at the Musée de la Mode et du Textile, Les Arts Décoratifs, Paris, 2012.
Overleaf: A selection of popular handbags that reinvent Louis Vuitton's iconic monogram, 'Louis Vuitton – Marc Jacobs' exhibition at the Musée de la Mode et du Textile, Les Arts Décoratifs, Paris, 2012.

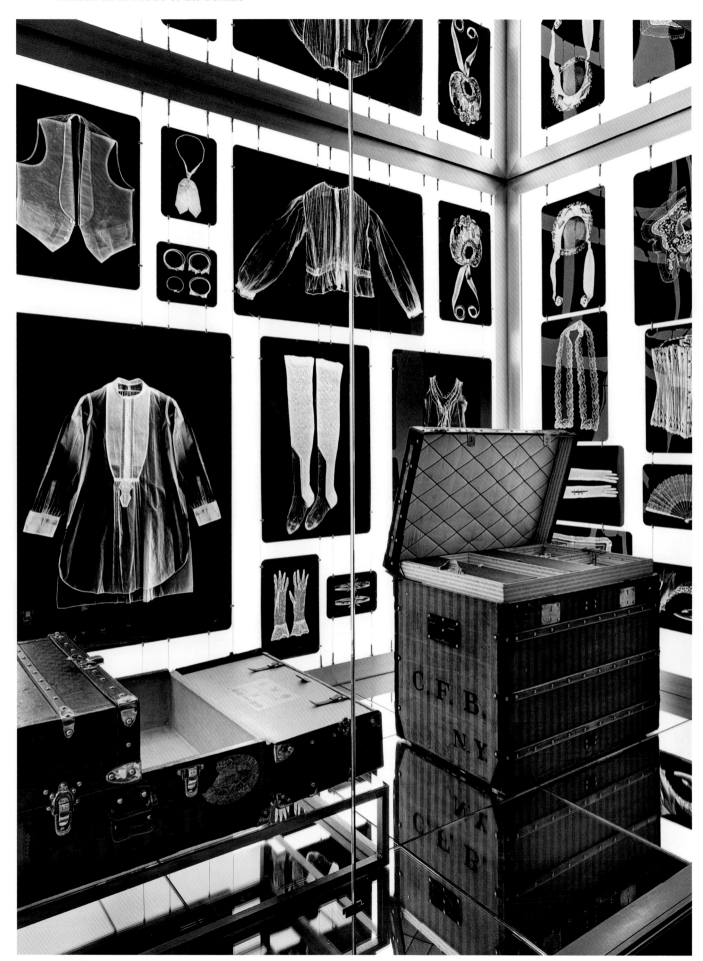

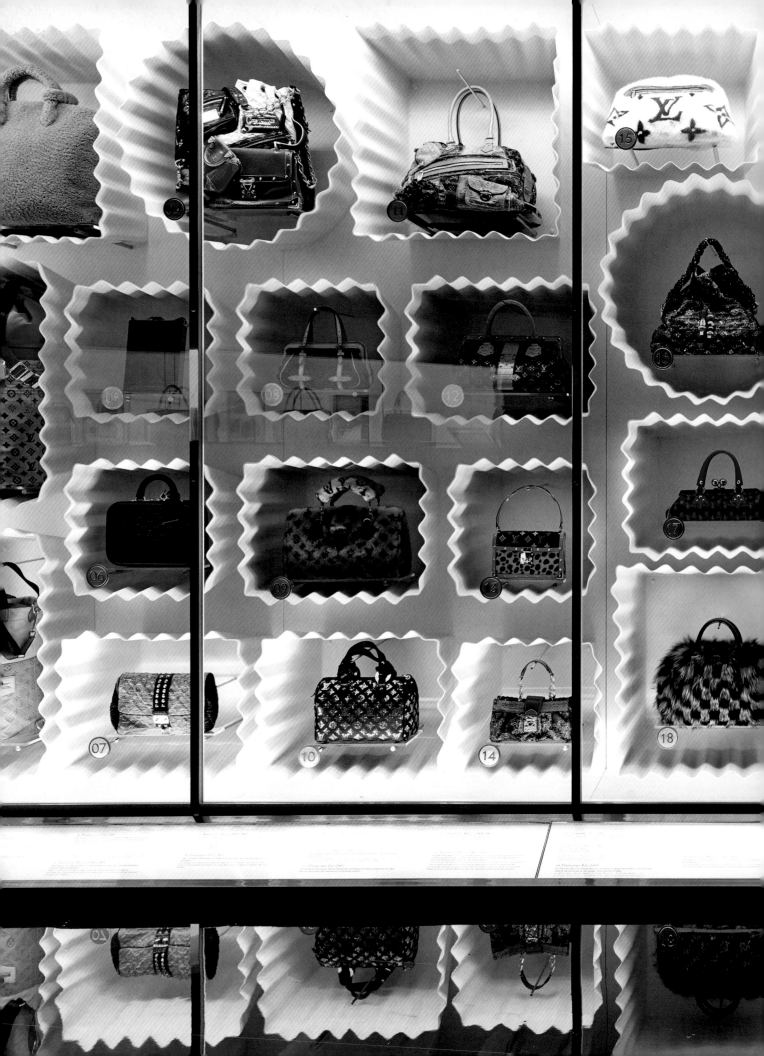

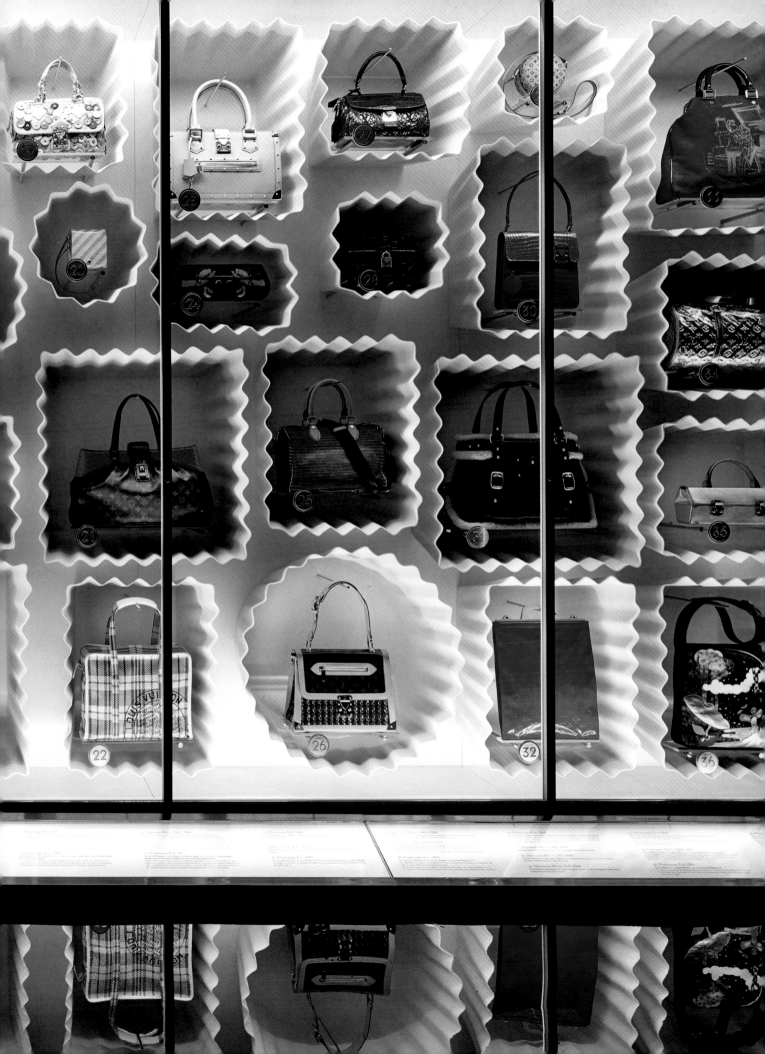

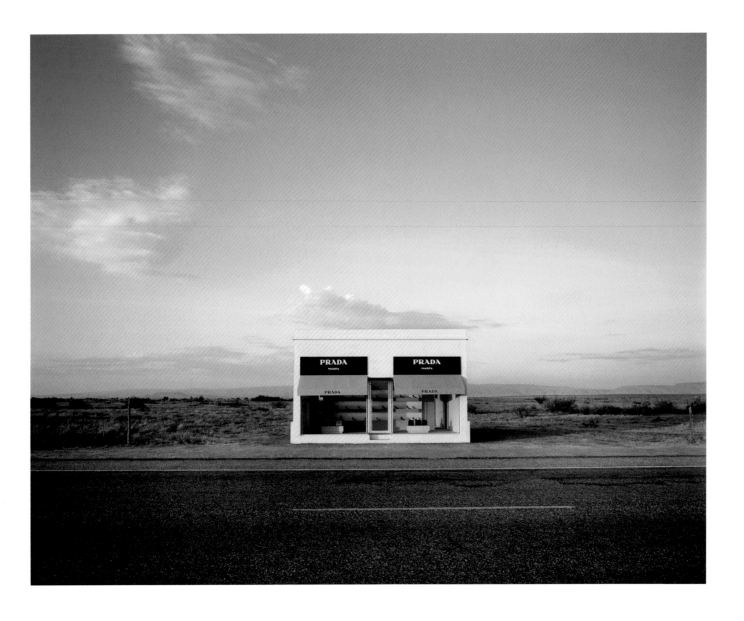

Above: Street view of *Prada Marfa*, the permanently sealed mock
Prada store created by artist duo Elmgreen & Dragset, outside
Marfa, Texas, 2005.

Prada Marfa

One of the most successful and striking examples of an artwork inspired by the collision of art and fashion is *Prada Marfa*, an installation created by Scandinavian artist duo Elmgreen & Dragset (Michael Elmgreen and Ingar Dragset) on the outskirts of the artistic community of Marfa, Texas, in 2005. The location of the work on the side of an interstate highway outside a small town in the middle of nowhere is conceptually significant, both as an incongruous juxtaposition of two radically different environments and as a play on the theme of pilgrimage, since visitors are required to make a long and difficult journey in order to view the installation. *Prada Marfa* was created to resemble a real Prada store, complete with a Prada-approved colour scheme, the brand's logo and real merchandise supplied by the label, which had previously collaborated with the artists on a project in New York in 2001.

Prada Marfa is to all intents and purposes a shop, yet it cannot be accessed by shoppers. It is a hermetically sealed, full-scale museum vitrine displaying some of the most important cultural icons of the new millennium: Prada handbags and shoes (only the right shoe of each pair, although this didn't stop thieves from ram-raiding the work shortly after it was installed). The 'boutique' is

Prada Marfa is a museum that will become a cabinet of curiosities as it decays and falls into disrepair.

oblivious to the arrival of new collections and trends – the items inside will remain forever unchanged, subjects of unfulfilled, unrequited desires when they were first made and displayed. The hapless 'shopper' or art admirer is forced to window-shop for these items long after they have passed their commercial use-by date. *Prada Marfa* is a museum that will become a cabinet of curiosities as it decays and falls into disrepair. As a sculpture it functions as a contemporary memento mori, a meditation on mortality and the futility of existence.

Jean Paul Gaultier at the Montreal Museum of Fine Arts

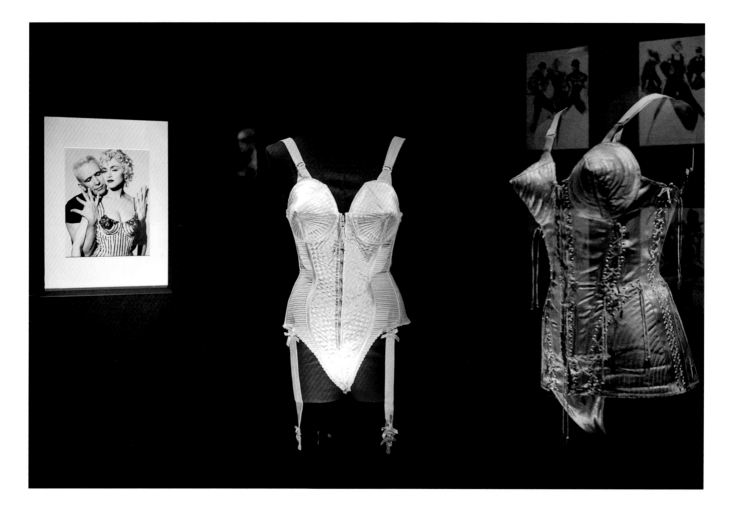

The Montreal Museum of Fine Arts is Quebec's leading art museum and holds one of the most important collections in North America. In 2011 Thierry-Maxime Loriot curated its groundbreaking exhibition 'The Fashion World of Jean Paul Gaultier: From the Sidewalk to the Catwalk', the first museum retrospective of the work of the French fashion designer, who had initially been reluctant to see a retrospective of his work because 'it would be like a funeral'.[5] Loriot, who had himself worked for over a decade as a runway model, drew on his own experience of the fashion industry to bring a sense of theatricality to the presentation. Work was borrowed from Gaultier's loyal celebrity customers, including Madonna and Kylie Minogue, and displayed on mannequins with animated faces projected onto them. The mannequins randomly spoke or burst into song, referencing Gaultier's reputation for performance as well as his penchant for defying conventions and breaking taboos. 'When you discover Gaultier's universe, you realize how open and generous his fashion is… empowering and giving freedom to a liberated contemporary woman in control of her life and her sexuality,' explained Loriot. The exhibition subsequently travelled throughout Canada, the United States and Europe, where it enjoyed large attendance figures.

Above: Bustiers made for Madonna displayed in 'The Fashion World of Jean Paul Gaultier: From the Sidewalk to the Catwalk', exhibition at the Montreal Museum of Fine Arts, 2011.

'Some fashion designers should be considered real artists. They are always in the process of creation and they always have to reinvent everything, every season, as with contemporary artists today with all the art fairs, like Basel, Fiac, Frieze – they must produce new works all the time for clients, and I think that is very similar to the fashion design calendar.'

Thierry-Maxime Loriot

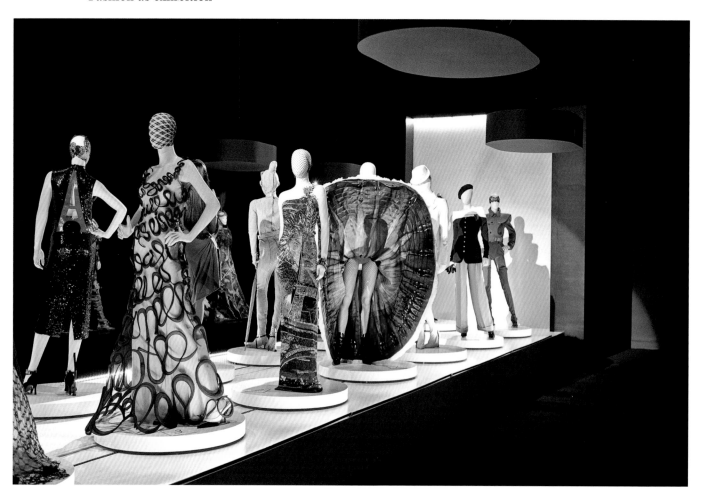

Above and opposite: 'The Fashion World of Jean Paul Gaultier:
From the Sidewalk to the Catwalk', exhibition at the
Montreal Museum of Fine Arts, 2011.

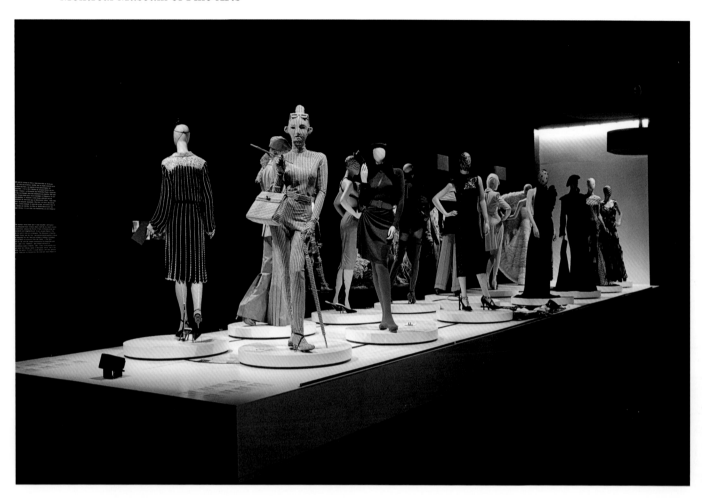

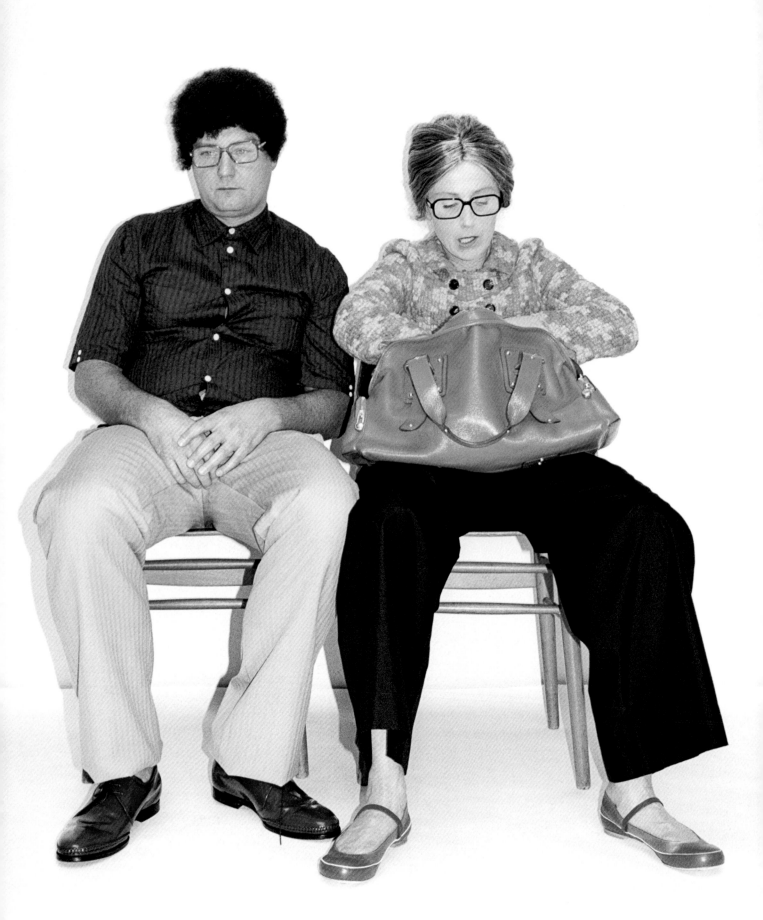

Beyond the photoshoot: New fashion media

Introduction:
Beyond the photoshoot

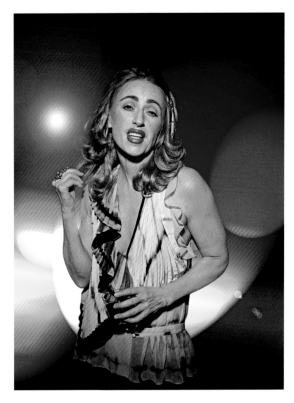

Cindy Sherman, *Untitled*, 2008,
created for Balenciaga.

Nowhere is the cross-pollination of fashion and art so evident as in fashion media, which, with the advent of digital technology and the concurrent revival of high-end traditional print publishing, has evolved significantly over the past decade in both form and content. The roles of fashion magazines, too, have changed as a result: their editors have become curators; fashion photographers are now also filmmakers.

The internet has challenged the traditional hierarchy of fashion media by providing an accessible and democratic platform for communication. The rise of fashion blogs and social media sites over the past decade has, as noted by Erik Torstensson and Jens Grede in *Industrie* magazine, rapidly transformed fashion media 'from an authoritarian business model to a democratic peer-to-peer quest for information'.[1] Scott Schuman, creator of blog *The Sartorialist*, has spawned a million imitators and demonstrated unequivocally the power of the blogger's voice. Although the quality and intellectual merit of some of these new blogs, forums and websites have been questioned by industry experts, there is no doubt that they have overturned the long-established system of fashion reporting in which trends were interpreted and summarized by a small group of elite editors who attended the seasonal runway shows, and then disseminated to the masses months later via print publications. Runway shows are now live-streamed online, where they can be viewed and reported on by anyone with an internet connection. Online versions of fashion editorials are posted moments after, and sometimes even before, print editions are released, negating the need to physically purchase and collect a publication.

Where it once had the power to make or break a collection with a single review, or by allocating or withholding page space in a magazine issue, the traditional mainstream fashion media no longer unilaterally controls the public perception of a particular label or designer. As a consequence of this shift, fashion brands have attempted to establish new communication channels that allow them to speak directly to their audiences. Many now employ moving images rather than still photography for this purpose, a trend also embraced by traditional art and fashion photographers who are increasingly experimenting with film as a medium. This transition has been aided by developments in digital technology that have made film equipment more accessible to photographers and films themselves more easily viewed by online audiences, as well as by the rise of platforms such as SHOWstudio.com, established by photographer Nick Knight in 2000, which champions moving image in the fashion industry.

Where it once had the power to make or break a collection...the traditional mainstream fashion media no longer unilaterally controls the public perception of a particular label or designer.

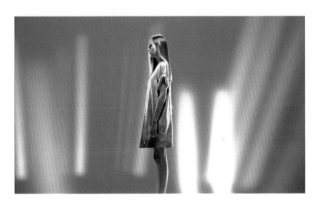

Still from an untitled short film created by Geoff Ang for ck Calvin Klein, Spring/Summer 2010.

Prada, for instance, often collaborates on short films, most memorably on *A Therapy* (2012) directed by Roman Polanski and starring Ben Kingsley and Helena Bonham Carter. The short film is in essence an ode to a fur coat: Bonham Carter plays a patient visiting her therapist (Kingsley) who becomes distracted by her luxurious Prada fur coat, swooning at himself in the mirror as he tries it on while she continues to talk, oblivious to his inattention. Importantly, the film premiered at the Cannes Film Festival in 2012, making it clear that *A Therapy* was intended to be viewed seriously as a work in its own right, not simply as an advertising short. As part of 'Schiaparelli and Prada: Impossible Conversations' (2012), at the Metropolitan Museum of Art, New York, Miuccia Prada herself starred in a series of eight short films directed by Baz Luhrmann in which she has conversations with the late Elsa Schiaparelli, played by actress Judy Davis, over a long dining table. The dialogue is a combination of paraphrased excerpts from Schiaparelli's autobiography *A Shocking Life* (1954) interspersed with Prada's own filmed interviews, creating the illusion of real-time dialogue between two true fashion originals.

This sort of intelligent insinuation of fashion into the narrative arc of a film reflects the historically significant role of fashion in film since its inception in the early 20th century. Fashion and film are seemingly inseparable: witness, for example, the red-carpet parades at the Oscars or the Golden Globes that feature film stars wearing endorsed product. More broadly, since the turn of the millennium there has been a spate of films about the fashion industry produced and directed by highly regarded documentary filmmakers. *The September Issue* (2009), directed by R. J. Cutler, offered a rare behind-the-scenes entrée to the workings of the most influential fashion magazine in the world, *Vogue*, as well as its reticent editor Anna Wintour (often described as the most powerful person in fashion) and creative director Grace Coddington, who ultimately emerged as the real star of the film. *The September Issue* is important not only for the huge audiences it drew to the cinema, but also for its affirmation of the cultural importance and relevance of fashion. Similarly, *The Eye Must Travel* (2012), examining the influence of the late Diana Vreeland, former editor-in-chief of American *Vogue* and one-time curator of the Costume Institute at the Metropolitan Museum of Art, is part of a historical revision of fashion as the litmus test of an era. This genre also includes *Lagerfeld Confidential* (2007), an exposé of Karl Lagerfeld by Rodolphe Marconi; *Valentino: The Last Emperor* (2008), which documented the retirement of the Italian designer; and the charming documentary *Bill Cunningham New York* (2010) by Richard Press, about the long-serving fashion photographer for the *New York Times*.

Despite the apparent downturn in magazine subscription rates as consumers move to digital platforms, there has been a proliferation of new print fashion titles that emulate the layout and intellectual content of art journals. These publications operate at different ends of the marketing spectrum, ranging from the mass-produced *Pop* and *Love* launched by stylist Katie Grand to the high-end, limited-edition *Visionaire* and *Self Service*. Collectively, these titles aspire to a more intellectual presentation of fashion characterized by non-traditional fashion editorials and collaborations with artists in a curator-like capacity. In eschewing straightforward product placement, they reject the traditional commercial priorities of fashion magazines in favour of presenting a curated picture of fashion trends. This 'curatorial' approach has also been adopted by traditional publications, including leading fashion and society magazine *W*, which in 2011, under the direction of editor Stefano Tonchi, arranged for dissident artist Ai Weiwei to direct a photoshoot inside the Rikers Island prison in New York via video link while under house arrest in China.

These collaborative magazine editorials have helped to make contemporary artists the new celebrities within the fashion industry, a trend popularized by Russian art collector Dasha Zhukova who, while editor of *Pop*

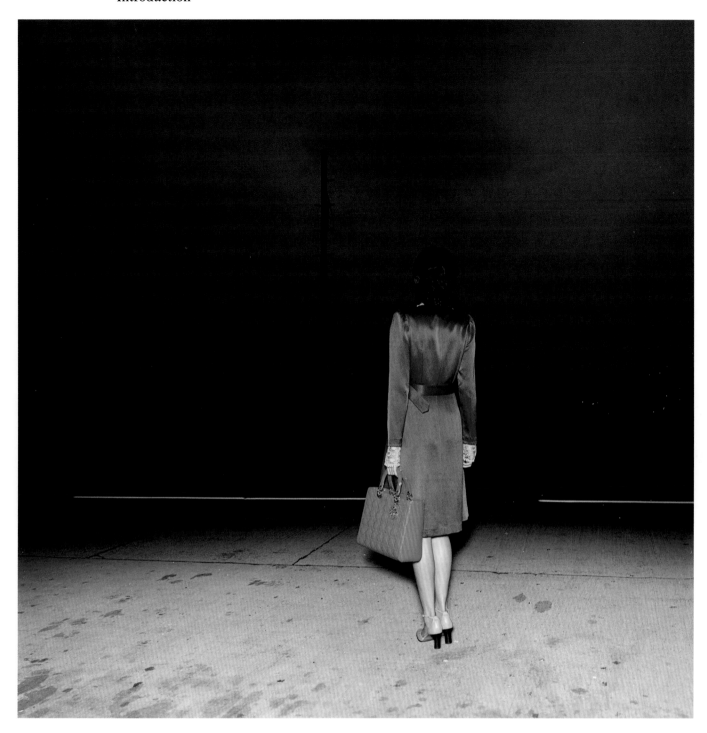

Above: Quentin Shih, *A Chinese Woman with a Lady Dior Handbag*, 2011, created for Christian Dior.

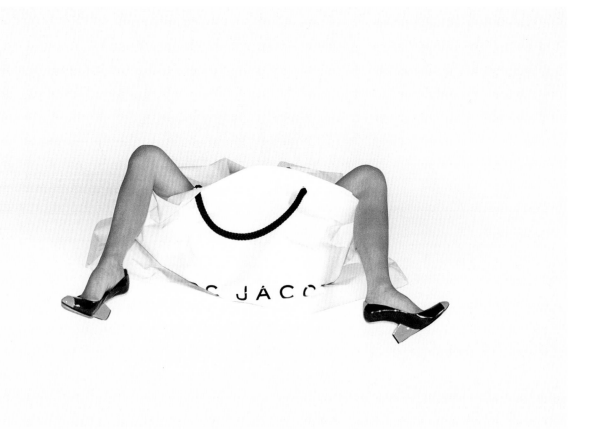

magazine, controversially expanded its remit by featuring the work of Richard Prince, Ed Ruscha and Takashi Murakami on special covers, and devoted content to both emerging and established artists, including photographer Cindy Sherman's reinterpretation of Chanel in 2010 (page 230). Meanwhile, fashion illustration, a more traditional form of art-based fashion editorial, has also made a comeback in mainstream print publications such as *Vogue*, which regularly features the work of a contemporary band of illustrators including David Downton, Daisy de Villeneuve and Richard Gray.

Another new development in fashion print media has been the proliferation of handsome hardcover publications produced by fashion houses such as Louis Vuitton, Gucci and Ermenegildo Zegna, documenting their art, fashion and architectural projects; the success of these volumes is indicative of the high level of public interest in the marriage of fashion, art and architecture. The practice has also been adopted by fashion magazines, including *Another*, *Vogue* and *Harper's Bazaar*, which have published hardback collections of their archival imagery in an attempt to ensure longevity for what has historically been perceived as a transient, throwaway print medium. As free and even more ephemeral websites increasingly supplant physical magazines, the re-publication of a selection of curated images in a glossy, expensive, artistically designed tome is a way of restoring a sense of value – both monetary and intellectual – to fashion media.

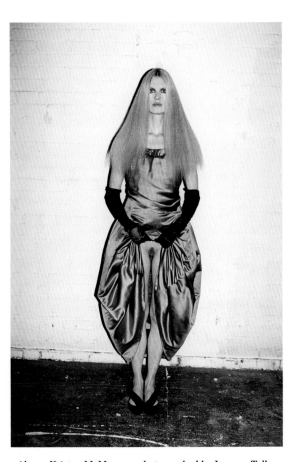

Above: Kristen McMenamy photographed by Juergen Teller
for Marc Jacobs, Autumn/Winter 2005.
Opposite: Victoria Beckham photographed by Juergen Teller
for Marc Jacobs, Spring/Summer 2008.

The current generation of fashion photographers – like their influential 20th-century predecessors Richard Avedon, Herb Ritts and Helmut Newton who first established the reputation of fashion photography within the art world – enjoy a high level of public recognition. The work of fashion photographers such as Mario Testino, Steven Klein, Tim Walker, Deborah Turbeville, Terry Richardson and the partnership of Inez van Lamsweerde and Vinoodh Matadin is taken seriously by the art world and is regularly exhibited in mainstream art museums and galleries. Meanwhile, other photographers who work primarily in fine art – including Juergen Teller, Sam Taylor-Johnson and Quentin Shih – have also produced many high-profile fashion shoots and advertising campaigns. Teller's ongoing collaboration with Marc Jacobs, for instance, has even been the subject of an illustrated monograph. In many cases such fashion work threatens to eclipse an art photographer's wider practice, due not only to the wide public exposure afforded by advertising campaigns, but also to the large budgets typically provided by the fashion labels that commission such projects, which allow for an especially grand realization of a photographer's vision.

Jefferson Hack, founder and editor of *Another* magazine, characterizes the 21st-century fashion-media landscape as an arena in which 'Photographers have become brands, stylists have transformed into artists and many magazines have emerged as contemporary exhibition spaces.'[2] Accordingly, the new forms of fashion media that have emerged over the past decade are adopting the presentation styles and editorial practices of the art world in an attempt to record and lend gravity to fashion projects that are inherently ephemeral. Fashion monographs, for instance, increasingly resemble art exhibition catalogues, as do the new fashion print periodicals, which challenge the format of mainstream commercial magazines by championing high design and production values, eschewing traditional forms of product placement and seeking out artists themselves as collaborators. Meanwhile, the fashion labels themselves turn to art photographers and filmmakers in an effort to reach the widest possible audience through new forms of media. Ultimately, however, all the journals, films, books and photographic campaigns discussed in this chapter share a common aim: to offer a richer and more authentic way of communicating and experiencing fashion.

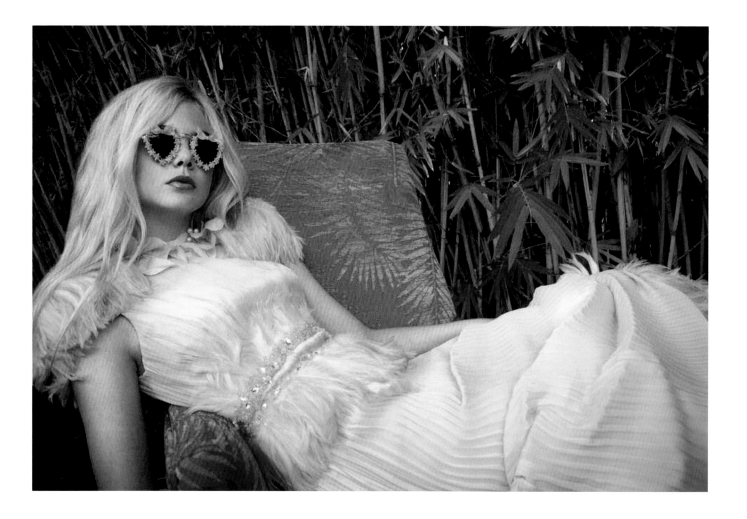

Above: Actress Elle Fanning photographed by
Bill Owens wearing Rodarte, Spring/Summer 2012,
for *A Magazine Curated By Rodarte.*

In conversation: Daniel Thawley, *A Magazine*

Biannual publication *A Magazine* is devoted to showcasing the creative output of individual designers and fashion brands who are invited to 'curate' each issue in collaboration with its editorial team, lending it a criticality that is often lacking in commercial fashion magazines. Past issues have been curated by Yohji Yamamoto, Haider Ackermann, Rodarte, Maison Martin Margiela and Martine Sitbon, among others. *A Magazine* aspires to artistic dialogue that, in the words of editor Daniel Thawley, 'leads to beautiful projects, special friendships and a fusion of explosive talent to create work that transcends the ordinary.'

'I think the reason that art, fashion and publishing work together is that they all tend to inform each other to different extents.'

Daniel Thawley

MITCHELL OAKLEY SMITH *What was the intention of* A Magazine *when it was launched, and what is it today?*

DANIEL THAWLEY Beginning its life in 2001 as Belgium's first true fashion magazine, *A* started as a look into the world and aesthetic of a different Belgian fashion designer with each issue. This quickly broadened into an international concept, and has since provided a 'carte blanche' platform for fashion designers to explore and expose the inner workings of their design processes, their personal journey, and the friends and heroes who inspire them.

MOS *The publication is an incredible fusion of art, fashion and publishing. Why do these forms sit so well together?*

DT *A Magazine* is a very honest publication in the way we give such freedom to a designer to dictate what is printed within it. I think the reason that art, fashion and publishing work together is that they all tend to inform each other to different extents. Many designers research art when designing a collection, just as they may also look at imagery – be it historical, artistic, ethnic, political – in beautiful books... The end result of each issue is a publication that accounts for a designer's singular vision in these three spheres combined, elevated by the contribution of their chosen peers and our established framework.

MOS *It must be a challenge, then, to select the curator of each issue.*

DT The members of our team all have different perspectives: our director also worked in film; our graphic designer comes directly from a graphic design point of view; and I myself am the member of the group most fully immersed in the fashion world. As such, our propositions and politics vary, and our choices, too, between issues. We like to plan ahead, to work with both established and emerging designers and celebrate a diverse mix of nationalities and styles. A good curating designer is one whose universe runs deep, traversing multiple disciplines away from the monotony of face-value fashion imagery. We are intrigued by designers who diffuse their own aesthetic and have a signature [look] in all facets of their garments, stores, shows, invitations, events, collaborations and communications.

MOS *What, then, is your role?*

DT My role differs to that of a traditional editor because I am more involved in shaping, guiding and realizing the vision of the curating designer than in selecting content myself. I consider my own knowledge of the *A Magazine* concept and history invaluable to the curator, assisting them in what to include and what not include when filtering their ideas, tastes, obsessions, idols and fantasies into a tangible and cohesive magazine format.

MOS *Do you provide the curators with a framework or guideline?*

DT We call it a white card – a 'carte blanche' – which means total free reign for the designer. The few restrictions that we have include the large 'A' on the cover, a 200-page limit, specific dimensions of the page size and the inclusion of an editor's and curator's letter to introduce each issue. Otherwise we offer suggestions and examples of how other designers have tackled this blank canvas in the past.

MOS *Who do you think is the typical reader of* A Magazine*? Is it an art reader or a fashion reader?*

DT I would say that we have quite a variety of archetypal readers, all of whom are open-minded and creative people with a keen interest in higher culture. There will always be the designer's loyal fan base who are eager to discover what makes them tick, and likewise a certain cult following of *A Magazine*, many of whom have collected issues since the beginning.

'A good curating designer is one whose universe runs deep, traversing multiple disciplines away from the monotony of face-value fashion imagery.'

Daniel Thawley

Overleaf: Valentino, Autumn/Winter 2010, photographed by
Erik Madigan and styled by Giambattista Valli for *A Magazine*
Curated By Giambattista Valli.

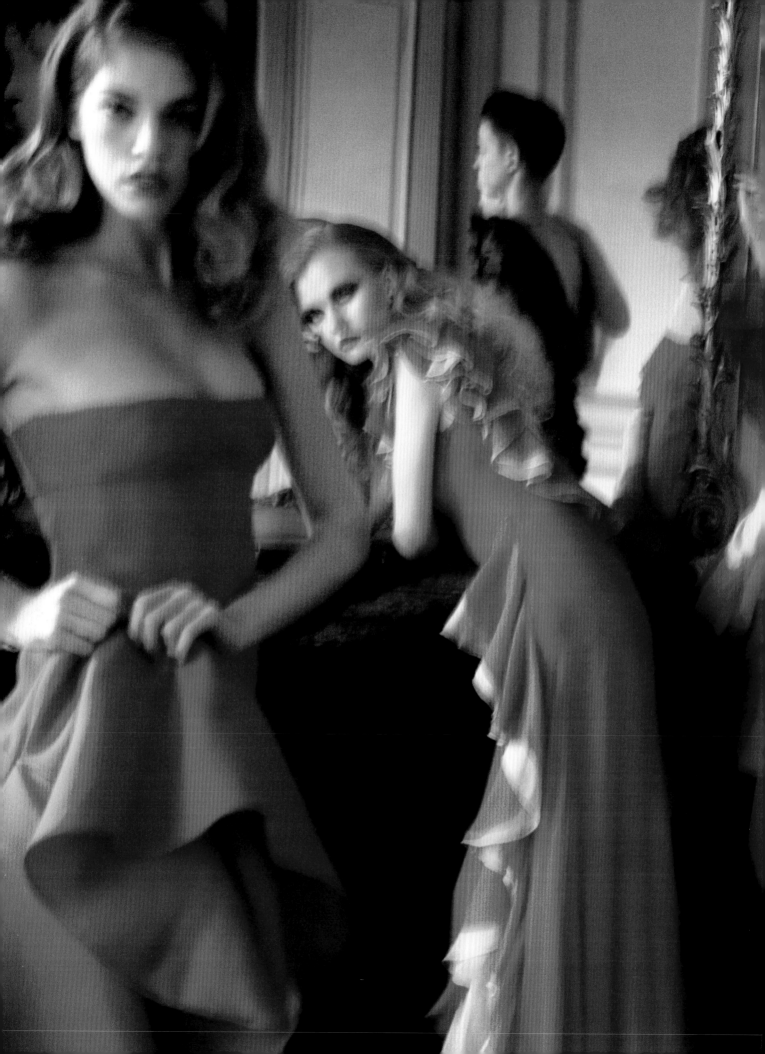

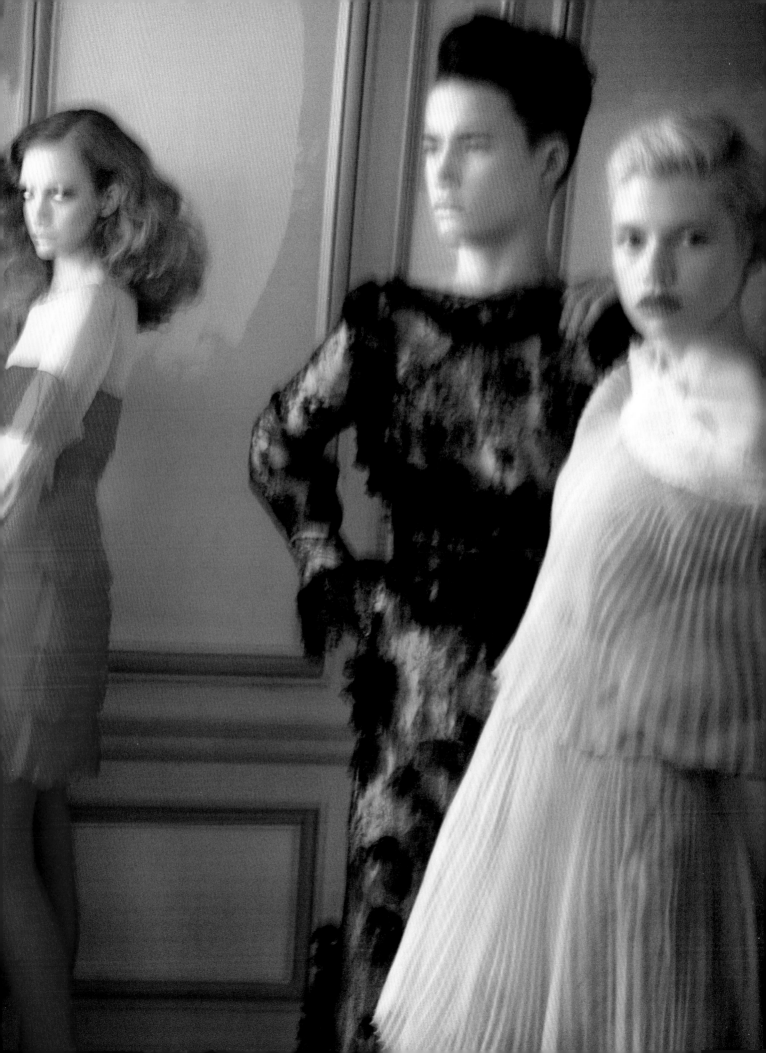

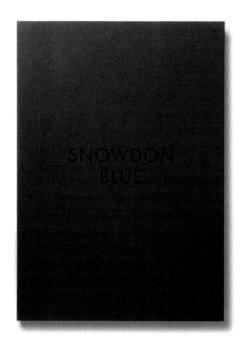

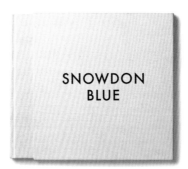

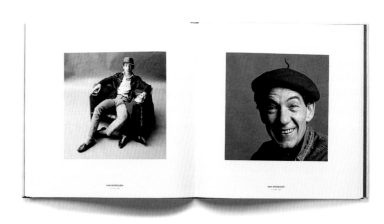

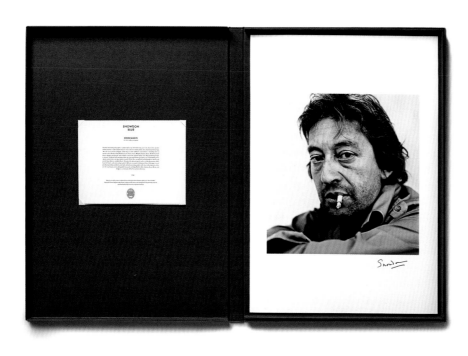

Acne & Lord Snowdon

In 2012, Swedish multidisciplinary label Acne launched a book, exhibition and capsule collection entitled 'Snowdon Blue' in collaboration with venerated society photographer Lord Snowdon, with whom Acne's creative director and founder Jonny Johansson has been working since 2007. The project comprised sixty-one portraits of iconic personalities such as David Bowie and Ian McKellen wearing a classic blue shirt, along with a series of eight limited-edition unisex blue shirts. What makes this seemingly incongruous meeting so relevant – Acne, with its reputation as an 'insider' brand and publisher of the influential journal *Acne Paper*; Snowdon, a relic of British aristocracy whose lens captures the wealthy and famous – is their mutual appreciation of the blue shirt, that most democratic and working class of items. 'Snowdon called the blue shirt "a kind of uniform",' explained Johansson.[3] The project injected Snowdon's original archival imagery with newfound relevance for a younger contemporary audience attracted by Acne's fashion cachet. Meanwhile, the collaboration elevated Acne to the status of royalty, imbuing it with a measure of style and elegance, and importantly, history, demonstrating the timelessness (some of the photographs are years old) of the blue shirt, but also echoing the adage that style is ageless.

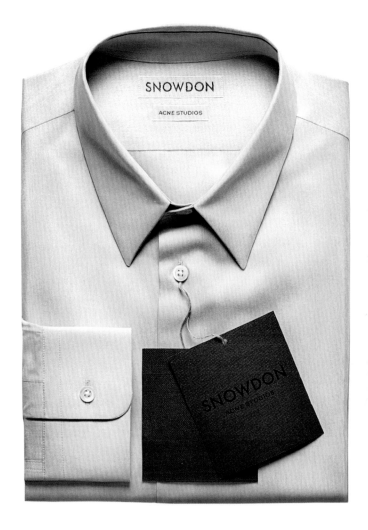

Above: Acne, shirt from the 'Snowdon Blue' project, 2012.
Opposite: *Snowdon Blue*, a monograph by photographer Lord Snowdon (Antony Armstrong-Jones), published by Acne Studios, 2012.

In conversation:
Daniel Askill

Daniel Askill is a filmmaker based in Sydney and New York. In addition to creating films, video installations, music videos and commercials, Askill has exhibited his work in both solo and group exhibitions at galleries including Prism, Los Angeles; Palais de Tokyo, Paris; and the Australian Centre for the Moving Image, Melbourne. As co-founder of multidisciplinary studio Collider, Askill has created works for fashion houses including Ksubi, Christian Dior and Acne, the latter for whom he worked with designer Michelle Jank in 2010 to create *Concrete Island*, a short film introducing its pre-collection presentation for Spring/Summer 2011 as suspended tableaux.

MITCHELL OAKLEY SMITH *To begin, what attracted you to work on a project with Acne?*

DANIEL ASKILL Acne has always been an interesting company to me, particularly because it branches out into disciplines beyond fashion – art, print, film, etc. – so I was immediately interested in working with them and the brief was also very open.

MOS *Some hold a critical view of working within fashion – do you see it as elevating or devaluing your broader oeuvre in any way, or is it simply a different form in which to work?*

DA Fashion has always been an interesting area to me. I particularly love it when it intersects with art. My brother [jewelry designer Jordan Askill] also works in fashion, so that has created a kind of bridge for me into that world. Working on films with fashion content is always of interest to me as long as the brief is not too prescriptive. I think there is a lot of interesting potential in the intersection between fashion and film, and the most exciting part is that it is only the beginning. For me, what is really key is the intention is to make good work, whether that be in the realm of film, fashion, art or some intersection of them all.

MOS *Conversely, do you think that a fashion house is elevated by working in a genre such as film?*

DA I think the key is that there is mutual respect and openness from both sides, and if that is the case, the work will be elevated by the collaboration.

MOS *You're part of a culture in which fashion films have become very popular – why do you think film has become such a big tool for brands?*

DA I think a really fundamental part of it is access to technology. Film is no longer such an elusive medium. With the emergence of digital SLRs with high quality video capabilities a lot of photographers are suddenly making short fashion films and a whole new generation of creative people are just getting into film without thinking twice, which wasn't really possible not so long ago. The flip side is that the quality of work coming out is a bit hit-and-miss since everyone can suddenly make moving images. Then again, it is great that so many people have access now, and it will no doubt lead to some revolutionary work in the future as the language evolves.

MOS *Another artist has noted that with the downturn of art sales, working with fashion brands is a viable financial proposition – what is your view on this?*

DA That is interesting, but I must say my personal experience is that I have never worked on fashion films for financial reasons. I have always approached them more like art projects. At the moment the budgets for fashion films are really much less than those for more mainstream commercial film projects, so I don't really see them as a viable source of income. For me it is more about an interesting mix of work that includes projects in the art, fashion, commercial and music spheres. I think the key is really just a desire to make good work and from that the rest will follow.

MOS *What was the process of creating the Acne film?*

DA The brief was really very open. I do remember that Jonny [Johansson] from Acne had referenced an old image of Halston's lover Victor Hugo fitting some mannequins. Beyond that, some clothes just arrived one day. I had a chat with [designer and friend] Michelle Jank and my brother Lorin about using a time-slice camera rig to create some imagery very loosely inspired by the photo, but recreated as suspended tableaux using very slow shutter speeds, and that is what we did.

This page and overleaf: Stills from the short film
Concrete Island, directed by Daniel Askill in collaboration
with creative director Michelle Jank and filmmaker
Lorin Askill for Acne, Pre-Collection, Spring/Summer 2011.

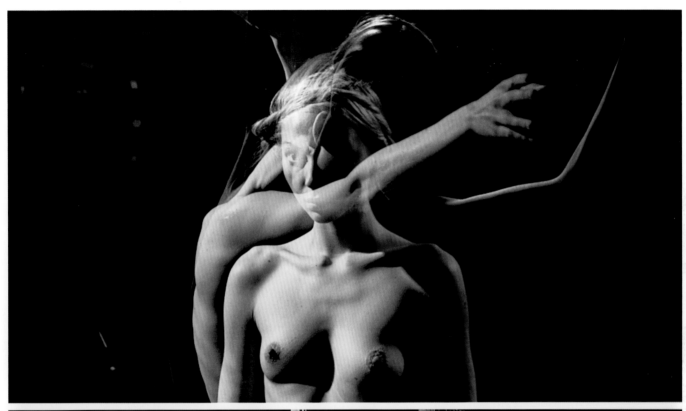

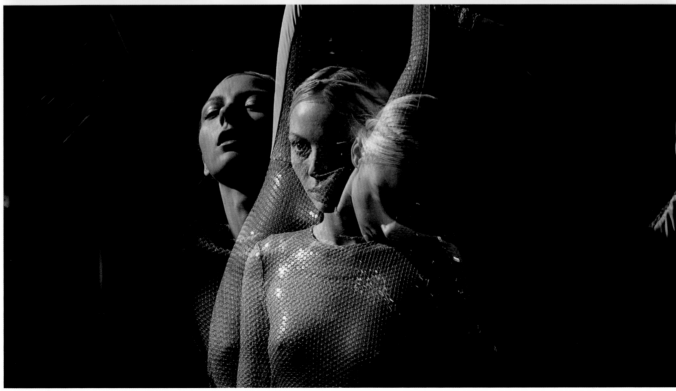

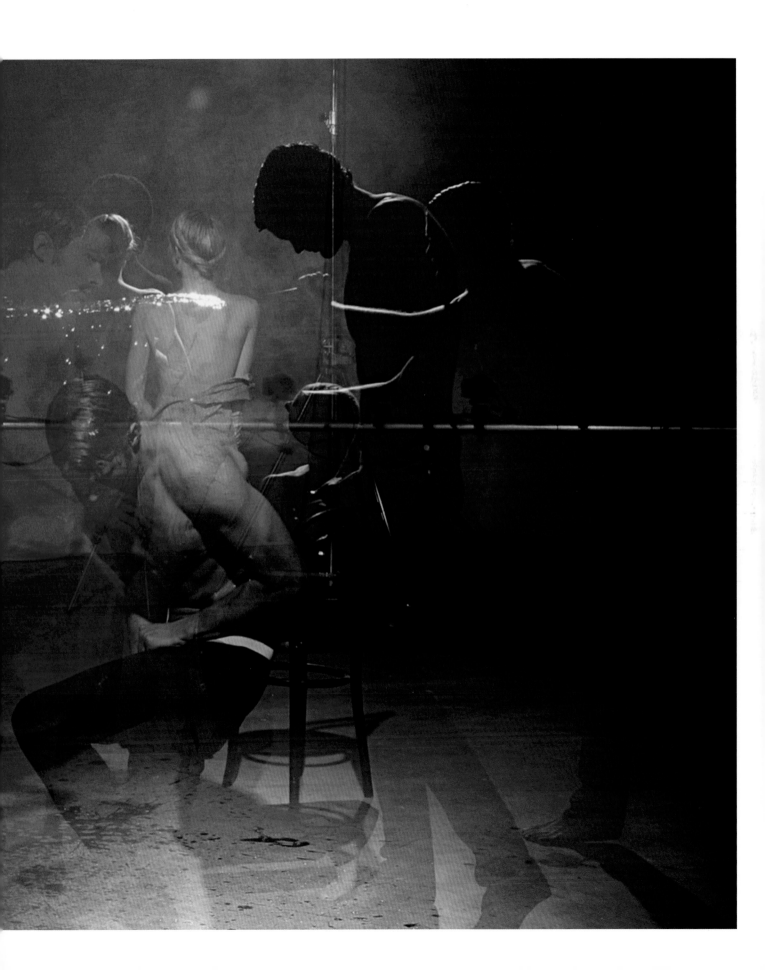

Inez van Lamsweerde
& Vinoodh Matadin

When Dutch collaborative photographic duo Inez van Lamsweerde and Vinoodh Matadin published a story in seminal fashion magazine *The Face* in 1994, it set in motion what has become a highly successful career that has spanned a quarter century. In contrast to the black-and-white, low-fi grunge aesthetic that defined the 1990s, Lamsweerde and Matadin's images, in which slick, polished models were digitally transposed against a rocket launch, a night-time cityscape and a disco dance floor, were precursors of 21st-century fashion photography.

Boasting an extensive body of commercial work that has included global advertising campaigns for Christian Dior, Gucci and Louis Vuitton, magazines such as *V*, French and American *Vogue* and the *New York Times Magazine*, Lamsweerde and Matadin have developed a much-imitated style in which digital technology is used to manipulate the human form, creating surreal and sometimes grotesque effects and offering an alternative view of beauty. While digital retouching is now common practice within fashion photography it was largely unheard of when Lamsweerde and Matadin pioneered the use of software program Paintbox in the early 1990s. As Lamsweerde explains, 'At that point it was used to straighten lines and shine up the wheels of a car for advertising. It hadn't really been used for fashion or for images of people...It just opened up the whole world for us.'[4] What defines Lamsweerde and Matadin's artistic output is the emotional integrity and personal quality that remains intact in their images and is amplified by the use of digital experimentation. Journalist Jochen Siemens describes their work as 'made up of many more layers than we are used to. These are pictures that give us more than mere views. Atmosphere is maybe the right word.'[5]

The photographers, who are represented by Gagosian Gallery in New York, choose not to draw a distinction between their commercial and artistic work, exhibiting and publishing both together. 'Sometimes our work that's been published as an advertising campaign ends up on the walls of a museum,' explains Lamsweerde 'The advertising and the editorials – everything sort of feeds together'.[6] Accordingly, the duo adapted one of their most famous 'art' photographic series, *Me Kissing Vinoodh* (1999), previously exhibited at the Whitney Museum, New York, for Lanvin Homme's Spring/Summer 2010 campaign, producing an image of the embracing couple in which the nude Lamsweerde is painted to look as if her skin is missing. The new image, entitled *Me Kissing Vinoodh (Eternally)* was later repurposed as a silkscreen in collaboration with renowned printer Eugene Licht. This ongoing melding of high-low artistic values is integral to the photographers' practice and is further evidenced by their presence, unlike the majority of their peers, on social media platforms such as Tumblr.

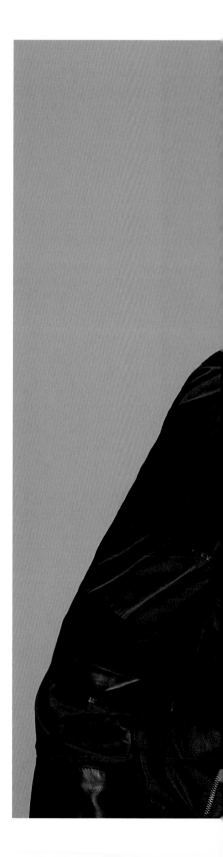

Below: Inez van Lamsweerde and Vinoodh Matadin,
Me Kissing Vinoodh (Eternally), self-portrait for Lanvin,
Spring/Summer 2010.

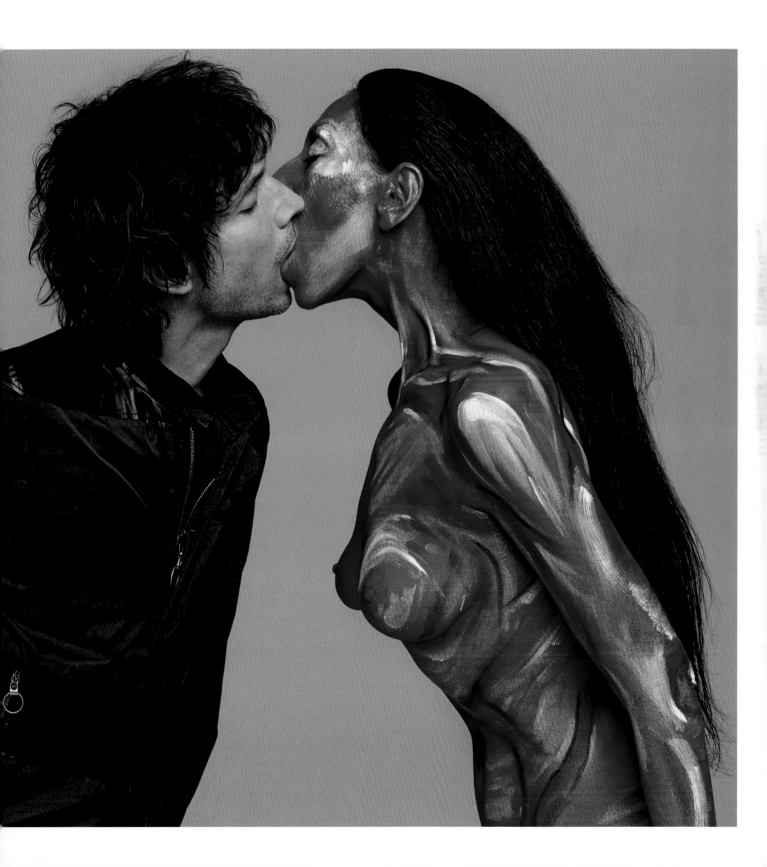

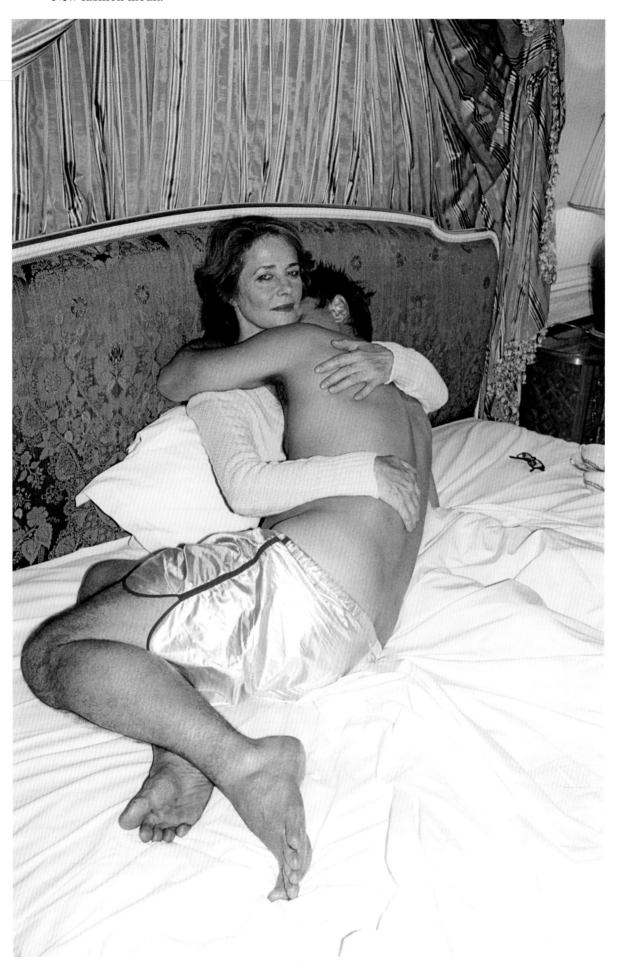

Marc Jacobs &
Juergen Teller

German photographer Juergen Teller's most recognizable campaigns, for Marc Jacobs's namesake label, have been ongoing since 1998. The photographer's style is best characterized by the aesthetic of the home snapshot. Teller artfully recreates the awkwardness of a random photograph with simple lighting, few props, plain backdrops and little post-production manipulation. The power of his images resides almost in their lack of artifice, which is, of course, their art. Teller's photographs for Jacobs's campaign have famously featured artists such as Cindy Sherman and Roni Horn alongside a roll call of actresses and celebrities. In one image, Sherman and Teller appear together, Teller dressed as Sherman's doppelganger; elsewhere, Teller appears in the arms of British actress Charlotte Rampling, in bed, wearing only a pair of shorts. In these images, which acquire multiple layers of meaning from the fact of being both artworks and photographs of an artist, the Marc Jacobs products themselves are almost an afterthought; the label simply acquires cultural credibility by association. According to the *New York Times* fashion critic Cathy Horyn, quoting the art dealer Barbara Gladstone, 'The ads are really for people who get it, and I think Marc and Juergen happily dispense with those who don't.'[7]

In these images...the Marc Jacobs products themselves are almost an afterthought.

Opposite: Juergen Teller and Charlotte Rampling photographed by Teller for Marc Jacobs, Spring/Summer 2004.

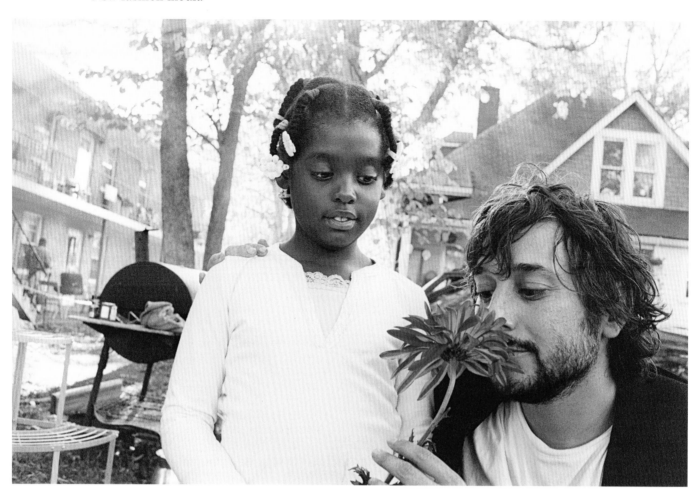

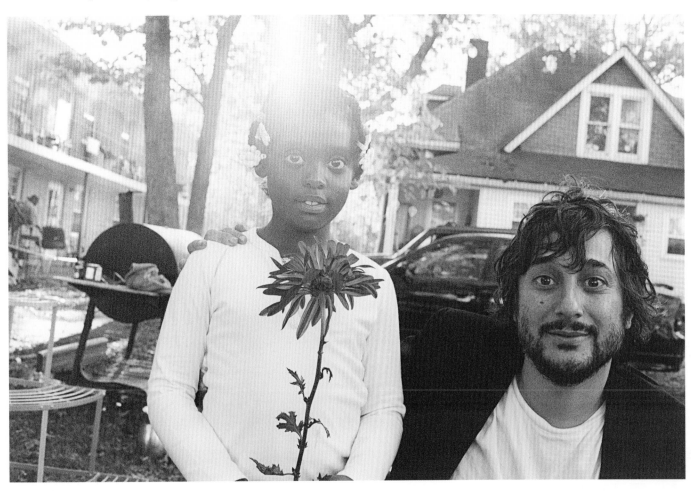

Above and opposite: Harmony Korine photographed by
Juergen Teller for Marc Jacobs, Spring/Summer 2008.

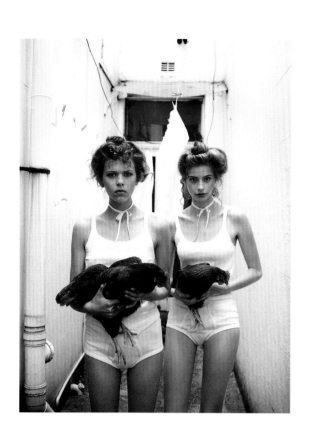

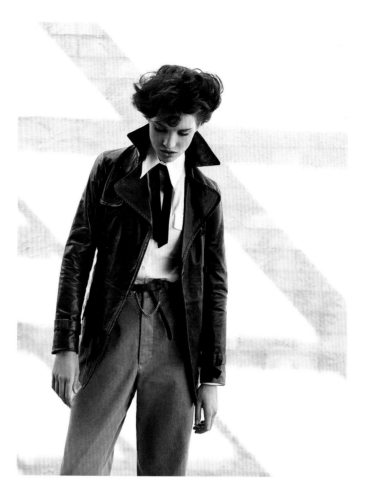

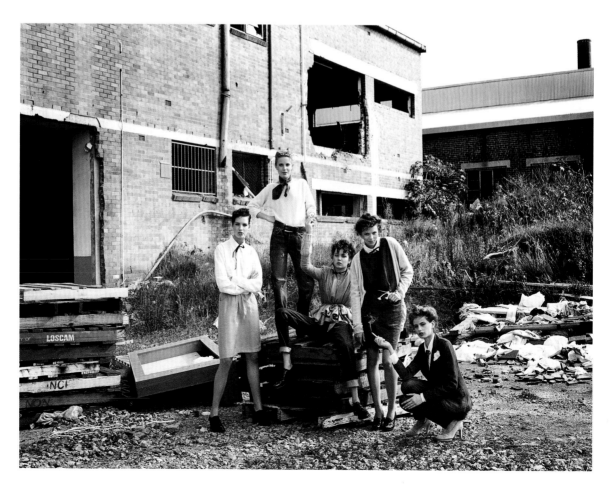

Liz Ham

There's nothing new in pointing out that portraiture can be a pretext for the self-depiction of the artist. Sydney-based photographer Liz Ham is well aware of the parallels she draws between herself and her subjects. Previously a punk, a goth, a raver and a hippie, Ham now explores the concept of 'otherness' through photographic portraiture and documentary. It's a concept that has been interrogated endlessly, so much so that the notion of exiting the mainstream isn't very radical at all. Nor is documenting it. Yet Ham, who works professionally as a commercial photographer, fuses traditional documentary with digital fashion photography, making for a rich and completely unique practice that finds more similarities in the work of wartime *Vogue* documentary photographer Lee Miller and in Karlheinz Weinberger's portraits of Swiss youth rebels than it does in that of her contemporaries.

Few other fashion shoots have garnered as much as attention as did Ham's 'Teddy Girls', published in *Oyster* magazine in early 2010. The project was inspired by the *Picture Post*'s 1955 documentary photographs of Teddy Girls, or 'Judies' as they were sometimes known, by British photographer and film director Ken Russell. Ham's 'Teddy Girls' brilliantly captures the spirit and activities of this small group of young girls who, working in offices or factories, spent their free time creating their own high style look to rival the fashion houses' revived interest in haute couture with pencil skirts, tailored jackets, rolled-up jeans and flat shoes, re-cut and re-styled with a streetwise, tomboy twist. Ham concedes that 2010 was a delicate time to present a shoot that explored the 'make do and mend' practice of wartime austerity, given the global financial crisis, but perhaps it was also an appropriate one. 'Fashion, no matter its subject, is lighthearted, and I like using it as a vehicle of education or way to have a little bit of fun with stories that are affecting us today.'[8]

'Teddy Girls' featured a group of five young Australian and New Zealand models playing in a vegetable garden, mending and hand-sewing clothing, arm wrestling and smoking: everyday activities that, although choreographed, make the project reminiscent of her early documentary photographs. The influence of Russell's work is apparent not only in the stylistic elements (clothing, hair and makeup, sets) but also in the composition of subjects, who are shown leaning against walls or sitting on each other's shoulders as if mimicking their male counterparts, and in the lighting, particularly the black-and-white shots that contrast light and shade. Ham uses light as part of her set, with shadows of buildings and railings cast against her characters; backlighting is used to create starkly white backgrounds, contrasting with the gritty setting and giving the images an aged appearance.

In a 2008 series, *Public Image Limited*, Ham explored the many different subcultures that evolved out of the fragmented post-punk scene in Sydney. The characters of Ham's youth are depicted by a cast of young men who were recruited from Ham's husband's former punk band, alongside professional fashion models, including the androgynous Serbian-Australian male model Andrej Pejić, who has since launched an international career modelling womenswear. The characters, whose outfits were assembled from contemporary garments rather than vintage clothing, included skinheads with their sideburns, tattoos, athletic shoes and trilby hats; poseur punks in leopardskin, fishnet stockings and black lace; New Romantics wearing frilly shirts, ripped denim and layered clothing; along with the androgynous styles of the Glam Rock era and Australia's homegrown Sharpies in their undersized knits and drainpipe jeans. In exploring these past eras through a contemporary lens, Ham offered a postmodern twist on fashion photography and highlighted the cyclical nature of fashion itself.

Opposite: Images from 'Teddy Girls', Liz Ham, 2010.

Cindy Sherman:
Balenciaga & Chanel

Cindy Sherman's ongoing artistic project involves photographing herself in myriad guises that explore stereotypical and non-typical tropes of the female as the subject of gaze. As both the subject and the photographer, Sherman creates self-portraits of her many suspended selves, appropriating elements of film and fashion photography. She has had several interactions with fashion in her work. In 1984 and 1994 she was commissioned by Comme des Garçons to produce its photographic campaigns. The resultant images, almost post-apocalyptic in nature, demonstrated both the avant-garde credentials of the brand and Sherman's ability to critique the medium of fashion photography. Sherman, too, has appeared as a photographic subject in Juergen Teller's advertising campaigns for Marc Jacobs (see page 202).

In 2010, Sherman was commissioned by French fashion house Balenciaga to create a series of six images incorporating its clothing. In the resulting project, *Cindy Sherman: Untitled (Balenciaga)*, which was unveiled at the *Vogue* Fashion's Night Out event in New York, the artist styled herself as the subject of mock newspaper society-page photographs in the vein of the work of the *New York Times*'s longtime street-style photographer Bill Cunningham. Sherman appears in the guise of a variety of socialites resembling everyone from Iris Apfel to Paris Hilton, in what is both parody and a celebration of Balenciaga's 'rebellious' image. Balenciaga, while under the creative direction of designer Nicolas Ghesquière from 1997 to 2012, built a loyal following as a result of its unfailing edginess and willingness to push the boundaries. To collaborate with an artist of Sherman's calibre demonstrated a cultural savvy that transcended the mere commercial viability of the brand. It was a recognition that Sherman, too, is a brand, highly collectable and coveted.

In 2012, the same year that a major retrospective of her work was shown at the Museum of Modern Art, New York, Sherman presented a smaller exhibition at Metro Pictures, the gallery in the city's Chelsea neighbourhood that represents her commercially. Based on an insert she had originally created for Dasha Zhukova's art and fashion journal *Garage*, Sherman photographed herself wearing the clothing of the French fashion house Chanel, which had granted her access to its archive of contemporary and vintage haute couture pieces, some dating back to the 1920s. Sherman then employed the stock fashion-magazine narrative device of photographing models in unexpected locations, mimicking their dramatic poses and digitally transposing the photographs of herself against exotic backdrops such as Capri and Iceland, infusing the photographs with a romantic, painterly quality; her lost expression, however, interrupted the conventional prettiness and perfection of traditional fashion images.

Opposite: Cindy Sherman, *Untitled*, 2008, created for Balenciaga.
Overleaf and pages 234–35: Cindy Sherman, *Untitled*, 2010/2012 (overleaf)
and *Untitled*, 2010/2011 (pages 234–35), featuring clothing from the Chanel
archive and altered from their original publication in *Garage* magazine for
an exhibition at Metro Pictures, New York, 2012.

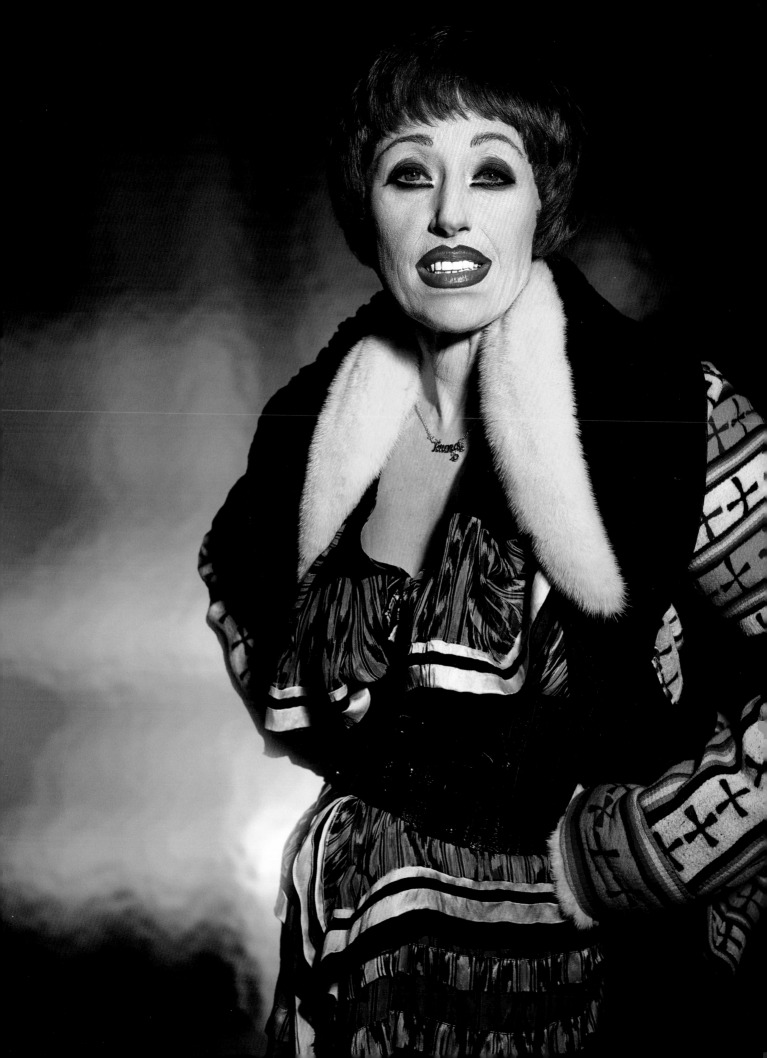

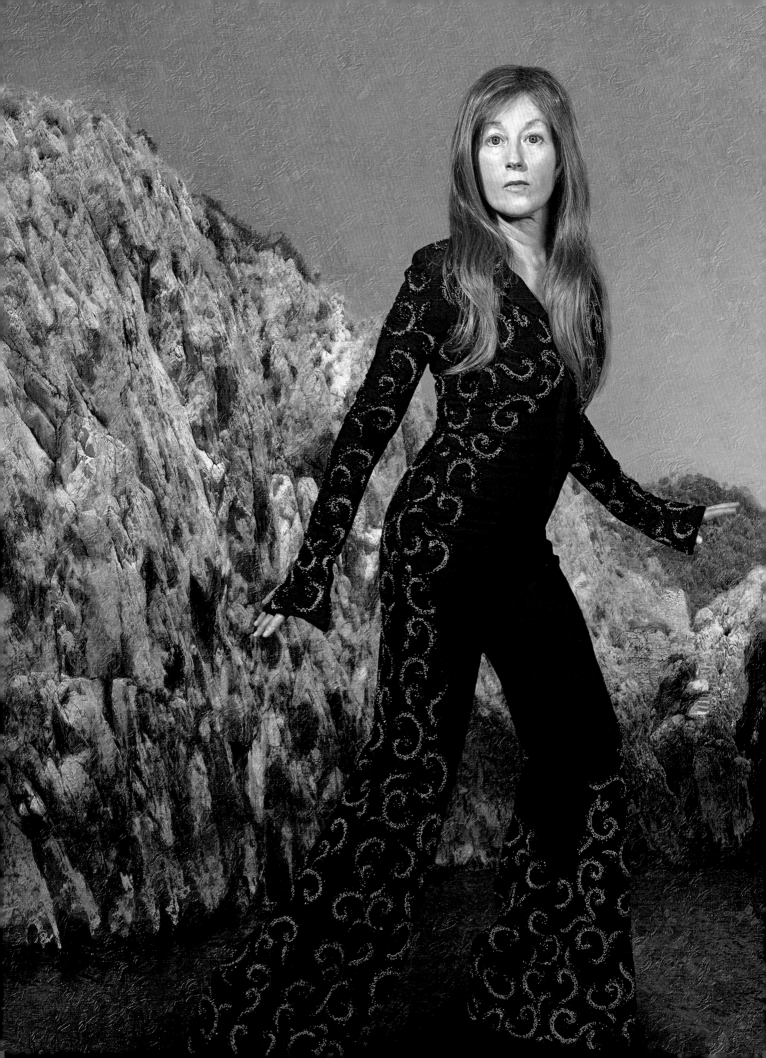

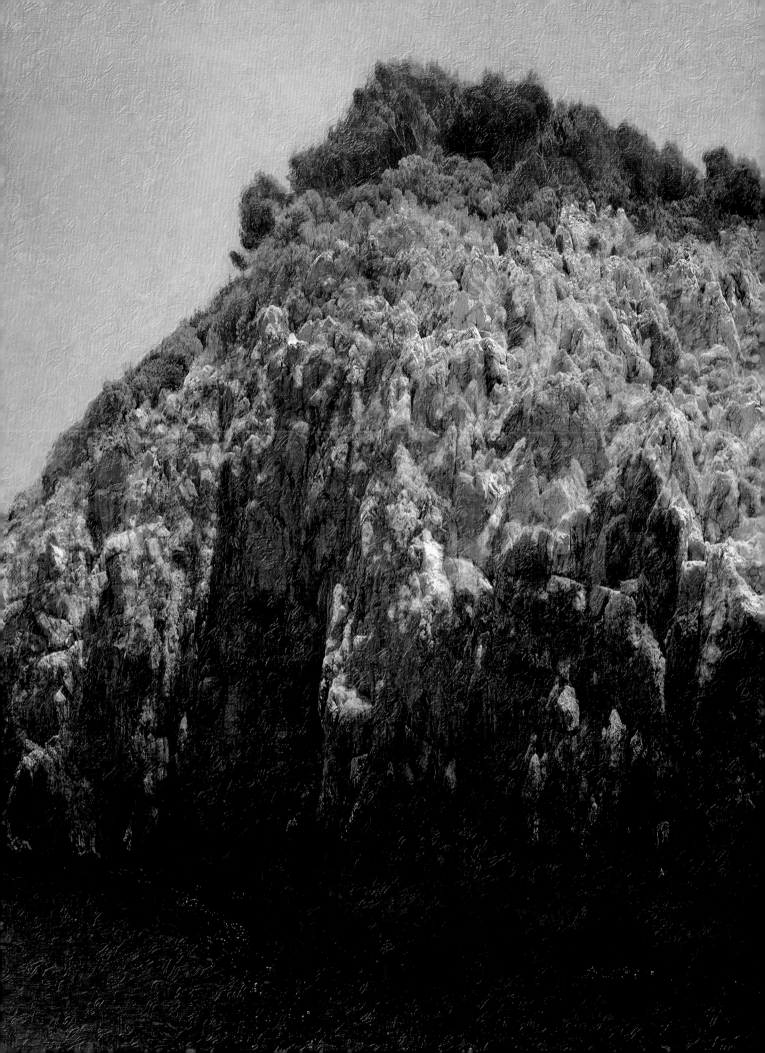

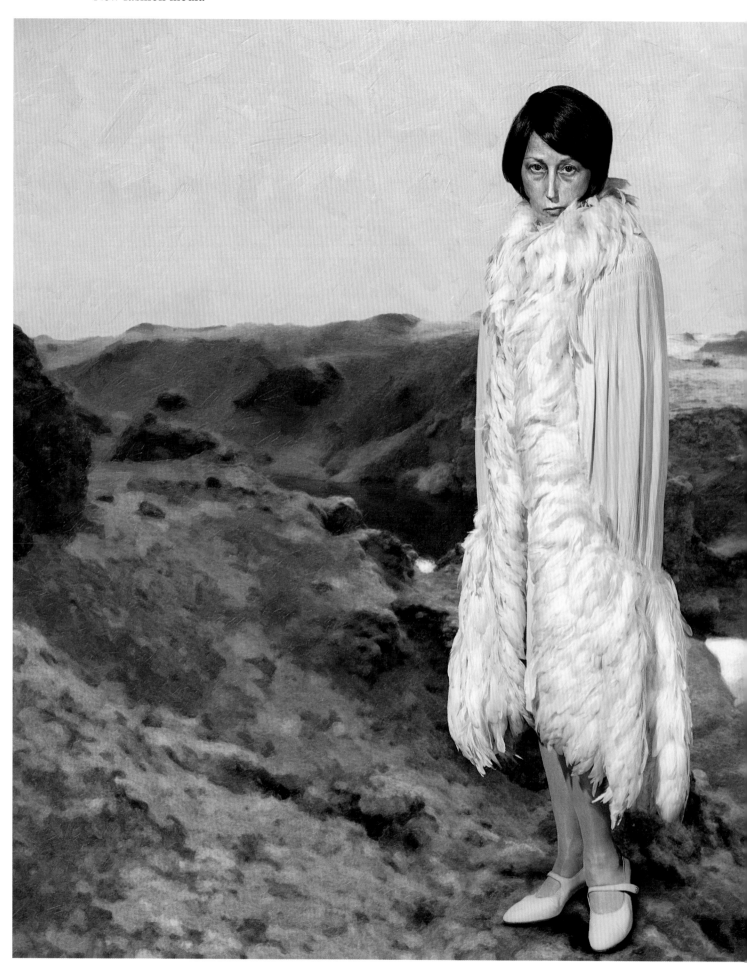

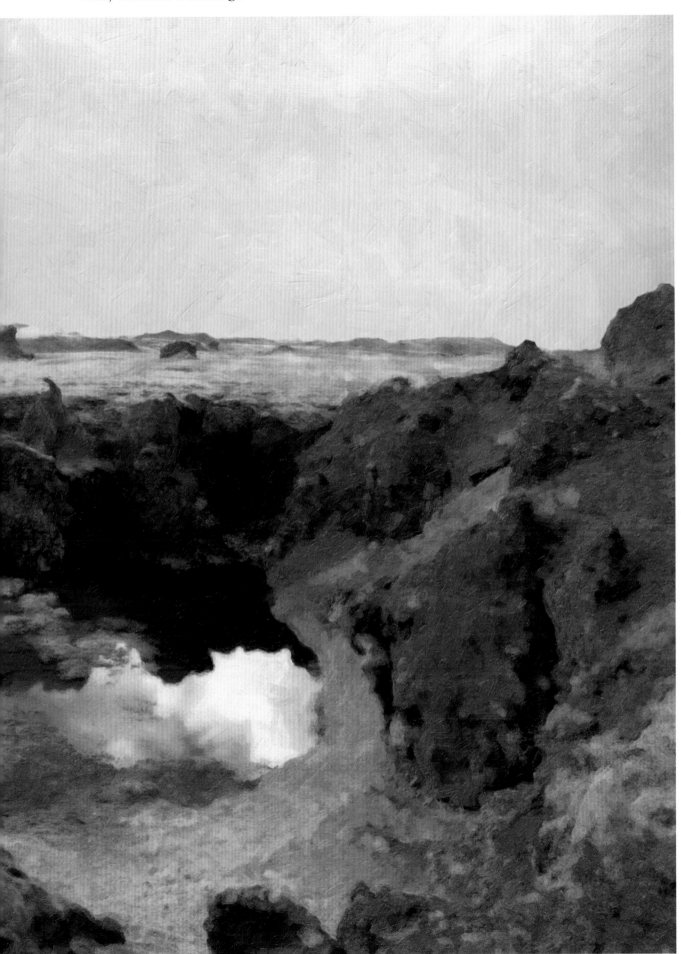

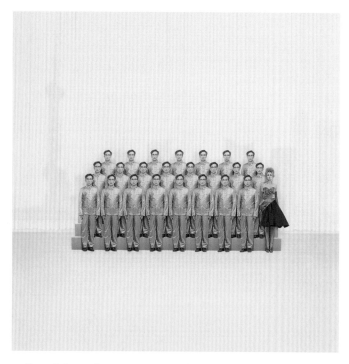

Christian Dior
& Quentin Shih

Above, below and opposite: Quentin Shih, *No. 06* (above), *No. 07* (below) and *No. 02* (opposite), from his *Shanghai Dreamers* photographic series created for Christian Dior, 2010.

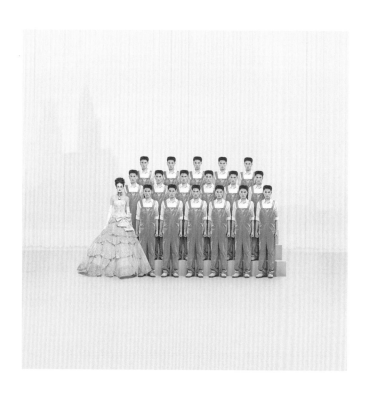

In 2008 Christian Dior mounted the exhibition 'Christian Dior and Chinese Artists' at the Ullens Center for Contemporary Art in Beijing to promote its position in the rapidly expanding Chinese luxury-goods market while tapping into the rising popularity of Chinese contemporary artists in the art world in tandem with the emergence of Hong Kong International Art Fair. One-off couture pieces by the house's then-creative director John Galliano were exhibited alongside a series of specially commissioned works by twenty of the country's leading contemporary artists, who had been asked to comment on what Christian Dior is or stands for. Among these works was photographer and filmmaker Quentin Shih's photographic series *The Stranger in the Glass Box* (2008) which was later included in 'Christian Dior: 60 Years of Photography' (2009) at the Museum of Modern Art, Moscow. In the series, fashion models wearing Christian Dior haute couture and sealed in glass boxes are inspected by small groups of identically dressed Chinese bystanders who resemble stereotyped characters from Communist propaganda posters, photographed against the backdrop of gritty industrial settings in northern China. The separation of the two cultures was, in fact, literal: the Dior models were photographed separately in Paris and then digitally inserted into the Chinese images. The series highlights the grotesqueness of each culture's image of the other, and gives visual expression to the impact of the arrival of affluent Western culture on the Chinese landscape.

Shih explored similar issues in two series he produced for Christian Dior in 2010, *Hong Kong Moment* and *Shanghai Dreamers*. The latter was commissioned by Christian Dior to mark the launch of the label's Shanghai store in 2010. In these images, which were produced using a complex photo-retouching technique, orderly rows of identical Chinese figures wearing 1970s or 1980s outfits, cloned from a single image, flank a single Western model in Dior haute couture. The Dior models literally stand out from the crowd. The arresting, dreamlike images were highly controversial: some critics accused Shih of perpetuating the racist myth that all Chinese people look the same, or of mocking the repression of his countrymen during the Cultural Revolution. Shih himself insisted that the series had been wholly misinterpreted. 'I wanted to show the power of Chinese people standing together and a kind of socialism in Chinese history,' he explained.[9]

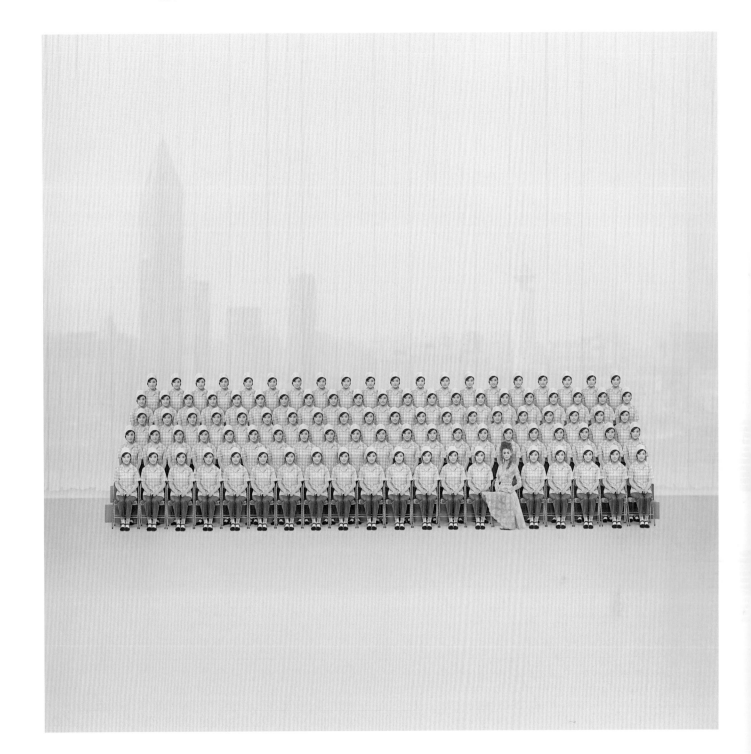

Overleaf: Quentin Shih, *No. 17*, from his *The Stranger in the Glass Box* photographic series created for Christian Dior, 2008.

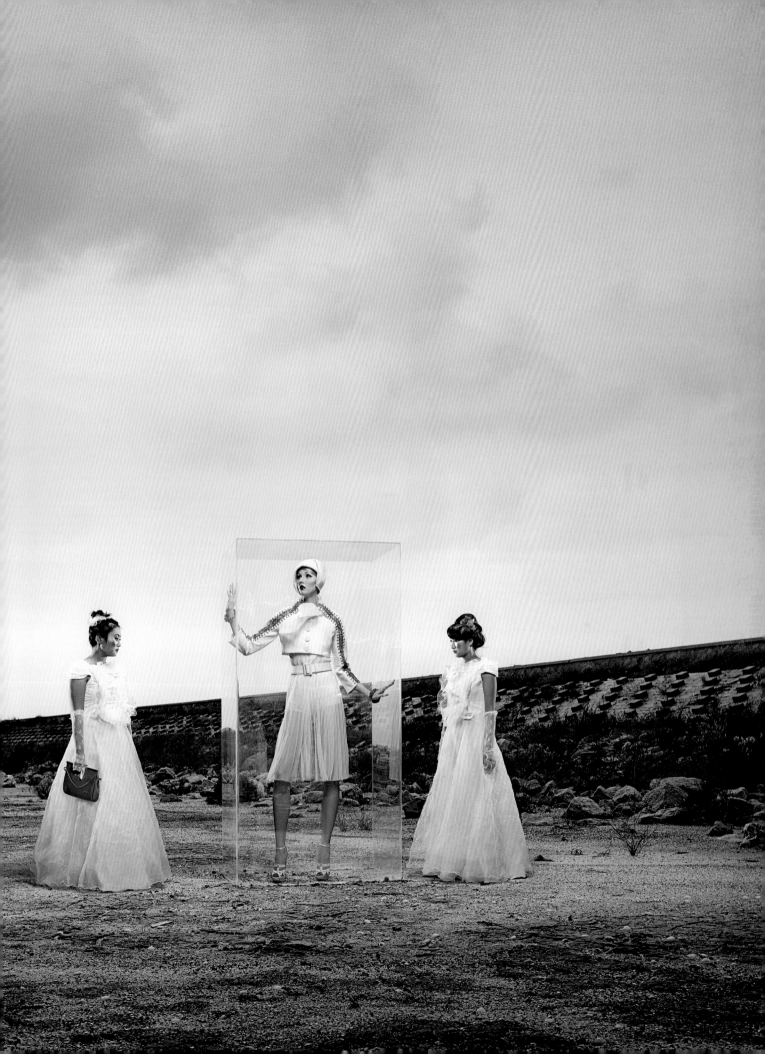

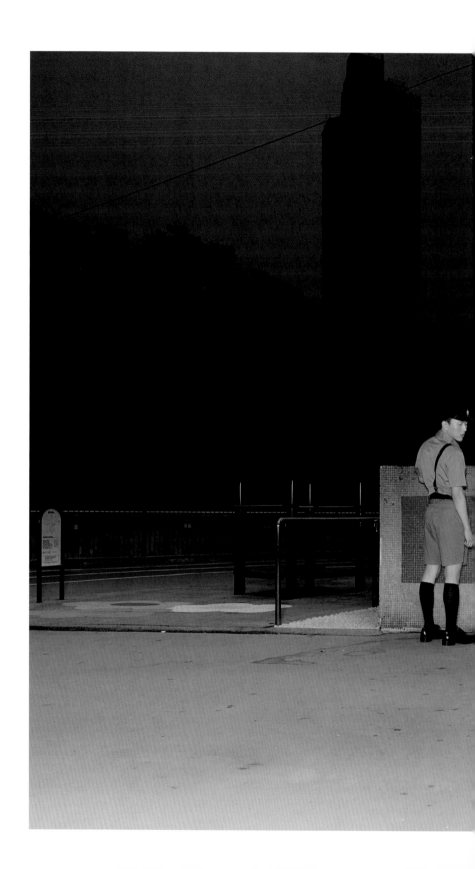

Quentin Shih, *No. 01*, from his *Hong Kong Moment*
photographic series created for Christian Dior, 2010.

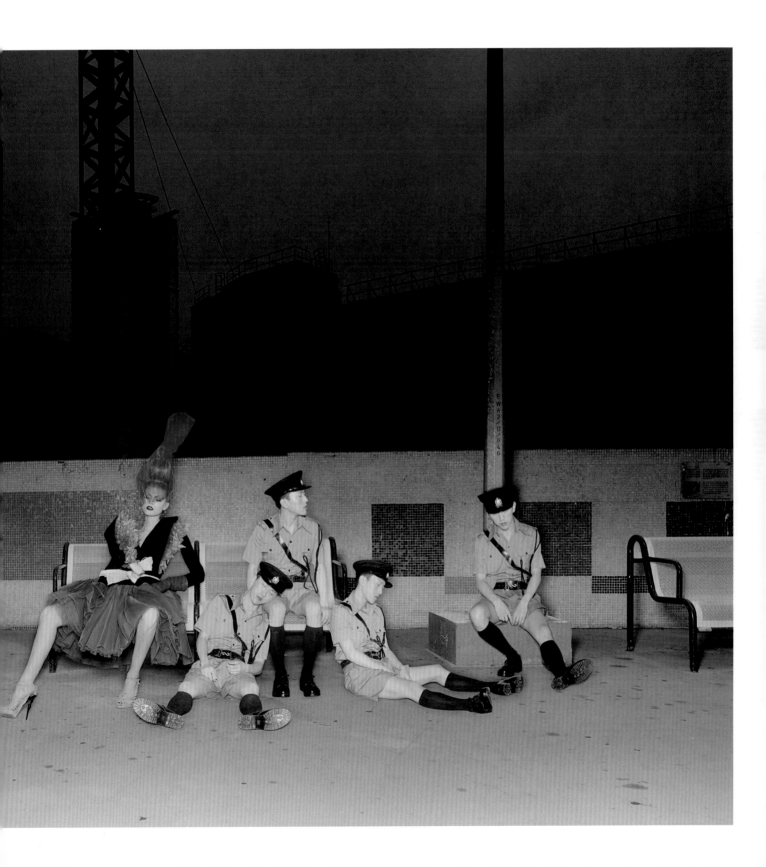

Scanlan & Theodore

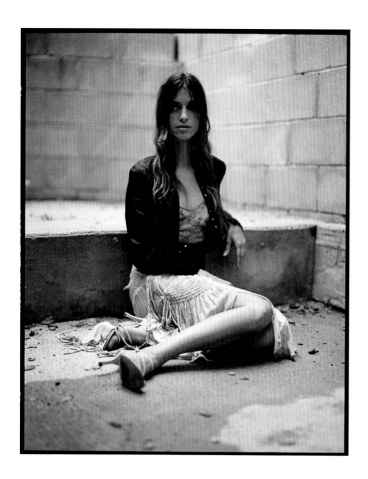

Australian label Scanlan & Theodore has engaged with artists across a variety of platforms, not only employing them directly on campaigns, but also facilitating exhibitions, including that of Louise Weaver in 2004, and collaborating with Dutch artist Daan Roosegaarde on an installation for the 2012 Biennale of Sydney and a companion video work for the brand's Sydney showroom. Most high profile, however, has been the work of photographers Bill Henson, Nan Goldin and David Armstrong for the label's advertising campaigns. Scanlan & Theodore is known for respecting the autonomy and creativity of the artists with whom it works, even in the face of controversy. Its collaboration with Bill Henson in 1997, on the back of the artist's lauded representation of Australia at the 1995 Venice Biennale, marked the brand's tenth anniversary and stirred debate about representations of young women in fashion and the sexualization of the photographer's gaze as it depicted a sixteen-year-old model with an exposed nipple.

Less controversially, from 2002 to 2004, renowned photographer David Armstrong captured some of the most intriguing faces in cinema and fashion, including muse Joana Preiss in 2002, Ann-Catherine Lacroix in 2003 and Diana Dondoe in 2004, for the label's campaigns. In 2010, Scanlan & Theodore worked with another provocative photographer, American artist Nan Goldin, who had already produced a series of blurrily romantic images for Bottega Veneta's Spring/Summer 2010 campaign. For the Scanlan & Theodore campaign Goldin depicted model and muse Erin Wasson as a well-dressed, dishevelled ingénue in a dilapidated mansion in upstate New York, photographed in the style of Goldin's intimate, voyeuristic, sometimes grubby studies of her close friends in her wider practice.

Above and opposite: Joana Preiss photographed by David Armstrong for Scanlan & Theodore, Spring/Summer 2005.

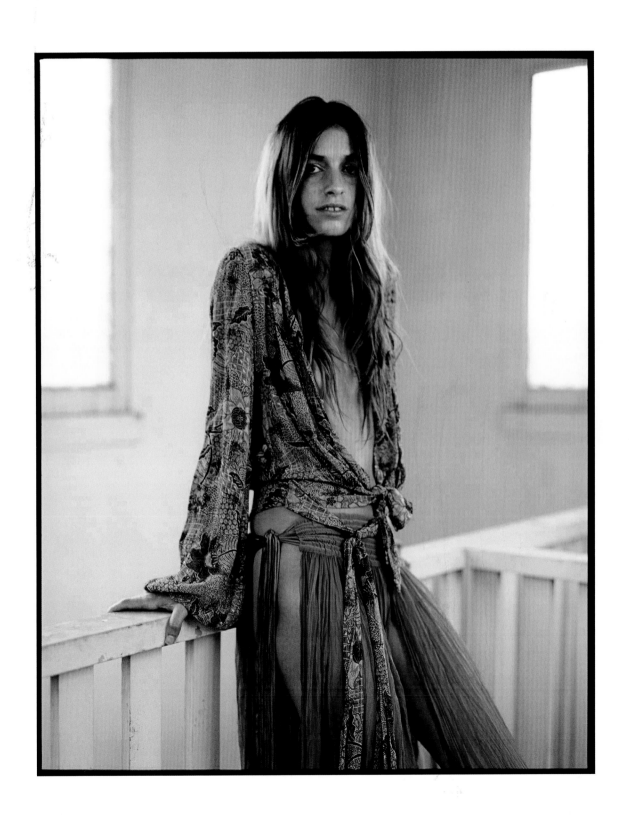

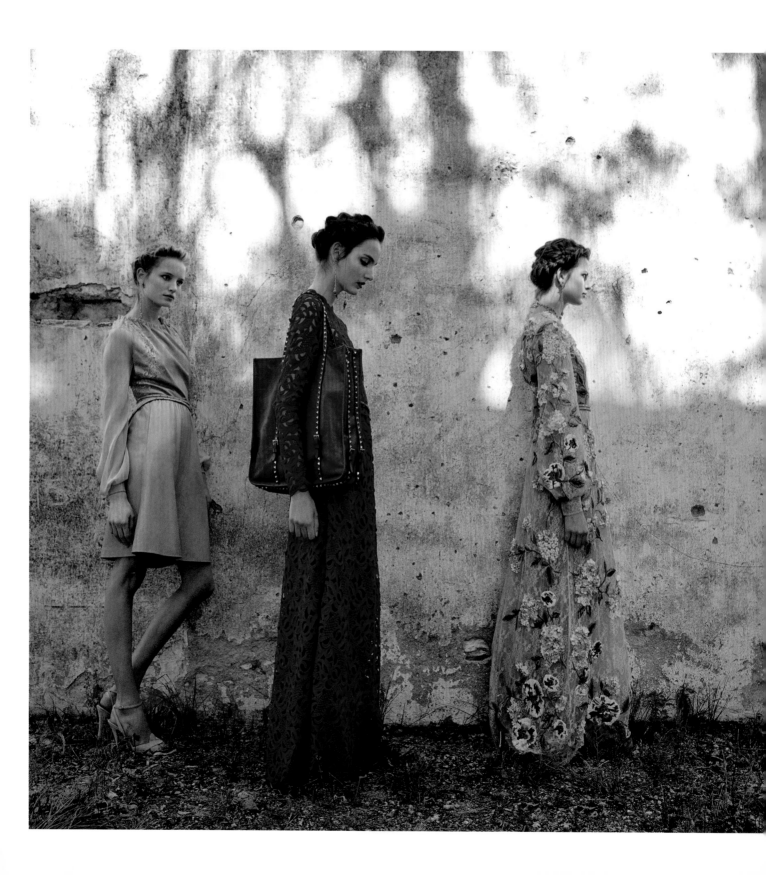

Valentino & Deborah Turbeville

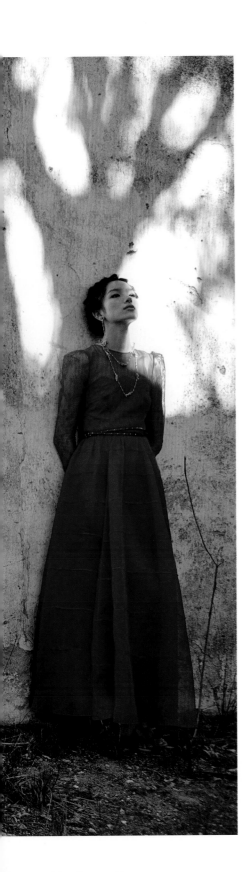

Revolutionary fashion photographer Deborah Turbeville has produced not only a considerable body of work over a career that spans nearly half a century, but also an entirely new style of photography that she continues to develop and perfect. She locates the inspiration for her distinctive artistic approach in her fashion work, rather than the other way around. 'I've developed a personal style through taking fashion photographs, and I think that I'm unique in that because most people put aside fashion when they go to shoot what they call their private work.'[10]

Turbeville's photography for fashion magazines and clients isn't conventional. She attracted the ire of some conservative readers for her groundbreaking *Bathhouse* series, which was published in *Vogue* in 1975. 'My fashion photography was [then considered] unorthodox', explains Turbeville of her early work. 'The girls weren't normal-looking fashion models and the environments were totally different to what photographers were using at the time.' Turbeville's advertising campaign for Valentino's Spring/Summer 2012 collection was designed to be 'more personal in the way the models look. They want an identity, to stand out, and for there to be a real woman behind the clothes.' The campaign was shot on location in Pozos, Mexico, in an abandoned mining town in the Guanajuato region. Valentino creative directors Maria Grazia Chiuri and Pierpaolo Piccioli described Turbeville as having a 'subversively elegant aesthetic vision', fitting well with the collection, which they aimed to capture in 'a fantasy setting for a new poetic femininity'.

Turbeville's signature style initially developed in opposition to that of her male contemporaries, most prominently Helmut Newton. 'I don't direct models in the way most photographers do, or at all,' she says. She rarely uses photography studios for sittings, and employs lighting, mist and smoke to create a sense of immobility and emotional distance. The natural palette that prevails as a result of Turbeville's avoidance of rich colour and photographic clarity adds depth and mystery to her work, further enhanced by her habit of scratching, taping and writing on negatives when shooting on film (although she increasingly uses digital photography for fashion commissions due to time constraints and the limited availability of traditional chemicals and papers). It is possible to view the mood of her work as nostalgic, but the emotional distance that Turbeville places between herself and her subjects – the result of which is a somewhat icy aesthetic – creates a sense not of nostalgia but of timelessness, of scenes without specific context, where one might discover real beauty in isolation. 'It's not as if I'm thinking specifically about a moment from the 1930s,' says Turbeville, explaining that because the magazines she works with – Italian *Vogue*, *L'Uomo Vogue* and the *New York Times Magazine* – understand her aesthetic approach 'the clothes I'm given [for the shoots] are sympathetic to my style, so generally they're things that do look a little out of their time.' Turbeville's unique aesthetic has never been successfully replicated, but it has certainly paved the way for contemporary practitioners to present more ethereal, even 'feminine' visions in fashion photography.

Valentino, Spring/Summer 2012 collection,
photographed by Deborah Turbeville.

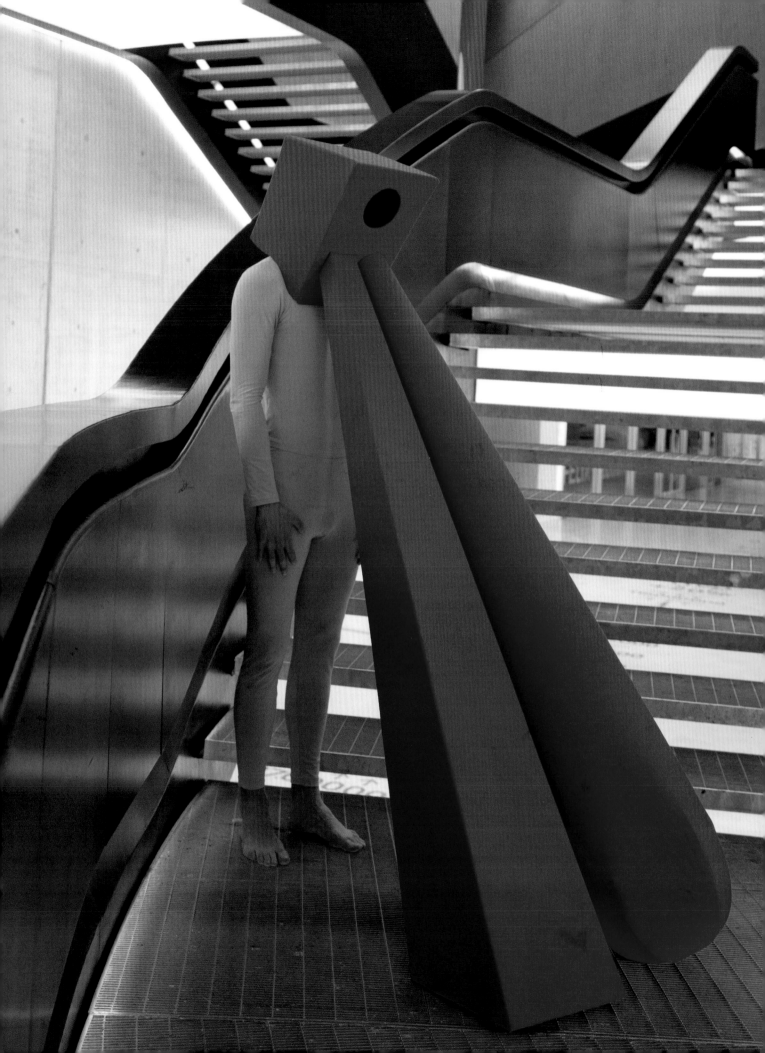

From boutique to gallery: Fashion, art and architecture

Opposite: Still from *Spirits – Fabulae Romanae*, Lucy + Jorge Orta, filmed video performance, 2012, commissioned by ZegnArt, an independent foundation of Ermenegildo Zegna.

Introduction: From boutique to gallery

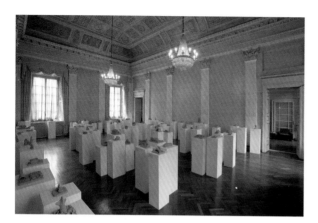

Peter Fischli and David Weiss, *Suddenly This Overview,*
ninety-two sculptures made from unfired clay, 1981–2006,
exhibited at Palazzo Litta, Milan, 2008, produced and
organized by Fondazione Nicola Trussardi in collaboration
with Tate Modern, London, and the Kunsthaus Zürich.

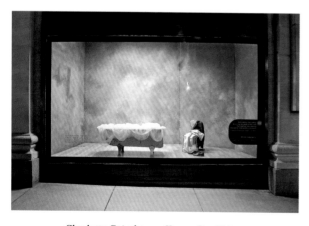

Charlotte Gainsbourg, *Heaven Can Wait,*
collaborative window installation for British department
store Selfridges 'Sounds of the Mind' campaign, 2010.

The close relationship between art and fashion is increasingly reflected in the built environment. Luxury fashion brands now regularly collaborate with award-winning architects to create unique retail stores, art museums and temporary structures to exhibit their goods. These architectural commissions are part of a wider 21st-century trend in which large luxury fashion conglomerates – most prominently LVMH (owner of Louis Vuitton, Givenchy and Christian Dior), Kering (Saint Laurent, Gucci and Balenciaga) and Richemont (Dunhill, Cartier and Montblanc) – are increasing their involvement in the art world, both financially as patrons and creatively as collaborators. Many have started their own foundations in support of the fine arts, assembling impressive art collections and building museums to house them, offering residencies and special commissions to contemporary artists, and funding and promoting innovative public art projects.

Just as fashion and art increasingly share a common audience and set of aesthetic values, so too do fashion and architecture. Design writer Bradley Quinn believes that the past decade's explosive combination of fashion, art and architecture, as exemplified by the proliferation of large-scale shopfronts and architecturally significant fashion emporiums, has deep historical roots and is an expression of the essential similarities between the two crafts. 'The relationship between fashion and architecture did not manifest itself suddenly or spectacularly; the two have been hovering on the margins of a mutual existence throughout history...The organization of space has always been the essence of both fashion and architecture; fashion's architectuality unfolds in its containment of space, while architecture continues to be fashioned by its relationship to the human form.'[1] Avant-garde designers such as Issey Miyake, Hussein Chalayan, Yohji Yamamoto and Junya Watanabe of Comme des Garçons frequently explore the architectural possibilities of fabric and the body, while major luxury fashion labels collaborate directly with leading architects and designers to produce innovative designs for retail and exhibition spaces.

Architecturally ambitious, the new fashion retail spaces are secular temples to good design and consumerism, places of worship for fashion's followers but also must-see sites for tourists. As such, they are evidence of an important change in the traditional architectural hierarchy in which retail spaces

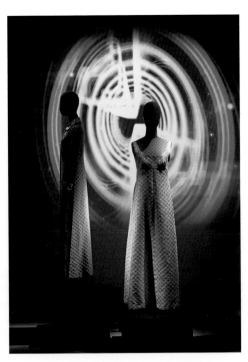

The Logomania exhibit at Gucci Museo, Florence, chronicles the evolution of the brand's double-'G' monogram.

enjoyed significantly lower status than public or civic buildings, as noted by academic Taro Igarashi: 'In architectural history, traditional structures such as temples, churches and palaces were the principal typologies since the dawn of civilization through the 19th century. With the advent of modernity, public and commercial institutions such as museums, city halls, train stations and office towers – as well as private domiciles became the locus of change, but retail design was paid scant regard.'[2] In the 21st century, however, some of the biggest international architectural projects have involved the construction of retail spaces, or offshoot projects by fashion houses (such as foundations). Fashion houses have the financial resources to hire the same high-profile architects who design landmark art museums: in New York, for example, Rem Koolhaas, who was responsible for the Guggenheim Museum in Las Vegas, designed Prada's SoHo Epicenter on the site of the now-defunct downtown New York Guggenheim Museum; and Frank Gehry, architect for the Guggenheim in Bilbao, designed Issey Miyake's Tribeca store in New York. Moreover, these fashion companies, with their private and independent funds, often have the fiscal freedom to throw caution to the wind in their pursuit of the ultimate architectural statement, knowing that an edgy, innovative and controversial design will become important creative capital for the brand. The resultant buildings would perhaps never make it through the bureaucratic red tape required of the public purse.

Paradoxically, however, the worldwide proliferation of these innovative, monumental bricks-and-mortar luxury fashion emporiums has been commensurate with the rise of online retail in the 21st century. The phenomenal success of internet-only retailers such as Net-A-Porter, ASOS and Moda Operandi has made leading fashion labels recognize the importance of establishing an online presence; yet at the same time, the established brands are conscious of their consumers' desire for a 'luxury' experience that transcends the ordinary shopping transaction. Large-scale and architecturally innovative bricks-and-mortar boutiques therefore provide an important complement to the increasingly dominant online retail sector as the public faces of digital labels; customers are drawn to these mansions of style so that they may experience a brand in way not approximated by a visit to either a website or

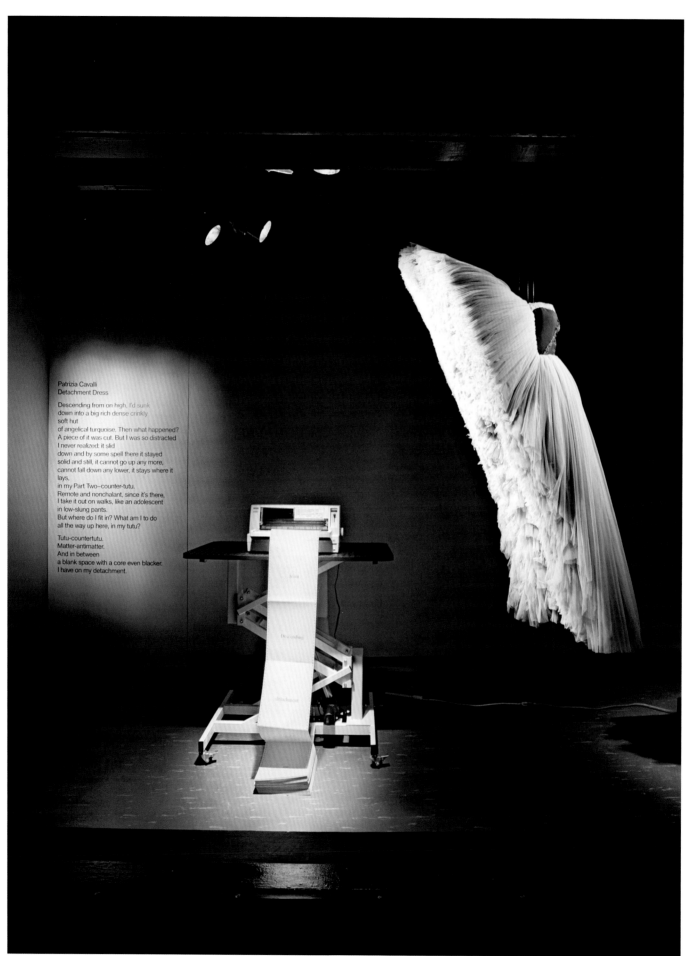

Patrizia Cavalli
Detachment Dress

Descending from on high, I'd sunk
down into a big rich dense crinkly
soft hut
of angelical turquoise. Then what happened?
A piece of it was cut. But I was so distracted
I never realized: it slid
down and by some spell there it stayed
solid and still, it cannot go up any more,
cannot fall down any lower, it stays where it
lays,
in my Part Two–counter-tutu.
Remote and nonchalant, since it's there,
I take it out on walks, like an adolescent
in low-slung pants.
But where do I fit in? What am I to do
all the way up here, in my tutu?

Tutu-countertutu.
Matter-antimatter.
And in between
a blank space with a core even blacker.
I have on my detachment.

'Art has become a central vocabulary for narratives now attached to fast-moving consumer goods, a competitive amenity, an aspect of design.'

James B. Twitchell [3]

Opposite: Poet Patrizia Cavalli's window installation for the 'destefashioncollection' project, displayed at Barneys New York in 2012, involves an ode to a dress from Viktor & Rolf's Spring/Summer 2010 collection. Cavalli's poem is displayed on the rear wall, played in audio form through speakers outside the window and continually spooled by a computer printer.

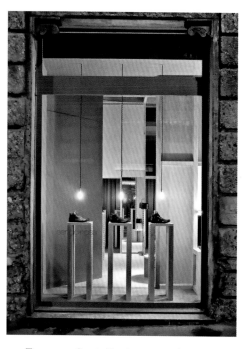

Temporary Sergio Rossi menswear boutique,
designed by architect Antonino Cardillo as part
of the Salone del Mobile, Milan, 2010, in
collaboration with *Wallpaper** magazine.

a traditional retail establishment. If you are going to spend a lot of money on clothing and accessories, it may as well be a memorable experience. Inspired by the success of the new fashion megastores, existing traditional boutiques and department stores are competing to attract customers via similar means, working with innovative architects, installation artists and art curators on a myriad of approaches that include pop-up stores, curated retail spaces and unique store windows that, according to cultural critics Gilles Lipovetsky and Veronica Manlow, 'have become canvases for avant-garde artists'.[4] In these newly art-informed retail spaces, 'Inaugurations are now performances. Original works are commissioned from contemporary designers and artists and displayed in the stores. This is a period for mixing genres and for hybridizing art and fashion.'[5]

As traditional art museums and galleries increasingly engage with the fashion world via blockbuster surveys of visionary designers, several of the industry's leading economic powers, including Prada, Louis Vuitton, Hermès and Cartier, have begun investing in and supporting the fine arts through the establishment of their own art foundations dedicated to the collecting and presentation of contemporary art. Many of these not-for-profit foundations are housed in buildings designed by well-known architects, boasting highly regarded, significant international contemporary art collections. These foundations are often informed by a fashion designer or CEO's personal artistic interests. Miuccia Prada, for example, established Fondazione Prada with her husband (and Prada CEO), Patrizio Bertelli, in 1993, two years later employing Guggenheim Museum senior curator Germano Celant as artistic director. Fondazione Prada now operates across two spectacularly Koolhaas-designed sites in Milan and Venice, hosting and developing offsite and independent projects with artists such as Anish Kapoor, Damien Hirst and Jeff Koons. Meanwhile, head of aforementioned Kering, François Pinault, is one of the world's most powerful art collectors. The François Pinault Foundation in Venice shows work from his extensive collection as well as standalone exhibitions curated by a team of professional art staff, and operates across two historically important sites. These major foundations have a reputation for staging exhibitions on a scale that rivals that of public institutions and, importantly, retain critical autonomy and engage leading international curators

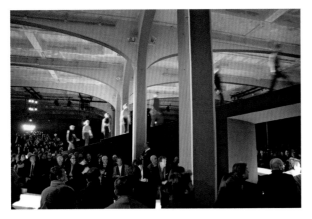

Show space at the Fondazione Prada in Milan, which is
redesigned for each season's runway presentation
by architect Rem Koolhaas's firm AMO.

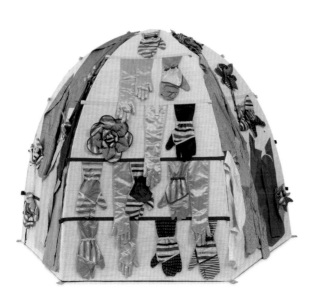

Dome Dwelling, Lucy + Jorge Orta, 2012, a commission
for ZegnArt incorporating Zegna fabric.

and consultants. Many of the foundations sponsor art prizes, a practice also embraced on its own by some luxury brands in the absence of a foundation, as with the Max Mara Art Prize for Women, the Bulgari Art Award, the Hugo Boss Prize and the Furla Art Award.

As fashion houses build these foundations, museums and architecturally significant retail spaces, the traditional division between store and museum is fast disappearing. As advertising critic and cultural historian James B. Twitchell explains, 'The modern department store and the art museum are now joined at the hip...They are all about vaunting things, branding things...We gaze at the framed object and floodlit *objets d'art* behind glass. We gawk at the decorated and elegant mannequin in the store window. We peer at the label beneath the painting just as we inspect the label on the object. We need to know provenance, the brand, *s'il vous plaît*, before we can consume.'[6] Twitchell sees this growing lack of distinction between museum and retail store as a result of specific cultural changes that began in the 1960s, when 'as our culture started moving from a gatekeeper to a ticket-taker culture, from a custodial culture to an entertainment culture, the museum was forced to compete for what became the modern patron, the shopping tourist. At the same time, the high-end retail marketplace was making its way uptown toward the museum, bringing with it the complementary form, the touring shopper.'[7]

An architecturally innovative retail store commissioned by a luxury house not only gives the fashion items offered for sale a perceived value akin to that of fine art displayed in a museum, but also becomes part of the brand's own identity, associating the label with cutting-edge architecture and reinforcing the sense of artistic 'authenticity' that its consumers crave. Meanwhile, the gallery shop has become an essential revenue stream for traditional art museums and galleries, offering the opportunity to take home a small piece of art at a more affordable price point. Like 21st-century Medicis, the fashion houses promote their brands and extend their influence by amassing significant international contemporary art collections and supporting the arts via foundations, museums, exhibitions and special commissions. With all these developments, Andy Warhol's famous prediction that 'All department stores will become museums, and all museums will become department stores' seems to be coming true in the new millennium.[8]

Sergio Rossi
& Antonino Cardillo

As part of the 2010 Salone del Mobile in Milan, the annual international design fair, Sicilian architect Antonino Cardillo was engaged to create a temporary men's boutique for Italian footwear maker Sergio Rossi at the initiative of design magazine *Wallpaper**. The ephemeral shop, built within the brand's permanent store in Milan, remained open for two seasons before embarking on a world tour to promote the Sergio Rossi men's collection. Each stage of the tour was marked by a unique store configuration, such as in the Galeries Lafayette Casablanca in Morocco, where Sergio Rossi commissioned local firm Younes Duret Design to create a three-dimensional shelving system in which to display the footwear.

Cardillo's design centred on the concept of superimposition, the insertion of one building into another, a recurring theme in architecture of the past, seen, for instance, in the medieval schola cantorum of the Basilica di Santa Maria in Cosmedin in Rome, and in the miniature replica Holy Sepulchre that the 15th-century architect Leon Battista Alberti installed in the Tempietto in Florence. For the first incarnation of his temporary structure in the Sergio Rossi boutique in Milan, Cardillo made use of the existing store space, articulated by a grille of exposed wooden beams to create a rhythmic sequence of vertical planes suggestive of cathedral vaulting, employing light grey tones and velvet curtains in the decor. A marriage of the sacred and profane, the design was intended both to augment and disrupt the reverence with which fashion products are presented and viewed in shops. The shoes themselves were displayed sparingly on tall plinths, lit theatrically with downlighting, emphasizing the museum-like quality of the space and bringing additional gravitas to the shopping experience.

Opposite and pages 256–57: Temporary Sergio Rossi menswear boutique, designed by architect Antonino Cardillo as part of the Salone del Mobile, Milan, 2010, in collaboration with *Wallpaper** magazine.

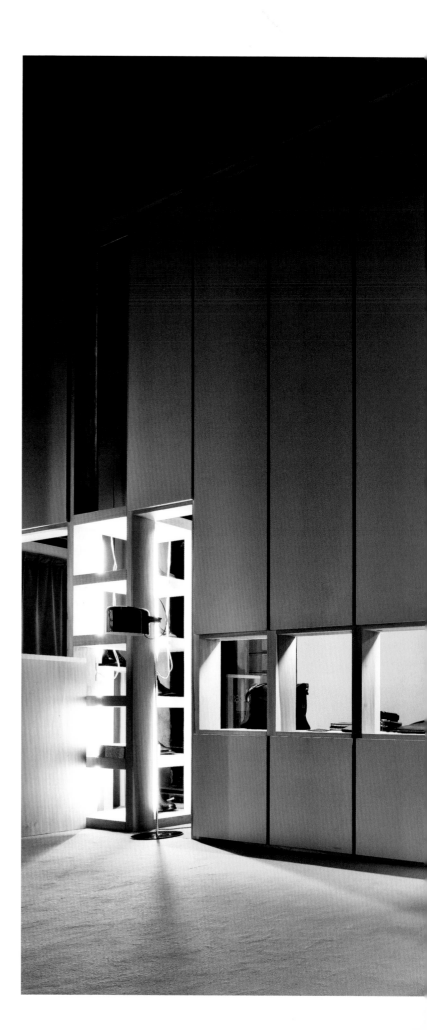

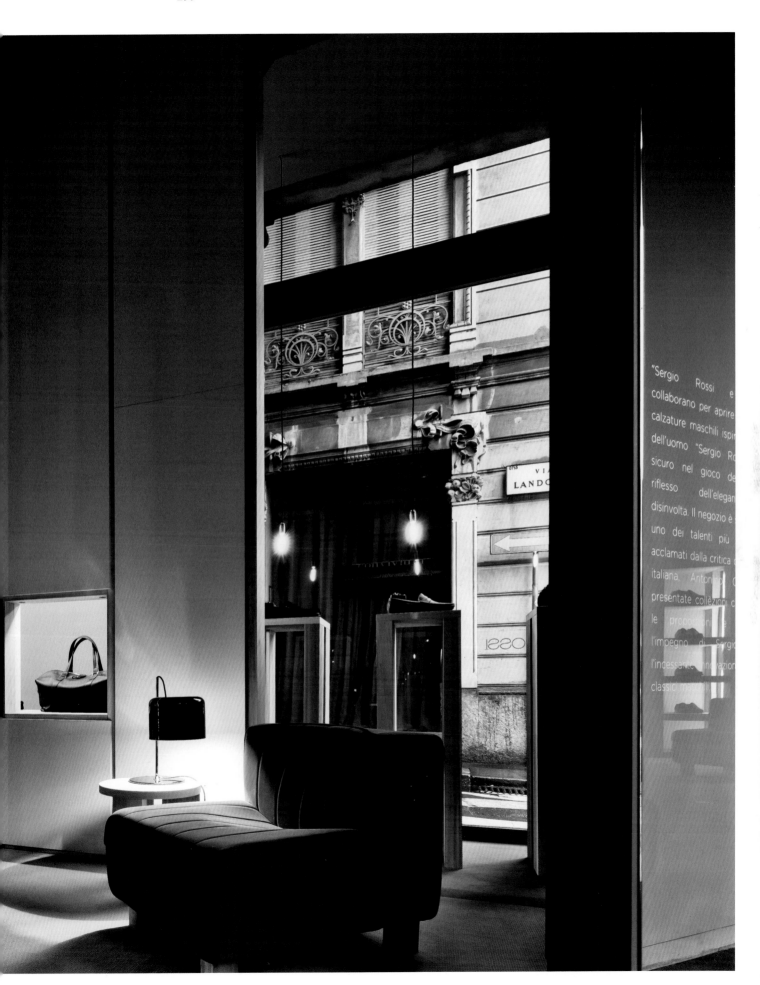

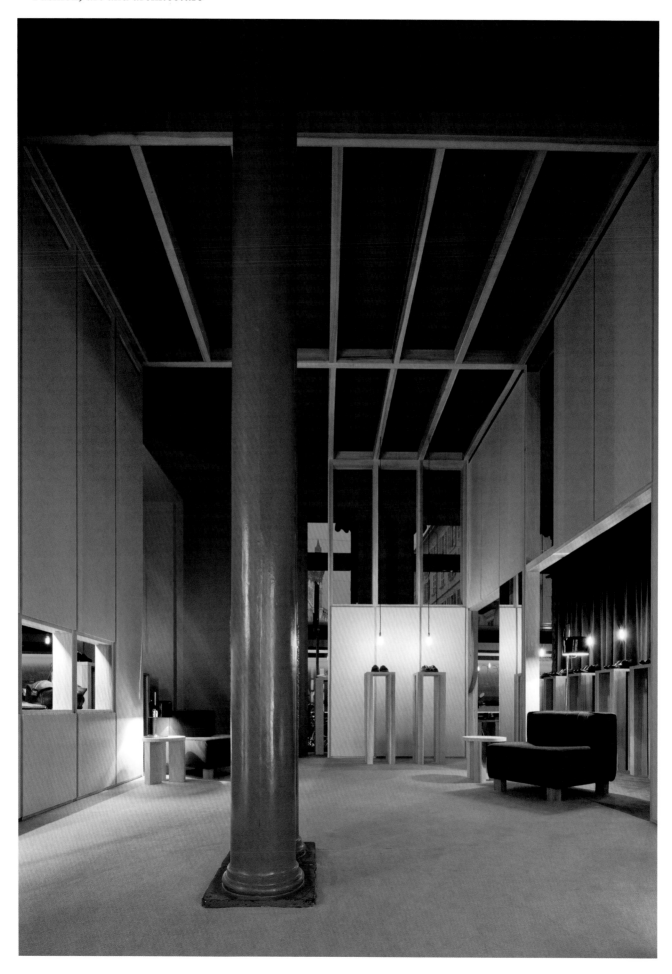

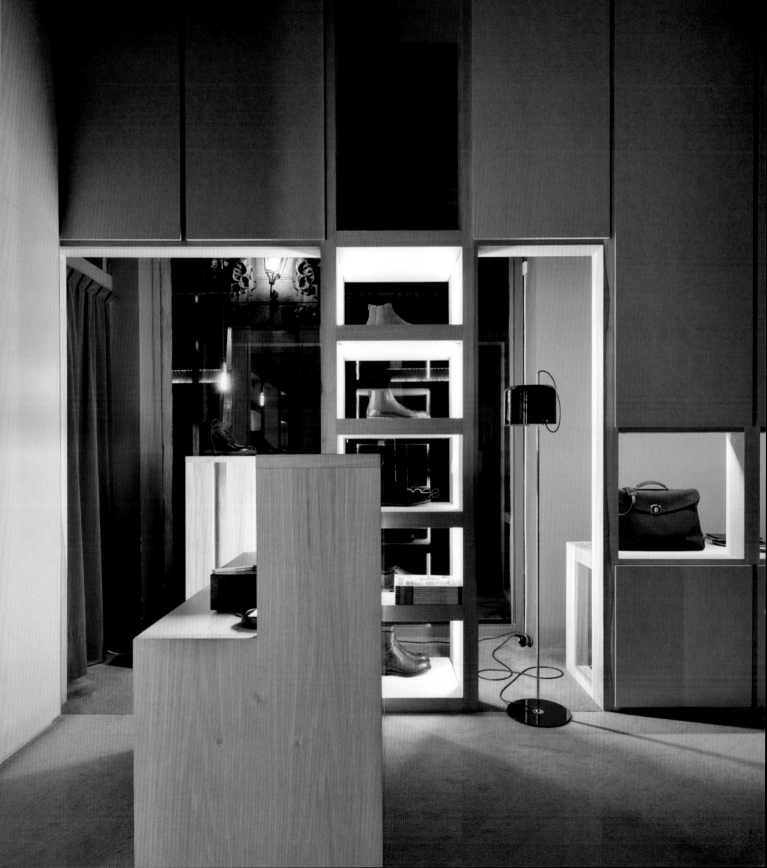

Bless Shops

Below: Bless Number 45, installation at the Arnhem Mode
Biennale, 2011, showcasing the label's *Metalstringcurtain*.
Opposite and overleaf: Bless Shop Home, Berlin.

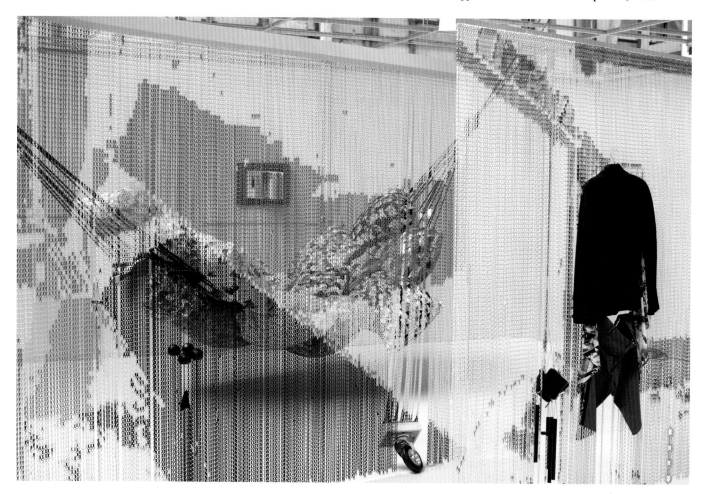

Given the inherently artistic nature of Bless, the avant-garde design and clothing company founded by Parisian Desirée Heiss and Berliner Ines Kaag in 1996, it seems natural that the label should receive regular invitations to participate in art exhibitions. The designers have mixed feelings about showing their work in an artistic setting, however: 'From our fashion point of view, it's irrelevant to show old products over and over again, since they were created for the present moment and not with an exhibition in mind.'[9] In 2000, in response to the constant invitations to exhibit, they launched Bless Shops, combined temporary retail shops and installation pieces that could be set up in museum spaces. Heiss and Kaag have since created close to twenty-five such pop-up stores in cities including Beijing, Berlin, Paris, New York, Brussels, Tokyo and Toronto. Each incorporates site-specific installations and modes of clothing presentation that challenge the traditional retail institution. For the Festival International des Arts de la Mode in Hyères in 2000, for instance, the Bless Shop comprised a series of tables installed in three rooms; products were displayed alongside press clippings about them. In Amsterdam, in 2001, the designers entirely covered the window of the vacant boutique in which the Bless Shop was installed, leaving the interior completely empty. At the Werkleitz Biennale in 2000, Bless products were arranged and sold in shops throughout the host city – a hairdressing salon for the hairbrush and fur wig; a shoe shop for the Bootsocks and customizable footwear; a furniture shop for the 'chairwear' – with the intent of bringing the Biennale audience into 'direct confrontation with the economic reality of a region devastated by unemployment'.[10]

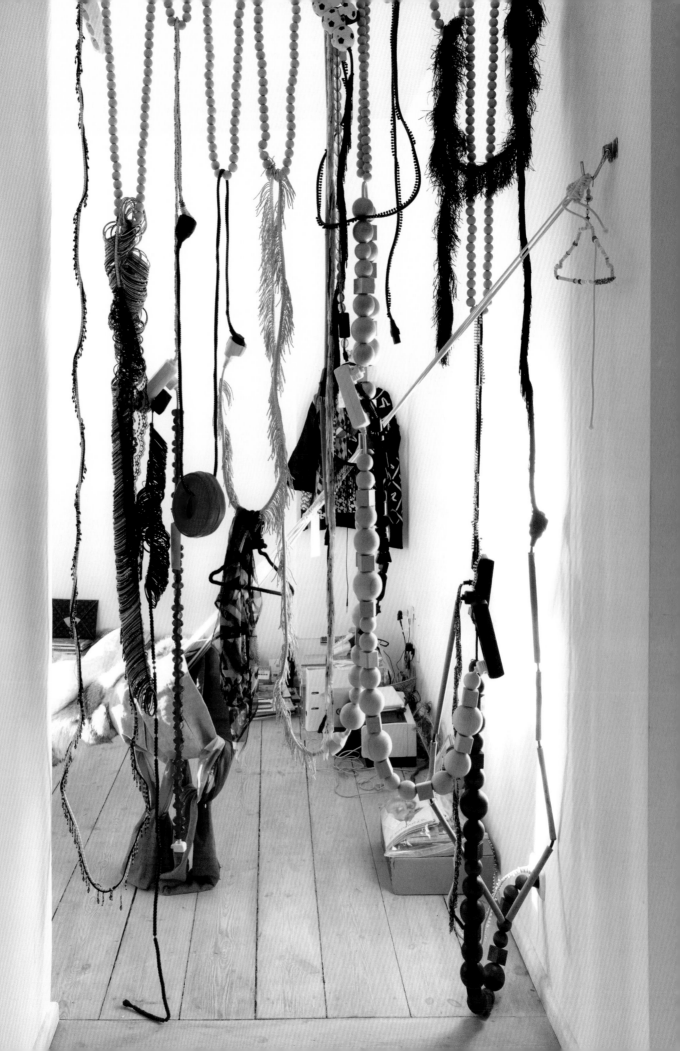

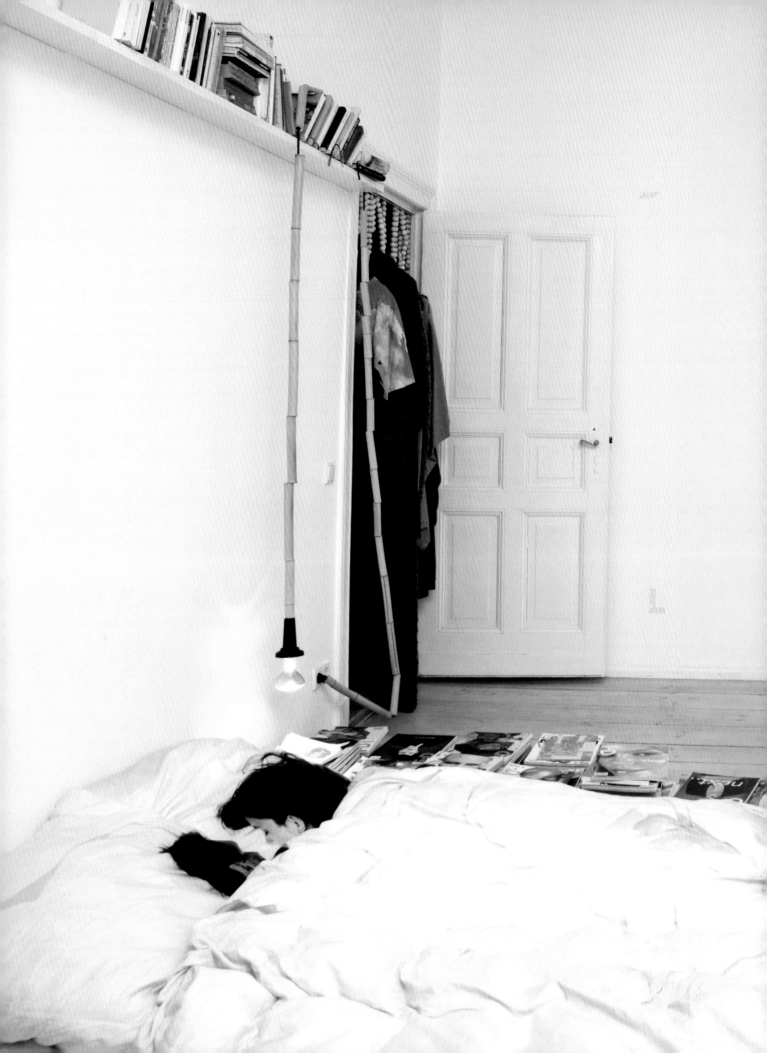

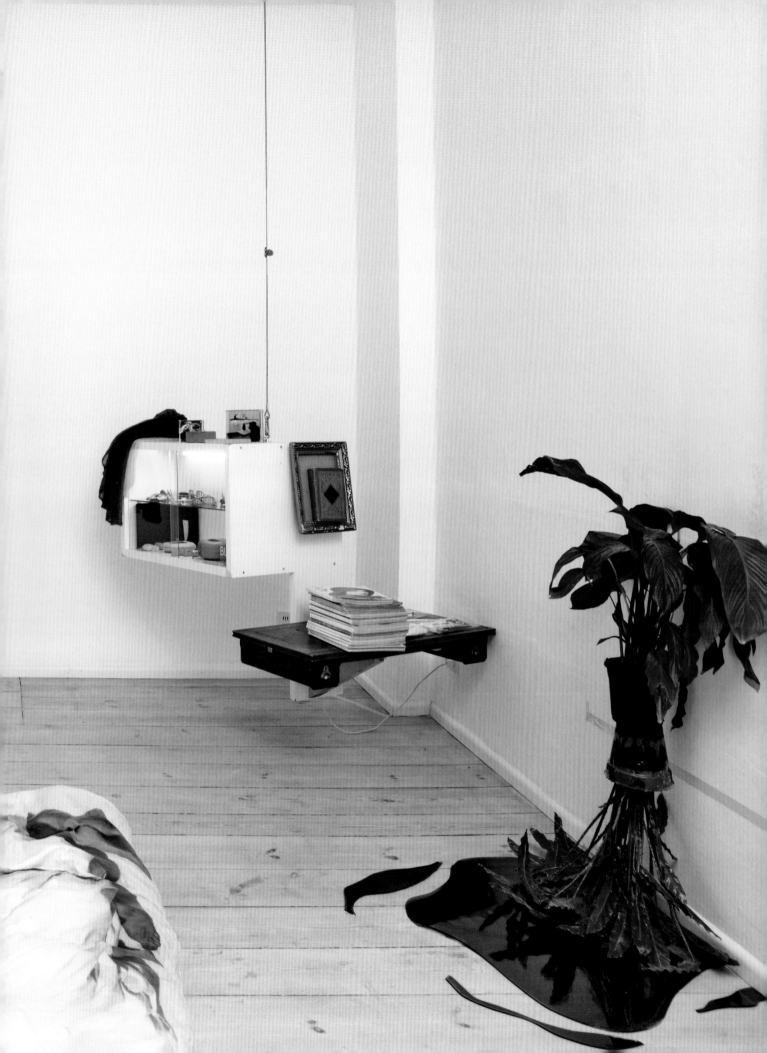

Louis Vuitton store design

The standalone boutiques of Louis Vuitton have revolutionized store design in the 21st century with their seamless fusion of fashion, art and architecture. Armed with the financial resources to employ the world's most respected architects, the historic French luxury brand has led the way as the fashion industry begins to overturn traditional notions of the shop floor, ushering in an era in which, according to Harvard University professor Mohsen Mostafavi, 'the luxury retail store has become a crucial forum for architecture,' a development he credits in large part to Louis Vuitton.[11] 'Through the realization of numerous projects, the architecture department at Louis Vuitton has been involved in establishing this new territory, and continues to pursue the exploration of architecture in a continually changing present.'[12]

The monograph *Louis Vuitton: Architecture & Interiors* (2011) displays the sheer breadth of the house's architectural collaborations, which have involved leading practitioners such as Peter Marino, Eric Carlson and Jun Aoki. Often Louis Vuitton works with local architects, for instance in Japan, where five of its six stores were designed by Aoki. What defines Louis Vuitton's stores, beyond their sheer size, however, is their incorporation of the label's innovative multimedia branding operations, which in a single store can include animation and video displays, temporary art installations and semi-permanent exhibitions. The development of digital manufacturing technology over the past fifteen years has made possible the incorporation of figuration and ornamentation into the structure at the inception of the building's design. Given that Louis Vuitton has been using its signature *damier* pattern since the 1870s to mark its goods as authentic, it makes

sense that all-encompassing branding should be so intrinsic to the house's architectural productions as well, with its logo and *damier* pattern embossed on the walls of some of its flagship stores.

Louis Vuitton regularly uses this comprehensive multimedia branding to transform its stores to promote its collaborations with contemporary artists. For the release of its Takashi Murakami collaborative products in 2002, store exteriors were covered in large reproductions of the artist's brightly coloured reinventions of the 'LV' monogram, while their interiors featured installations of his large 'plushie' toy sculptures. In 2012, coinciding with the release of its collaborative line with Yayoi Kusama, the house set up six global pop-up stores stocked exclusively with the accessories and ready-to-wear goods decorated with the artist's signature dot patterns, while its existing store windows were given over to major installations of dot-patterned tentacles and miniature dolls of the artist, eschewing any display of the products themselves; the exterior façade of Louis Vuitton's Fifth Avenue store was covered in dots to coincide with the artist's retrospective at the Whitney Museum in July of 2012.

Opposite and overleaf: Interior views of the Peter Marino-designed Louis Vuitton Maison, Rome.

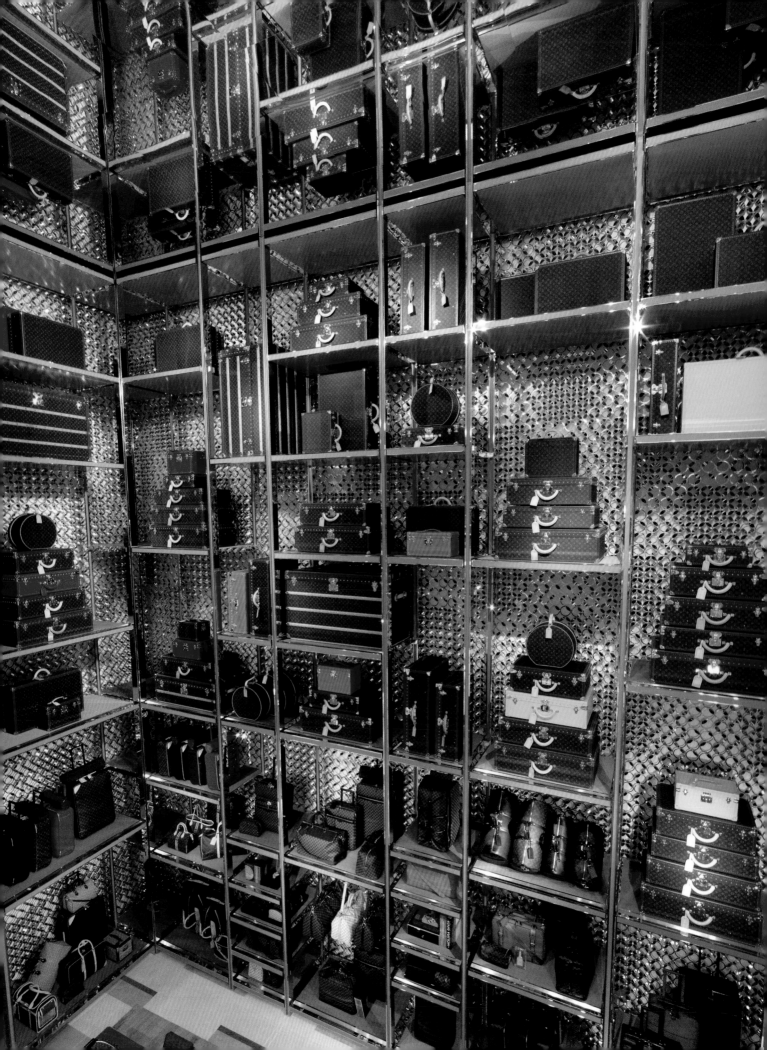

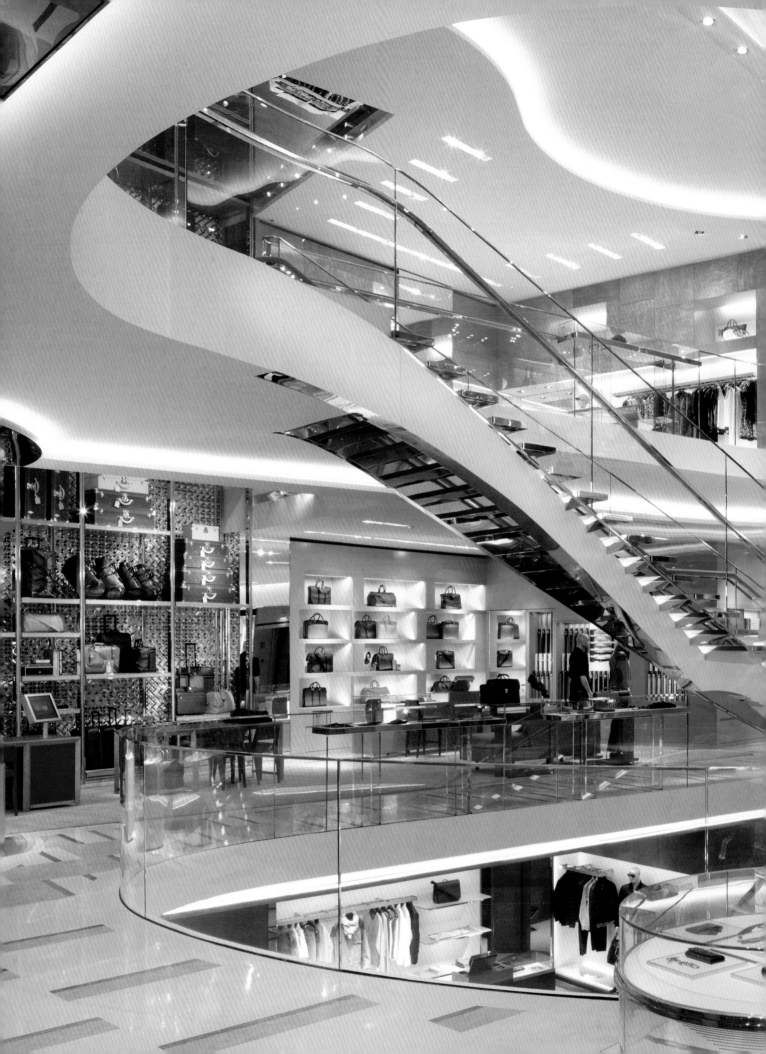

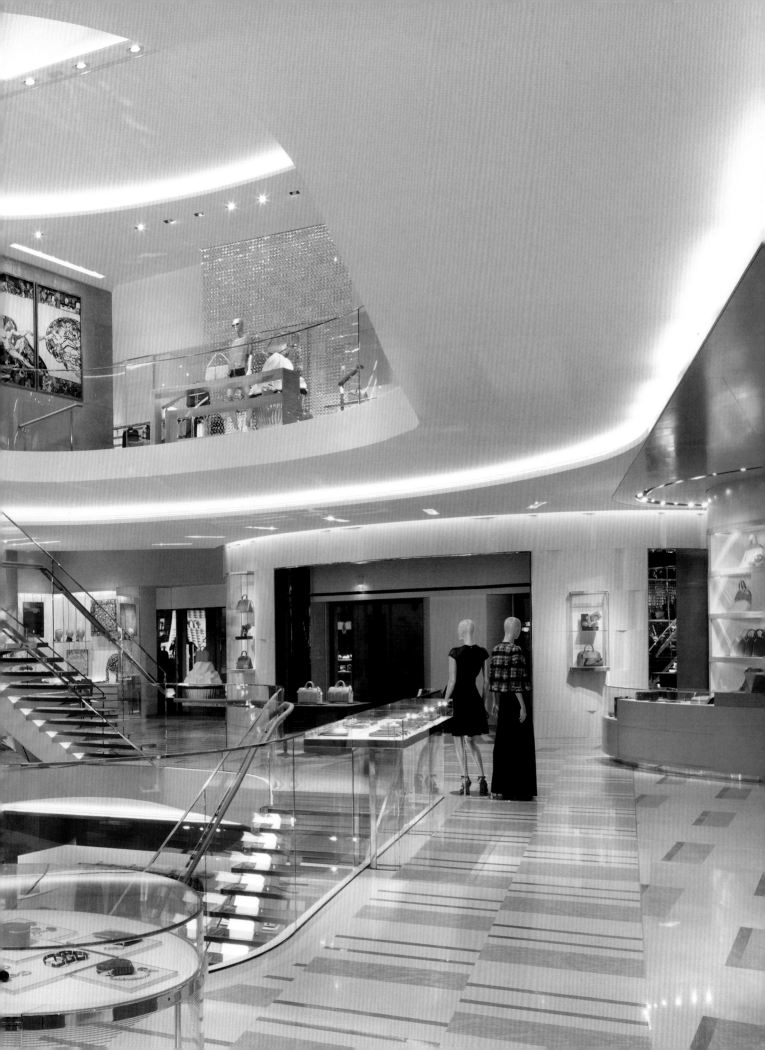

Fondation Louis Vuitton
pour la création

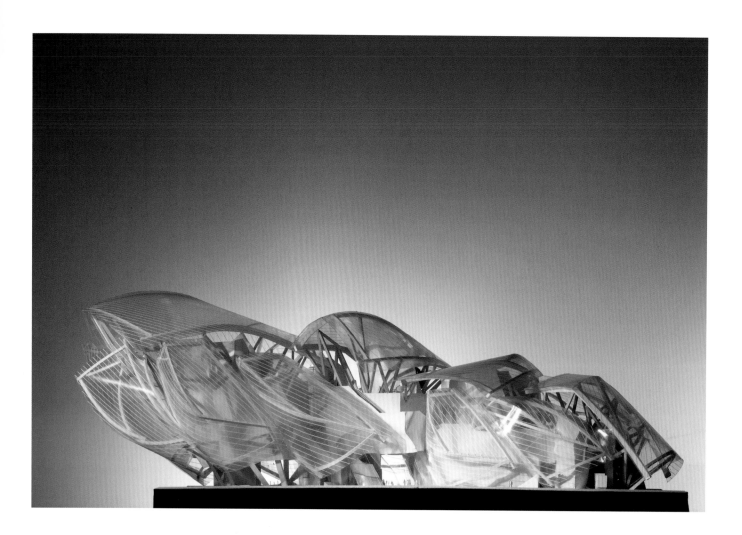

Above: A three-dimensional model of architect
Frank Gehry's design for the Fondation Louis Vuitton
pour la création in Paris.

'The museum has to invite young people playing in the park to come inside...and say "Hey! I wanna go there".'

Frank Gehry

Louis Vuitton views its extensive involvement with the visual arts as patronage. Creative director Marc Jacobs famously initiated a long-running programme of high-profile collaborations involving contemporary artists (see pages 122–29 and 224–27), but Louis Vuitton also engages with the art world in a number of other ways. In 2006, the company inaugurated an exhibition venue on the seventh floor of its Paris headquarters on the Champs-Élysées with a presentation of previously unseen photographs and videos by Vanessa Beecroft.

Louis Vuitton has further cemented its connection to the art world through the creation of an ambitious contemporary arts space in Paris, the Fondation Louis Vuitton pour la création. The building is a contemporary architectural icon in its own right, designed by renowned Pritzker Prize-winning architect Frank Gehry, whose previous commissions include the Guggenheim Museum in Bilbao, Spain. According to Bernard Arnault, chairman and CEO of Louis Vuitton's parent company LVMH, the goal of the Fondation Louis Vuitton pour la création is to 'introduce the widest possible audience to 20th- and 21st-century art,' through exhibitions of works of the period's great masters.[13] The hope of engaging the younger generation in particular encouraged LVMH to select the site near the Jardin d'Acclimatation, a leisure garden for families that welcomes approximately 1.5 million visitors a year, as the location for the museum. As Gehry explains, 'The museum has to invite young people playing in the park to come inside...and say "Hey! I wanna go there".' Gehry took inspiration for the building's physical design from the surrounding environment as well. 'Since the site is located between the Bois de Boulogne and the Jardin d'Acclimatation, it became obvious that a glass conservatory would make the most sense,' explained Gehry of the transparent structure, which also integrates a number of roof garden terraces that echo the parks' green spaces. Gehry describes the planned building as both playful and serious, in accord with the contemporary brand values of Louis Vuitton. When complete, it will be used to display artwork from the foundation's permanent collection as well as temporary exhibitions.

Montblanc: Cutting Edge Art Collection & Art Bags

Montblanc, the German-based purveyor of fine writing instruments, timepieces and jewelry, cannot constantly reinvent its offerings in the manner of historic luxury clothing and accessories brands such as Louis Vuitton, Hermès or Gucci. The market for Montblanc's specific products is more conservative than that of the wider accessories industry, so aesthetic change can only be introduced very slowly. As a historic company established in 1906, however, Montblanc has had to find other ways to appeal to a new generation of consumers, and patronage of contemporary art has been an important part of its strategy to accomplish this.

Since the start of the millennium, Montblanc has amassed an impressive permanent collection of contemporary art known as the Cutting Edge Art Collection. The collection, originally developed by Ingrid Roosen-Trinks, director of the Montblanc Cultural Foundation, now comprises over 160 works by artists including Thomas Demand, Liam Gillick, Sylvie Fleury, Jorge Pardo and Fang Lijun, and is accessible to the public on guided tours of the company headquarters in Hamburg, Germany. In addition, the Montblanc Young Artist World Patronage programme, established in 2005, commissions emerging artists to interpret the brand's star logo. Reproductions of these artworks are then displayed in Montblanc's stores throughout the world, giving the artists visibility with a broad international audience. This project was later expanded to include commissions from renowned Chinese contemporary artists, including Fang Lijun, Qin Yufen and Zhu Jinshi, reflecting the economic importance of China in the international luxury-goods market.

One of the brand's most high-profile contemporary art projects was its Montblanc Art Bags. To celebrate the opening of Montblanc's flagship store on the Champs-Élysées in Paris, artists Jean-Marc Bustamante, Sylvie Fleury, Gary Hume, David LaChapelle, Sam Taylor-Johnson and Anne and Patrick Poirier were each commissioned to decorate 3-metre (10-foot) aluminium shopping bag installations, incorporating the Montblanc star logo. The bags were later displayed around the world at art events and in front of Montblanc stores. In 2011, Montblanc added a seventh shopping-bag sculpture by Marcel van Eeden. On the occasion of its art collection's tenth anniversary in 2012 the company presented a new commission, *Montblanc Target Orange*, consisting of thirty-one drawings by artist duo Eva & Adele, as well as three new art bags by Chinese artists Zou Cao, Ma Jun and Huang Min.

Opposite: *Amanda as Marilyn*, 2003, designed by David LaChapelle for the Montblanc Art Bags project. The 3-metre (10-foot) aluminium bag depicts transgender model Amanda Lepore styled as Marilyn Monroe.

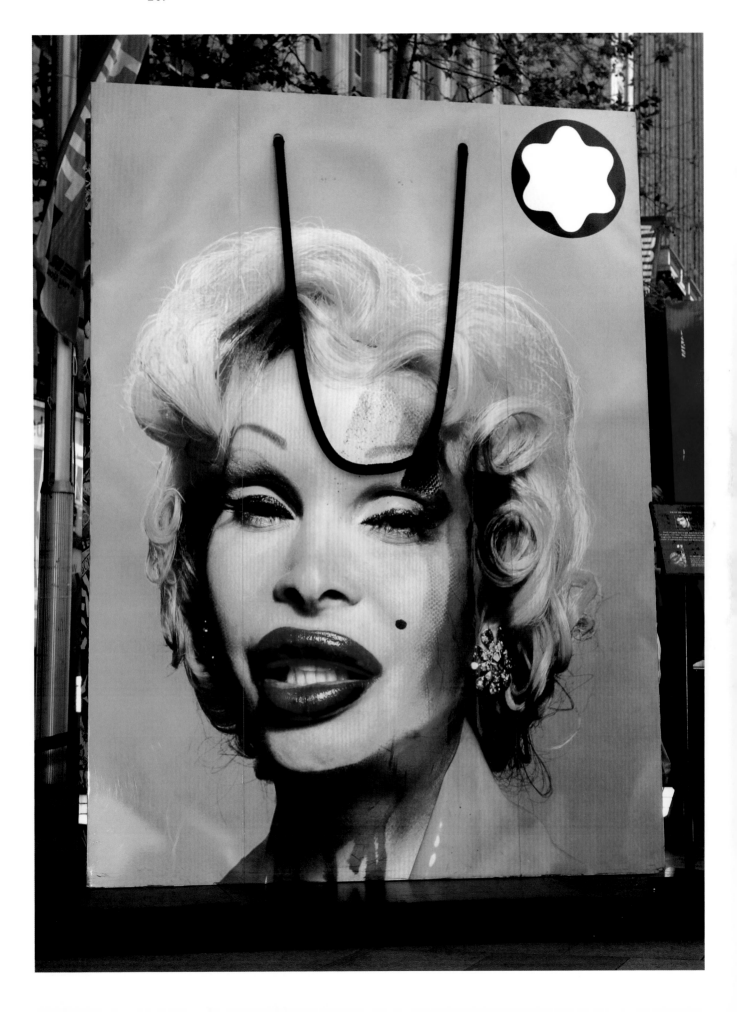

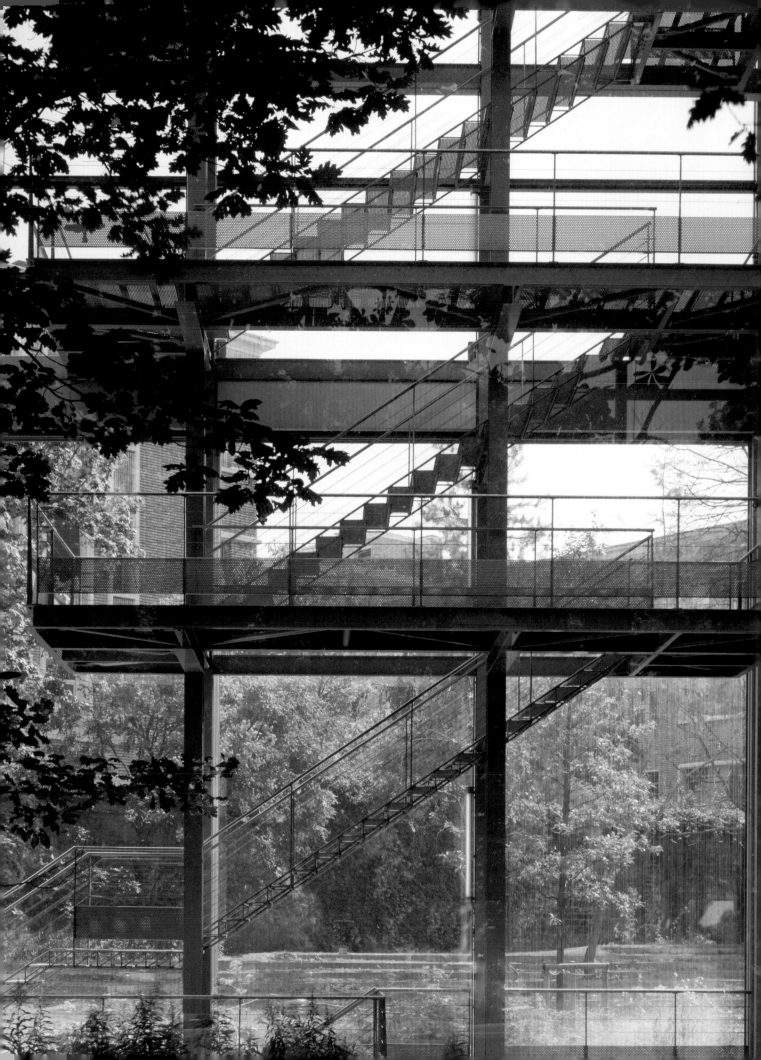

Fondation Cartier pour l'art contemporain

Housed within a striking, semi-transparent glass building designed by Pritzker Prize-winning architect Jean Nouvel and surrounded by wildflower gardens, the Fondation Cartier pour l'art contemporain was inaugurated in 1994 and is now one of the best-loved museums in Paris. The project, initiated in the 1980s by Alain-Dominique Perrin, then head of French jewelry house Cartier, at the suggestion of French artist César Baldaccini, represents corporate philanthropy on a most elegant scale. The foundation is dedicated to promoting contemporary arts across a wide range of genres and media, and boasts a collection that is regularly borrowed by other institutions. Importantly, the foundation supports the creation of new work, sponsoring residencies and commissioning pieces from artists such as Cai Guo-Qiang and Tatsuo Miyajima. Its Nomadic Nights programme focuses on the performing arts with a view to exploring links with other art forms.

The Fondation Cartier includes fashion within its curatorial remit, staging an important survey of Issey Miyake's work in 1998, 'Issey Miyake: Making Things', which featured Miyake's collaborations with Yasumasa Morimura and Cai Guo-Qiang, and in 2004 invited designer Jean Paul Gaultier to create an exhibition. The resulting 'Pain Couture' was a witty take on the grand French traditions of both couture and cuisine, featuring an installation of dresses designed by Gaultier, including his infamous conical corsets, made from bread. The dresses were outrageous; the entire show a delicious folly that evoked Marie Antoinette's famously misquoted 'Let them eat cake'.

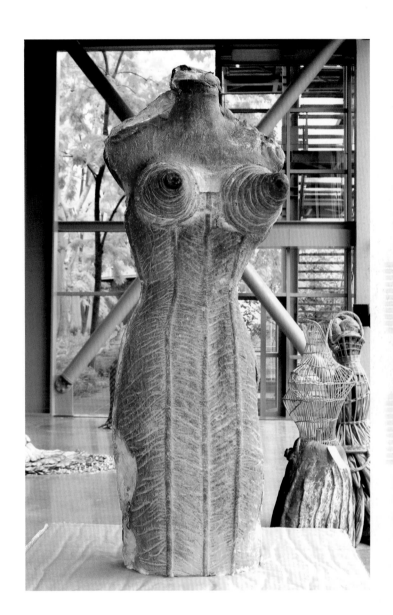

Above: Installation view of 'Pain Couture', 2004, an exhibition of the work of Jean Paul Gaultier for which the designer reproduced his signature pieces, including corsetry, in bread.
Opposite: External façade of the Fondation Cartier pour l'art contemporain, Paris, designed by architect Jean Nouvel.

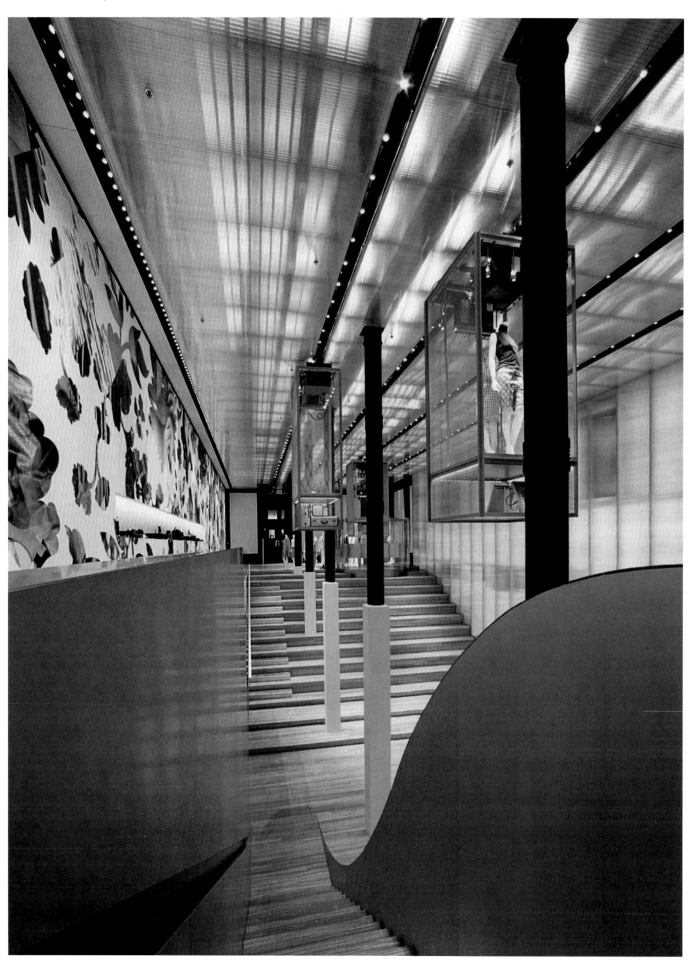

Prada store design

Prada's interest in avant-garde architectural design is one of its defining aspects as a company and has inspired the creation of an entirely new kind of retail store. The two studios of Rotterdam-based architect Rem Koolhaas, OMA (Office for Metropolitan Architecture) and AMO (Architecture for Metropolitan Office), worked with Prada to design its first $30 million (USD) Epicenter store in New York in 2001, followed by similar stores in Los Angeles and San Francisco. AMO is also responsible for the design of the show spaces for Prada's menswear and womenswear collections at Milan Fashion Week; this usually involves adapting the expansive Fondazione Prada space (see pages 278–79), a converted factory adjoining the company headquarters.

Prada's Epicenters offer a unique combination of retail and cultural space. The New York Epicenter, on the site of the now-defunct downtown Guggenheim Museum, for instance, has a space dedicated to temporary art installations; it features a deep timber staircase that is mirrored by a heavily sloped, skate-ramp-like wall. On the other side of the world, Prada engaged Swiss architecture firm Herzog & de Meuron to design an Epicenter in Tokyo's Aoyama district. The resultant building – a six-storey standalone structure whose walls are made of panes of glass arranged in a diagonal grid – stands out as one of the most distinctive buildings in the area, and houses retail space, storage and offices. Fondazione Prada director Germano Celant sees the building as an attempt 'to go beyond the form in order to project itself toward a dimension that does not yet exist.'[14]

Opposite: Prada's New York Epicenter features motorized display cages that hang from the ceiling.
Below: Temporary wallpaper created by design studio 2×4 covers a 60-metre (197-foot) wall at the New York Epicenter.

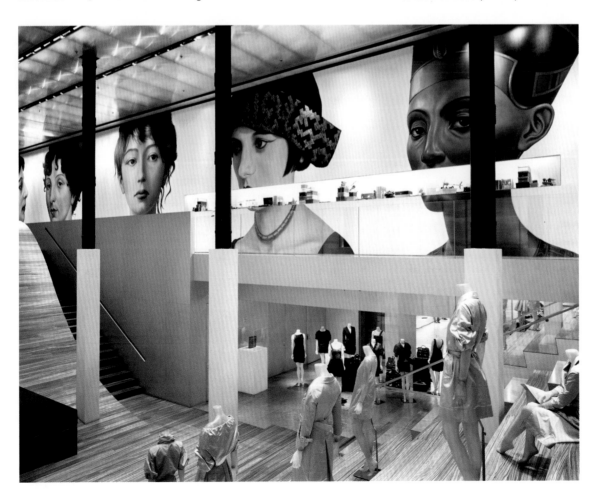

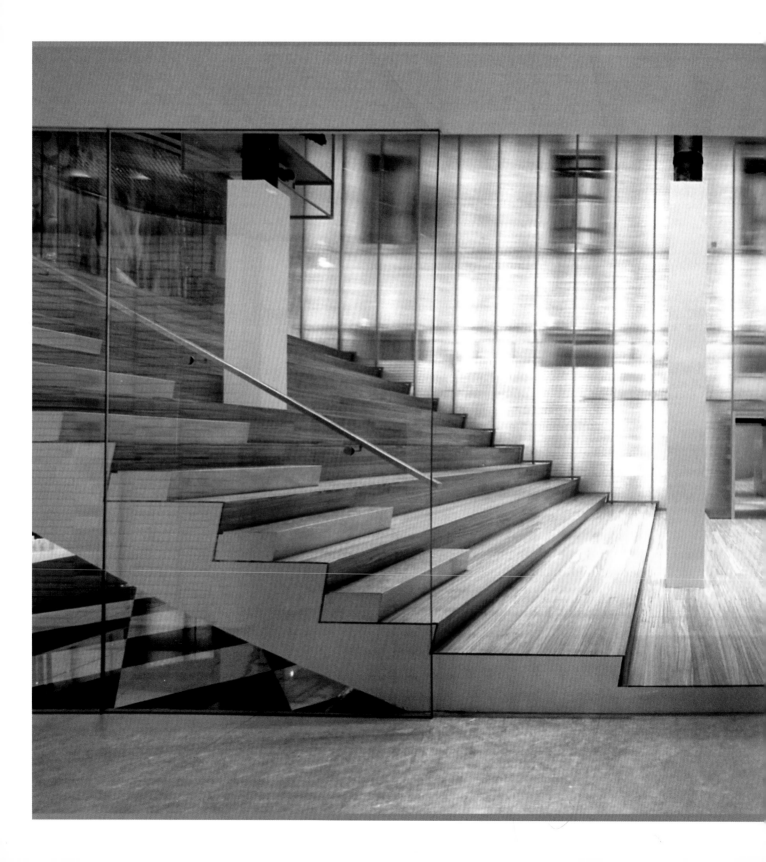

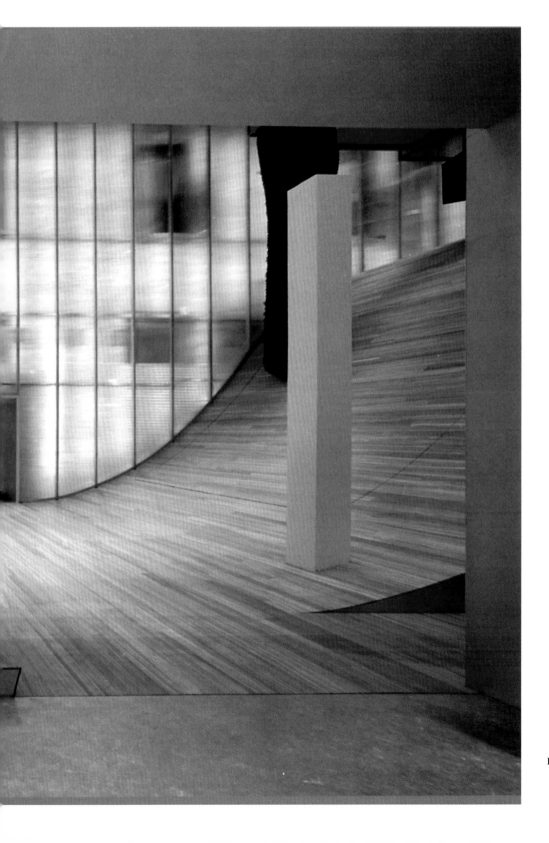

Prada's New York Epicenter, designed by
Rem Koolhaas of OMA/AMO, features
a zebrawood 'wave' that undulates from
street level to the floor below.

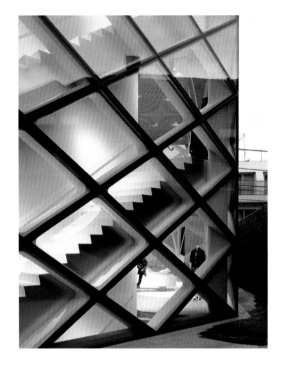

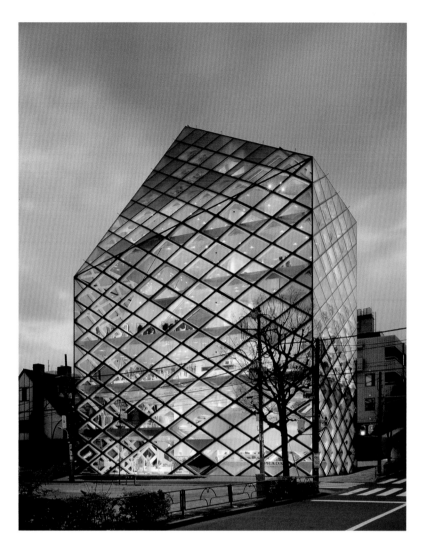

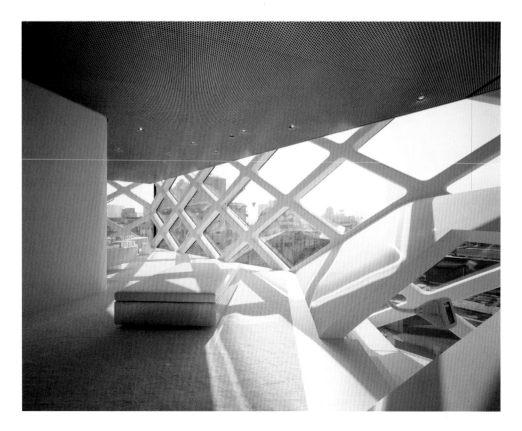

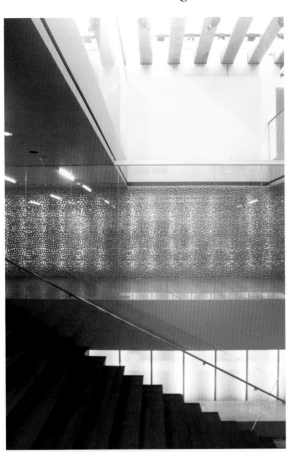

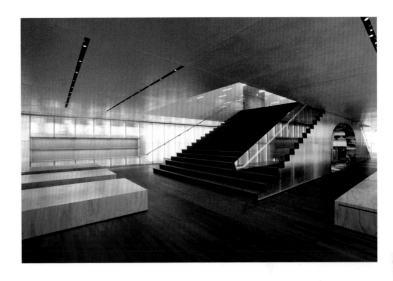

Opposite: Prada's six-storey standalone Epicenter in Tokyo, designed by Swiss architects Herzog & de Meuron.
This page: Prada's Los Angeles Epicenter, designed by Rem Koolhaas of OMA/AMO, features an unobstructed storefront (bottom) with an air curtain to maintain climate control and display windows submerged below the pavement.

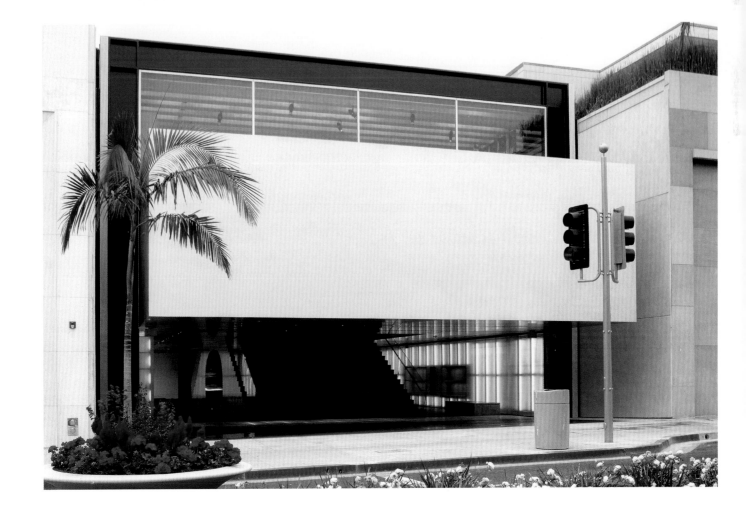

Fondazione Prada

Designer Miuccia Prada and her husband, Prada CEO Patrizio Bertelli, established the Fondazione Prada in Milan in 1993 as a non-profit organization to support contemporary art. Two years later internationally respected curator and art historian Germano Celant became its director. Under his guidance the foundation has grown in size and critical reputation, and has widened its remit to include sponsorship of projects in architecture, design and film, and even in the sciences. One of the most exquisite early projects supported by the foundation (in conjunction with the Dia Art Foundation) was the permanent large-scale fluorescent-light installation in the church of Santa Maria in Chiesa Rossa, Milan, in 1997. The work had been created by American minimalist artist and sculptor Dan Flavin shortly before his death in November 1996.

The foundation's original exhibition space in Milan hosts ambitious shows of major contemporary artists, and in 2011 an additional space opened in Venice, in the heritage-listed Ca'Corner della Regina on the Grand Canal. The renovation of the building was overseen by Dutch architect Rem Koolhaas, a longtime Prada collaborator. The inaugural exhibition at the new site included work from both the foundation's own permanent collection and other major international collections, with monumental sculptures by Anish Kapoor, Michael Heizer and Jeff Koons displayed alongside important works by Walter De Maria, John Baldessari, Charles Ray, Damien Hirst, Louise Bourgeois, Blinky Palermo, Bruce Nauman, Pino Pascali, Donald Judd, Francesco Vezzoli and Maurizio Cattelan.

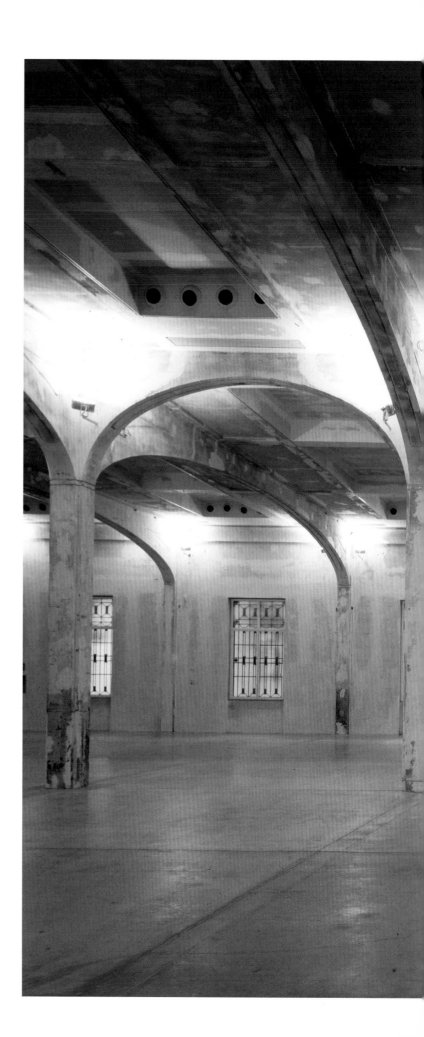

Fondazione Prada's permanent site in Milan.

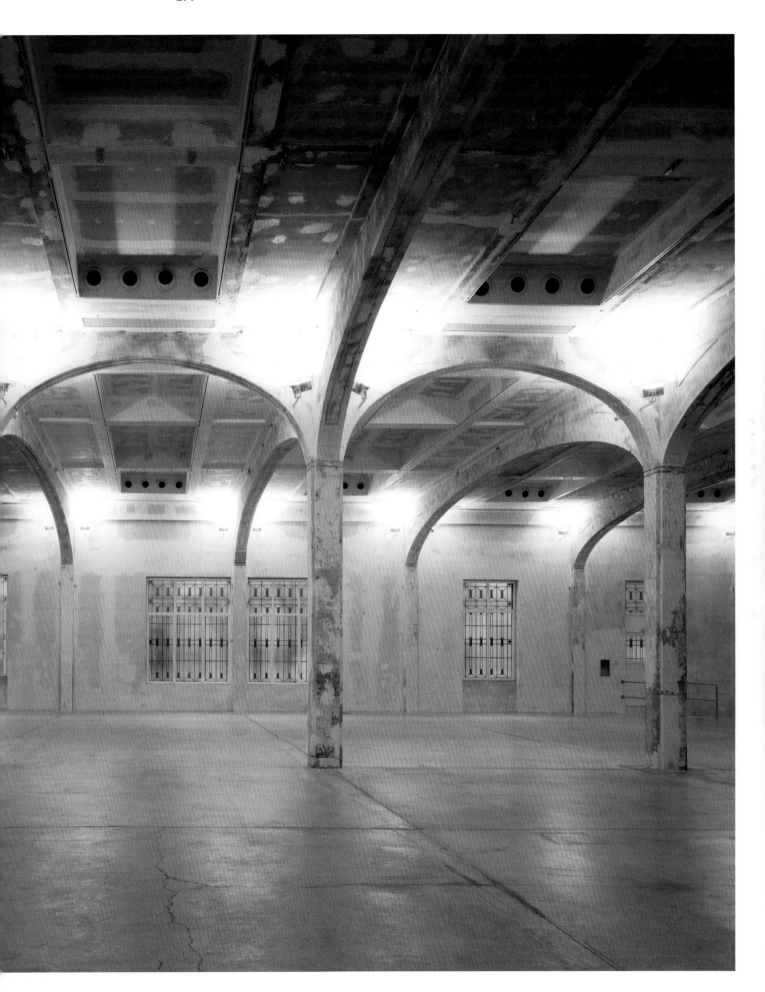

Prada Transformer

One of Prada's most significant architectural projects is the Prada Transformer, a temporary museum designed by Dutch architect Rem Koolhaas's firm OMA (Office for Metropolitan Architecture). The basic structure is a mechanical tetrahedron covered in an elastic membrane that allows its shape to be changed in order to suit the exhibition it houses. It can even be turned upside down by cranes. In 2009 it was installed next to Gyeonghui Palace in the centre of Seoul, where over the course of three months it flipped and shifted its shape to house a series of exhibitions intended 'to bring together, for the first time, the brand's diverse activities in the fields of culture, fashion, architecture, cinema and art in one space,' according to Patrizio Bertelli, Prada's CEO. The exhibitions in the Transformer included a cinematic programme selected by *Babel* director Alejandro González Iñárritu and co-curated by film critic Elvis Mitchell, and 'Waist Down – Skirts by Miuccia Prada' (see pages 166–67), an exhibition of Prada skirts. In the final stage of the structure's rotation, students from local universities produced independent events, performances and exhibitions across the fields of fashion, architecture, graphic design, film and multimedia.

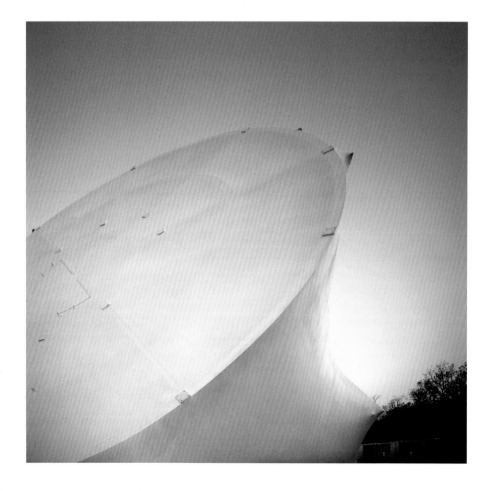

This page and opposite: Two different rotations of the Prada Transformer, designed by Rem Koolhaas of OMA/AMO, Seoul, 2009.

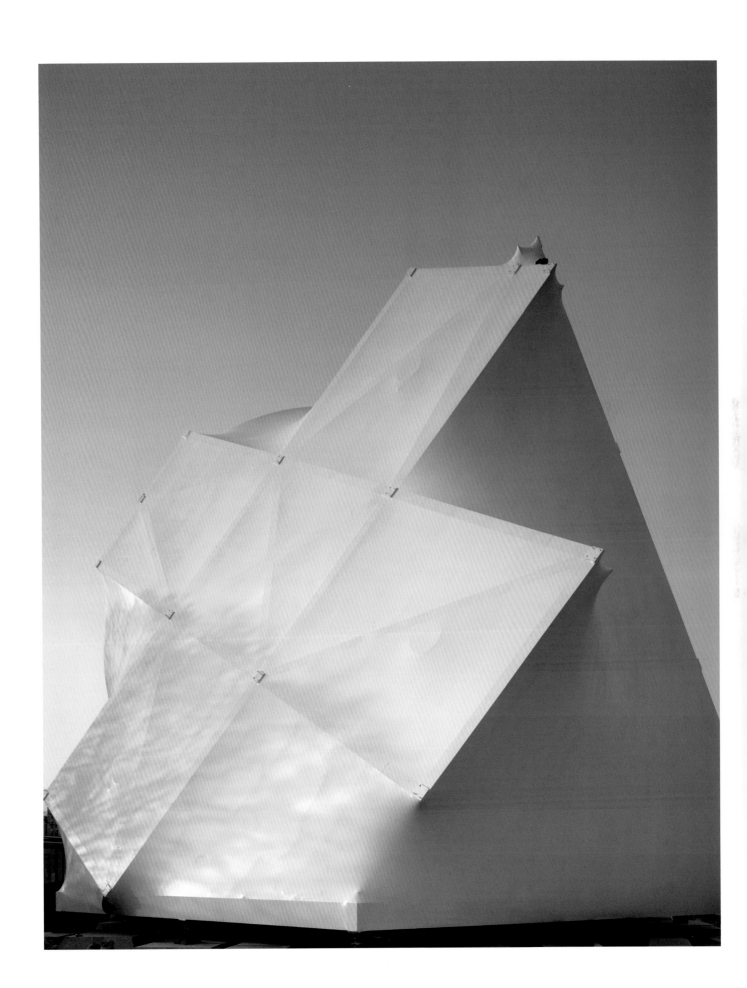

In conversation: Dennis Freedman, Barneys New York

American luxury department store Barneys New York has a long tradition of engagement with the arts. Its recent collaborative ventures include an exhibition in 2012 of 'destefashioncollection', an ongoing project of Greek art collector Dakis Joannou's DESTE Foundation for Contemporary Art, which each year invites a contemporary artist to select five fashion pieces of outstanding cultural significance to be acquired by the foundation, and then to create original artworks inspired by these objects. The exhibition, which was displayed in the windows of the Barneys flagship store on Madison Avenue in New York, featured work by design studio M/M, photographer Juergen Teller, artist Helmut Lang, poet Patrizia Cavalli and filmmaker Athina Rachel Tsangari.

As creative director of Barneys since 2011, Dennis Freedman oversees all of the company's photographic and video campaigns, graphic design, store design and visual merchandising. He also serves as 'curator' of its shop windows, engaging artists, designers and other collaborators to create unique installations, tableaux and dioramas. Prior to his role at Barneys, Freedman spent two decades at *W* magazine where, as founding creative director, he oversaw its groundbreaking melding of fashion and fine art content, working with photographers such as Steven Klein, Bruce Weber and Mario Sorrenti on innovative and award-winning editorials.

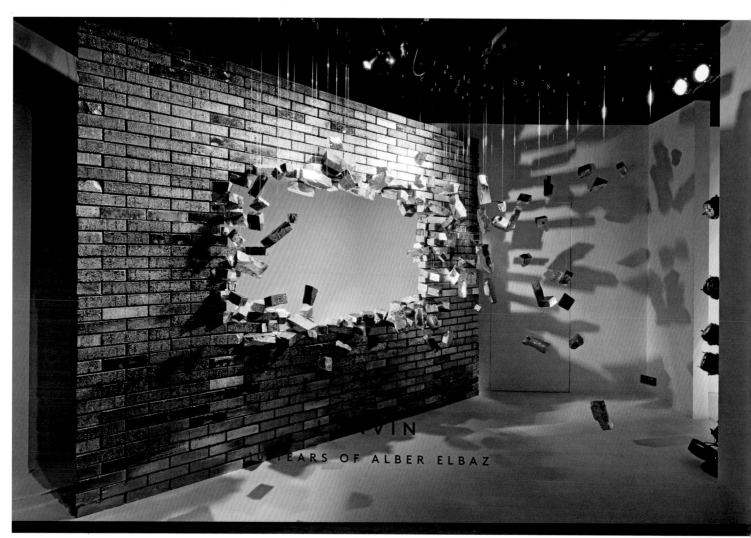

Below: Barneys New York window installations featuring
Lanvin designs in celebration of the tenth anniversary of the
brand's artistic director, Alber Elbaz, 2012.

MITCHELL OAKLEY SMITH *Have we arrived at a point where customers have come to expect an experience, so to speak, when shopping, such as Barneys offers with its artistic window displays?*

DENNIS FREEDMAN Yes, I think so. It is, in the end, [intended] to be commercially successful. Even with the DESTE project, 90% of the work is created with our merchandise.

MOS *Some of the artists that have created installations are very respected – can the windows therefore be considered art?*

DF This is not art. This is applied art, without a doubt. We are always focusing on the bags or the shoes, which form the basis of the installations. This is not art for art's sake.

MOS *The work with DESTE was really interesting in the context of a retail space. How did it come about?*

DF I don't think anything like that has been done before. I met Dakis [Joannou] through *W* when we did a piece [on him], and because we both share an interest in late 20th-century furniture, we stayed in touch. About

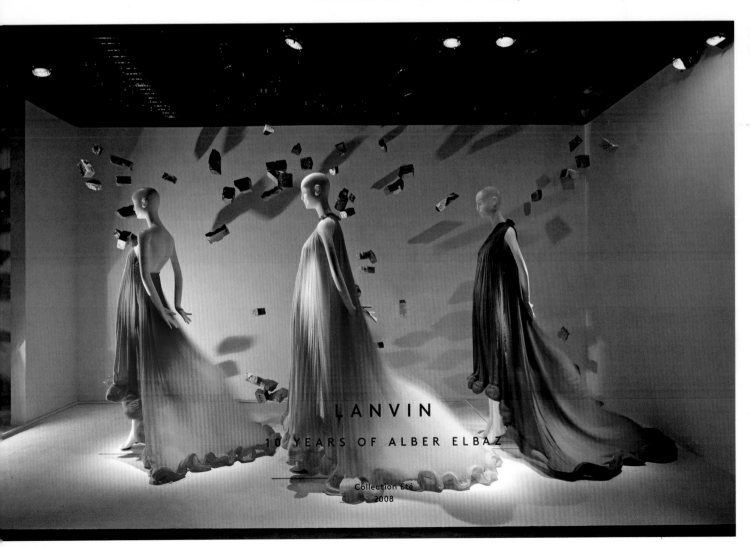

LANVIN
10 YEARS OF ALBER ELBAZ

Collection Été
2008

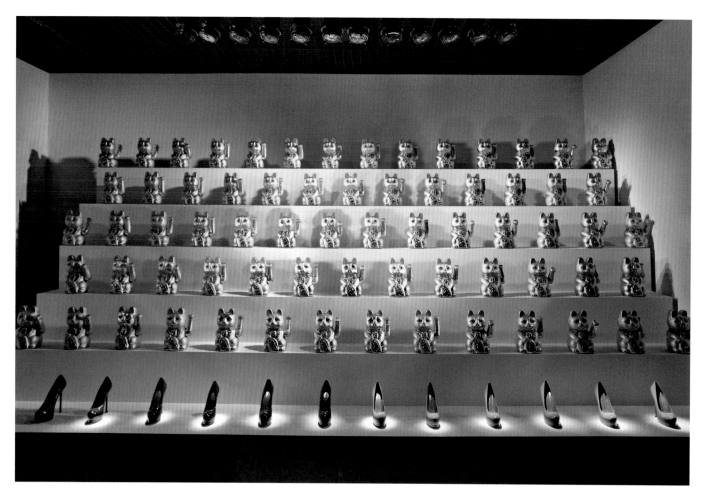

'This is not art. This is applied art, without a doubt. We are always focusing on the bags or the shoes, which form the basis of the installations. This is not art for art's sake.'

Dennis Freedman

Above and opposite: Barneys New York window installations
incorporating repetitive mechanical devices, 2012.

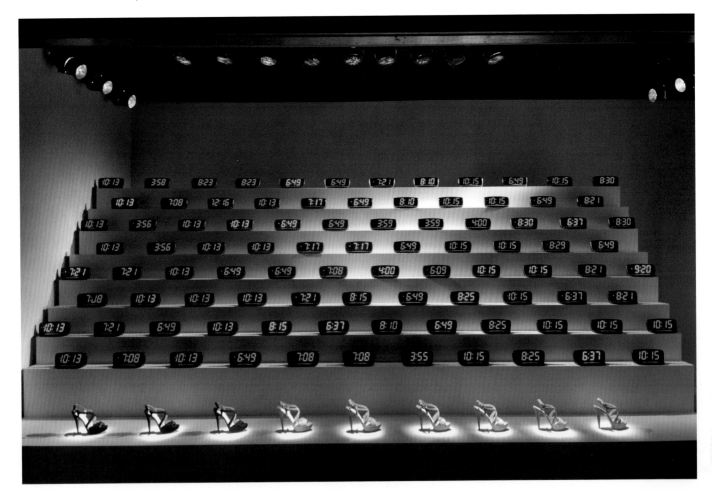

six years ago, Dakis remembered a cover of *Artforum* magazine from 1982 with an Issey Miyake dress, which had stuck in his mind, and he decided to venture into the world of fashion. Five years later, Dakis got in touch about the project and was looking for a museum in New York in which to show it. I said, 'I've got five windows on Madison Avenue,' and proposed we show it here. He was immediately into it.

MOS *How are the installations created?*

DF It's so inspirational to create work that relates not just to fashion, but also [to] art and theatre and technology, and is very much a way of defining our brand. I like moving parts but I'm tired of the slickness [of window displays] so we aim to use motors and inexpensive materials and contraptions. Videos are very influential: it's about seeing things in a way that is not necessarily employing the latest technology, as in some ways there's an honesty and power in the analogue [versions]. The other thing is that we use a lot of sound: we commission sounds and scores to go with the windows, and they become very important to the pieces and don't translate in photographs.

MOS *The DESTE project aside, is it a collaborative process when you commission someone to create a window display?*

DF It varies from collaboration to commission. In 2011 we commissioned [New York-based painter] Ella Kruglyanskaya to create five original paintings for our windows, because I thought her work is amazingly powerful. The paintings later sold and she had a big show at Gavin Brown's Enterprise. That project couldn't have had more to do with art. The collaboration is the basis of what we try to do, and we try to work with as many people in as many fields as possible. That extends to the commercial collaborations, too, like those with Nicolas Ghesquière, Hedi Slimane, Alber Elbaz – we always make clear it is a collaboration, something that we or they would never do on our own, because it results in far more interesting work.

Selfridges: Store windows, The Museum of Everything & Tracey Emin

Founded in 1909, Selfridges remains one of the world's leading multi-brand department stores and has been a prominent figure in the British retail landscape for over a century. The Selfridges flagship store on Oxford Street in London boasts an extensive frontage of glass windows that are regularly employed to house innovative product displays and installations by renowned artists, photographers, cultural figures and musicians. The windows, with their characteristic melding of luxury goods and pop-culture ephemera, have become synonymous with the Selfridges shopping experience.

The Museum of Everything, a travelling contemporary art project, became the largest installation in the history of Selfridges in 2011 when it filled

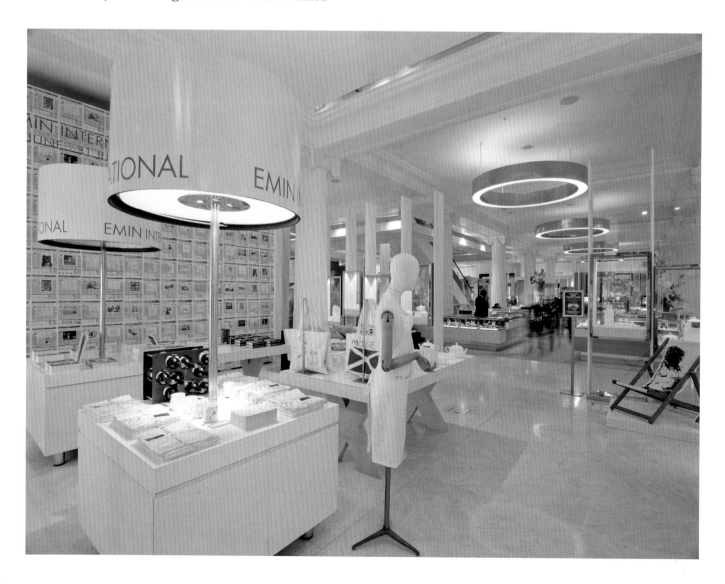

the department store's window displays and basement level with over two hundred never-before-seen artworks. The exhibition, the Museum of Everything's fourth, was accompanied by a pop-up store, the Shop of Everything, which sold a fashion collection designed in collaboration with Clements Ribeiro, as well as a line of bespoke products and accessories under the eponymous label Everything Ltd. The exhibition itself consisted of a major survey of the work of self-taught artists with developmental and other disabilities. Unlike most of the high-profile art projects sponsored by large retailers, this installation showcased only unknown artists, trading on the unconventional nature of their work which, according to a Selfridges spokesperson, 'reveals an astonishing visual language, which speaks for those who often cannot, and asks the audience to consider why these artists remain invisible.'[15]

Other art projects hosted by Selfridges in the 21st century have included 'Exactitudes', an exhibition in 2008 in collaboration with the Photographers' Gallery, featuring images of London-based fashion and cultural tribes by Dutch team Ellie Uyttenbroek and Ari Versluis; 'Vivienne Westwood Shoes: An Exhibition 1973–2010', in 2010; and, in 2009, 'Statuesque', a window display featuring Greek and Roman sculptures from the British Museum and the Victoria & Albert Museum displayed in tableaux vivants alongside drapery-inspired garments from the Spring/Summer 2009 fashion collections of Alexander Wang, Preen, Jil Sander and Alexander McQueen.

In 2011 British artist Tracey Emin collaborated on an installation for Selfridges. 'Walking Around My World' consisted of a space given over to the artist for her curatorial selection of goods from across the store, from brands as diverse as Aspinal of London, Vivienne Westwood and L'Atelier du Vin, interspersed with items from her own Emin International collection of limited-edition artworks, some of them commissioned exclusively for the Selfridges collaboration. The installation offered shoppers entrée to Emin's personal tastes with the option to emulate them via purchase, and demonstrated the blurring of boundaries between the spaces of art gallery and shop. As part of 'Walking Around My World' Emin was also invited to dress five of the internal store displays, while one side of Selfridges Oxford Street shopfront featured a life-sized cutout of the artist alongside one of her neon works. Importantly, the collaboration was timed to coincide with Emin's major retrospective at London's Hayward Gallery, 'Tracey Emin: Love Is What You Want', which was supported by Louis Vuitton.

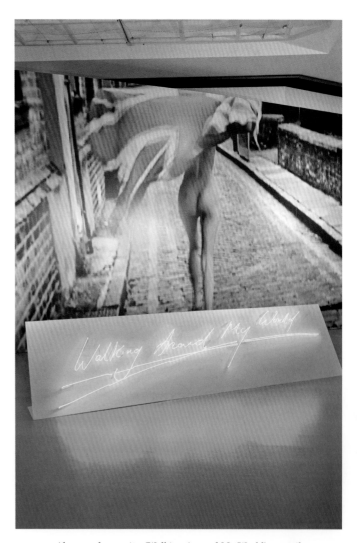

Above and opposite: 'Walking Around My World', a retail space within Selfridges curated by artist Tracey Emin in 2011. Overleaf: Window display reproducing artwork by Japanese artist Tomoyuki Shinki, as part of Selfridges 'The Museum of Everything' exhibition, 2011.

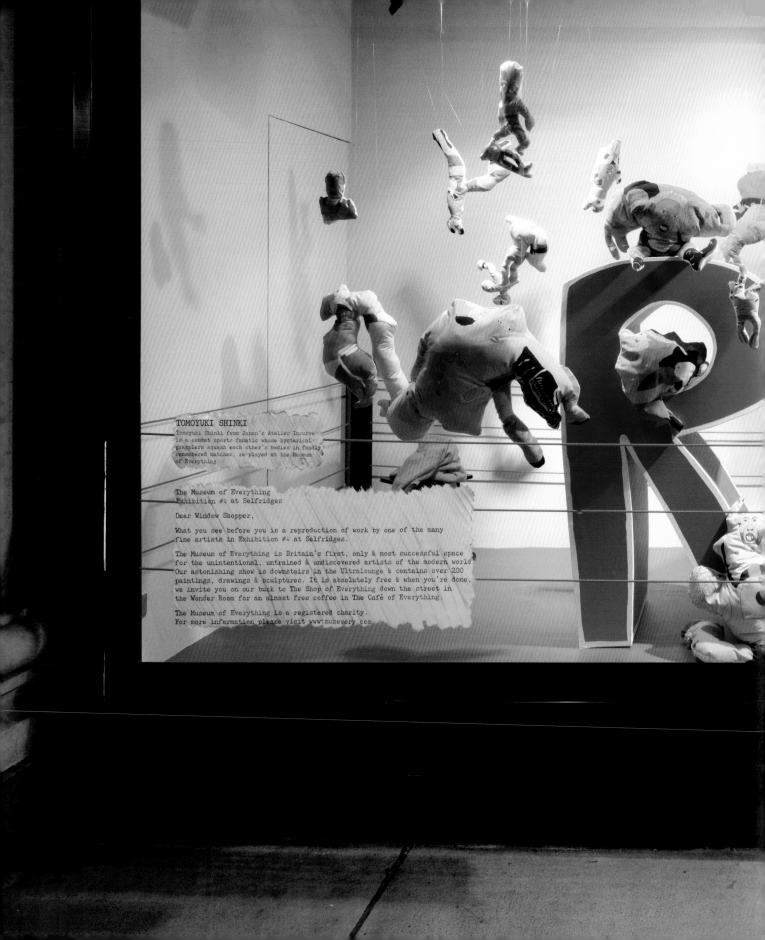

TOMOYUKI SHINKI
Tomoyuki Shinki from Japan's Atelier Incurve
is a combat sports fanatic whose hysterical
grapplers squash each other's bodies in fondly
remembered matches, re-played at the Museum
of Everything

The Museum of Everything
Exhibition #4 at Selfridges

Dear Window Shopper,

What you see before you is a reproduction of work by one of the many
fine artists in Exhibition #4 at Selfridges.

The Museum of Everything is Britain's first, only & most successful space
for the unintentional, untrained & undiscovered artists of the modern world.
Our astonishing show is downstairs in the Ultralounge & contains over 200
paintings, drawings & sculptures. It is absolutely free & when you're done,
we invite you on our buck to The Shop of Everything down the street in
the Wonder Room for an almost free coffee in The Café of Everything.

The Museum of Everything is a registered charity.
For more information please visit www.musevery.com

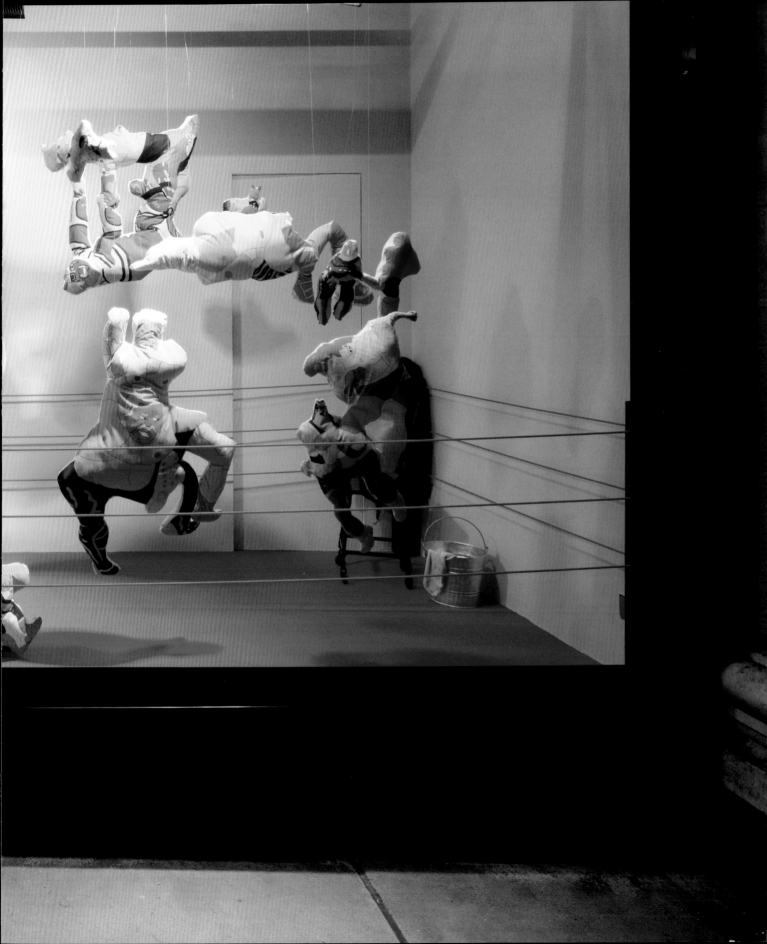

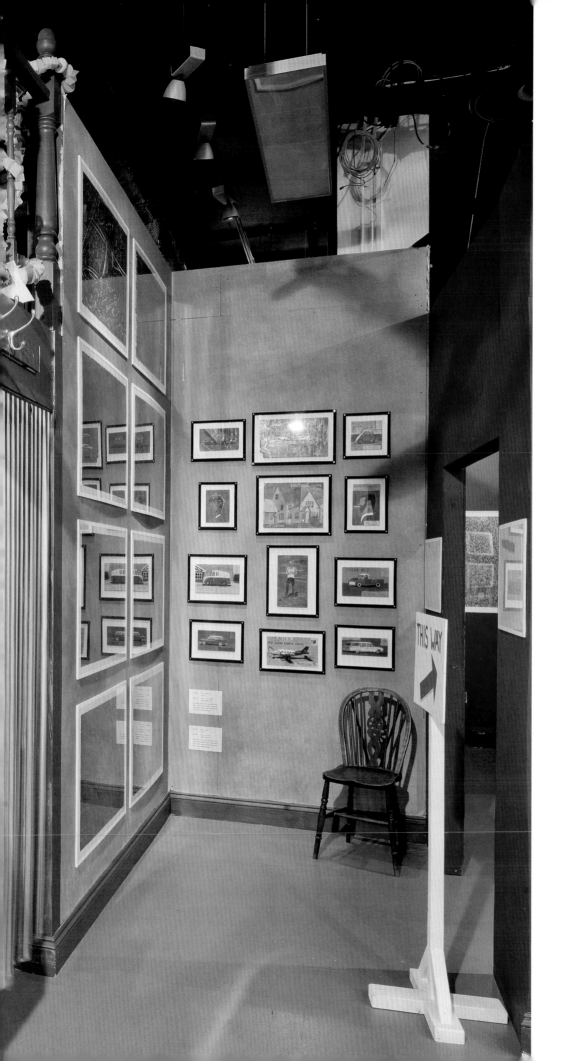

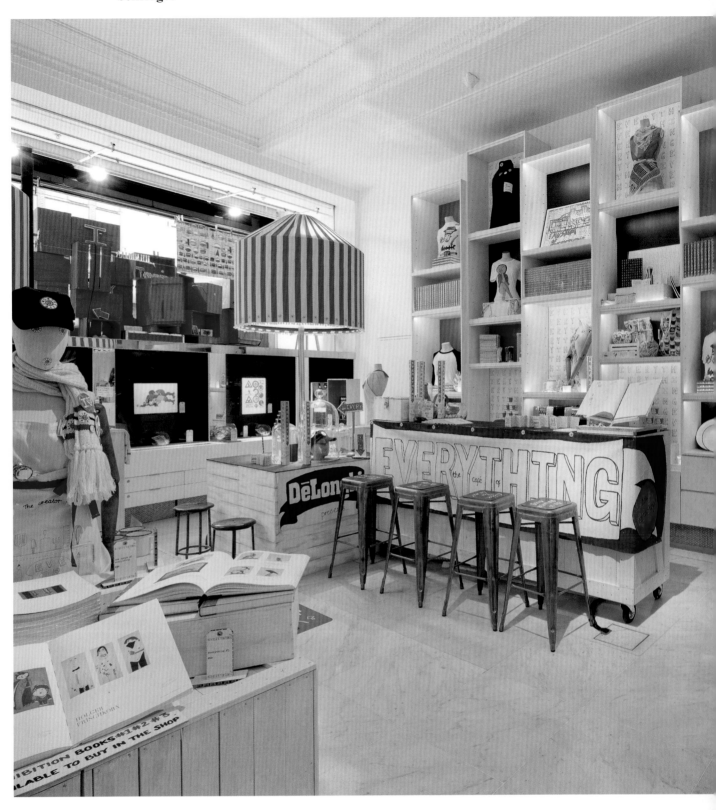

Above: The Shop of Everything, the retail component of
Selfridges 'The Museum of Everything' exhibition, 2011.
Opposite: 'The Museum of Everything', 2011, an exhibition
in Selfridges basement comprising over two hundred
artworks by self-taught artists with developmental
and other disabilities.

Fondation d'entreprise Hermès

French luxury brand Hermès's interest in the arts should come as no surprise, given its illustrious history of producing exquisitely handcrafted items. Hermès regularly collaborates with artists to produce designs for its iconic silk scarves, but it has also sponsored standalone art exhibitions and commissioned artists to work on projects for *Le Monde d'Hermès*, its in-house magazine. The Fondation d'entreprise Hermès, established in 2008, represents a more formalized approach to art patronage, as well as supporting traditional crafts, international educational initiatives and environmental biodiversity. It sponsors two art prizes: the Hermès Foundation Missulsang for contemporary Korean art and the Prix Émile Hermès for design. The foundation's activities also include artist-in-residence programmes at its French ateliers, six exhibition spaces worldwide (in Bern, Brussels, Singapore, Tokyo, New York and Seoul) and an ambitious performing arts programme.

An example of the foundation's unconventional approach to art patronage is H BOX, a programme that makes stipends available annually to four international artists who are selected to produce single-channel works in video. The videos are then displayed around the globe in a demountable screening room designed by architect Didier Faustino. The foundation describes H BOX as 'an object that blends references: a screening room, a travel kit, and a modern curio cabinet of sorts.'[16] Since the project's inception in 2006 more than twenty videos have been screened in the H BOX at major museums and art centres in Europe and North America.

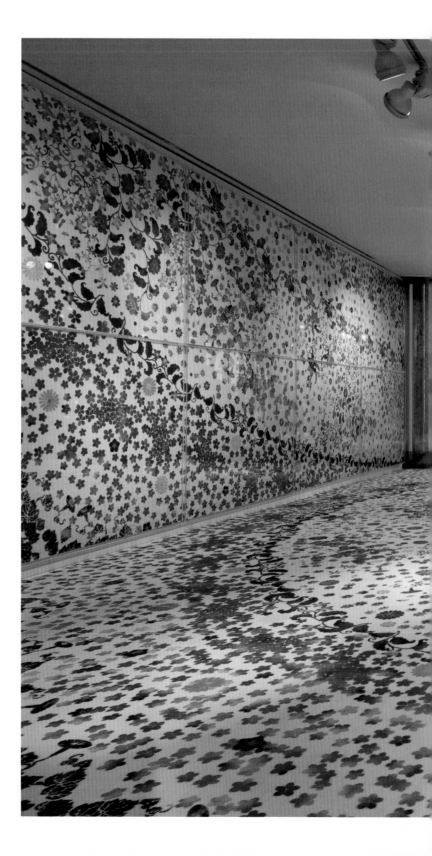

Shinji Ohmaki, *Moment and Eternity*, site-specific installation at Third Floor, Singapore, 2012, an exhibition of the Fondation d'entreprise Hermès.

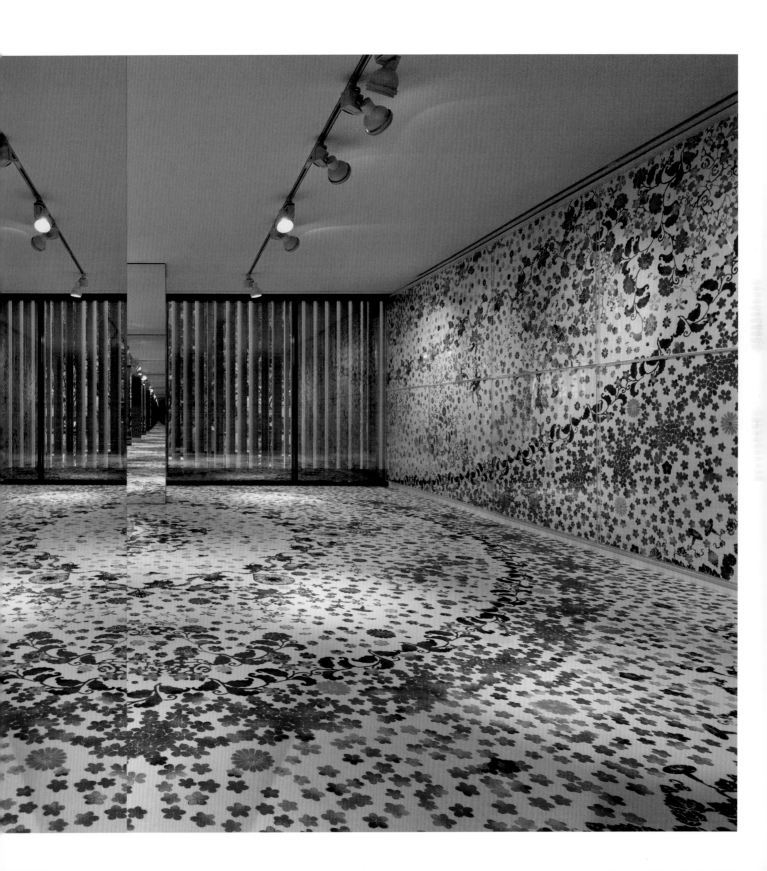

ZegnArt

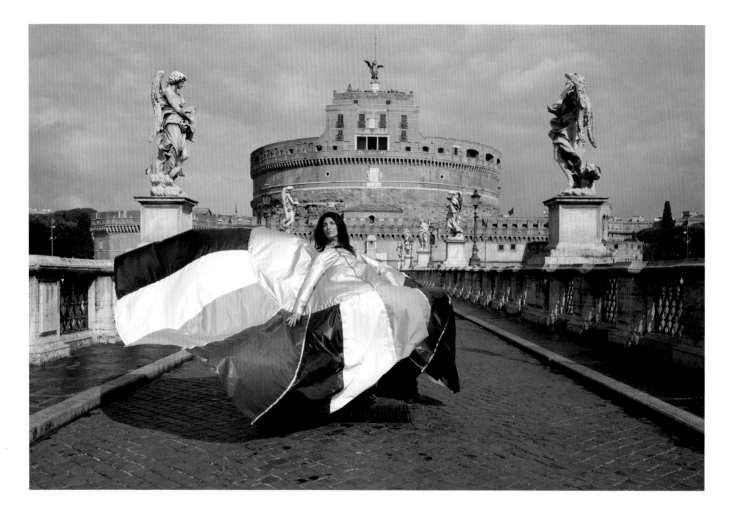

ZegnArt is an independent foundation established in 2011 by the Ermenegildo Zegna Group, owners of the historic Italian luxury menswear house. It commissions public art installations as well as works to be displayed in the brand's global stores. It also sponsors ZegnArt Public, in which it partners with art museums in the developing world to commission new public works from mid-career local contemporary artists, and offer young artists four-month residencies at the Museum of Contemporary Art in Rome. Organized by curators Cecilia Canziani and Simone Menegoi, the programme is based on 'a principle of dialogue and reciprocal exchange between countries'.[17] ZegnArt Public's first partnership was with the Dr Bhau Daji Lad Museum in Mumbai, through which new work was commissioned from artist Reena Saini Kallat in 2012.

ZegnArt's first commissioned special project, *Fabulae Romanae*, by British-based contemporary artists Lucy + Jorge Orta, was showcased at the MAXXI, Rome's National Museum of 21st-Century Arts, throughout 2012. The commission was conceived in association with curator Maria Luisa Frisa and was included in the museum's group exhibition 'Tridimensionale'. Zegna also commissions international artists – such as Mimmo Jodice, Frank Thiel, Emil Lukas and Michelangelo Pistoletto – to produce works inspired by the spirit and philosophy of the Zegna Group, which are then housed within the brand's stores around the world.

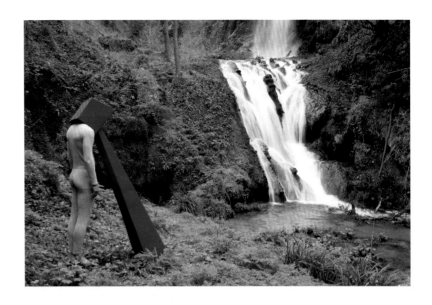

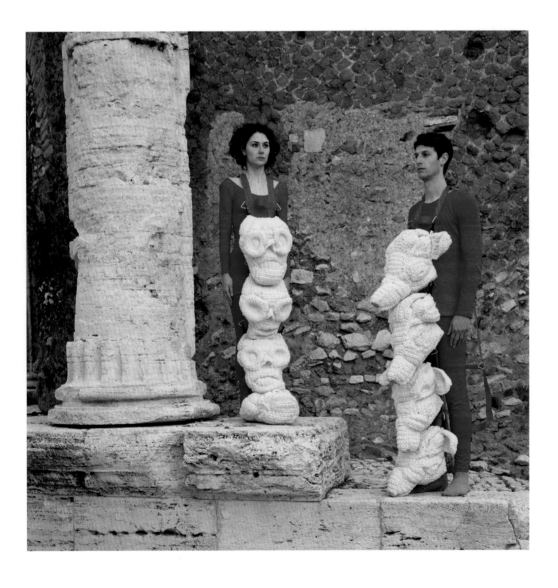

This page and opposite: Stills from *Spirits – Fabulae Romanae*,
Lucy + Jorge Orta, filmed video performance, 2012,
commissioned by ZegnArt.

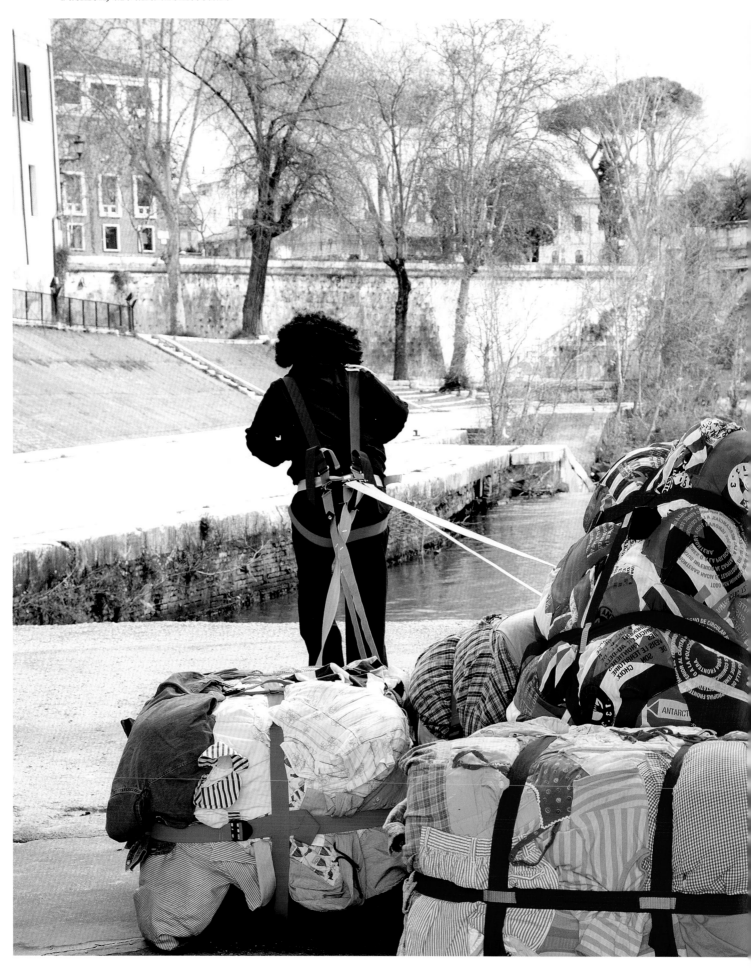

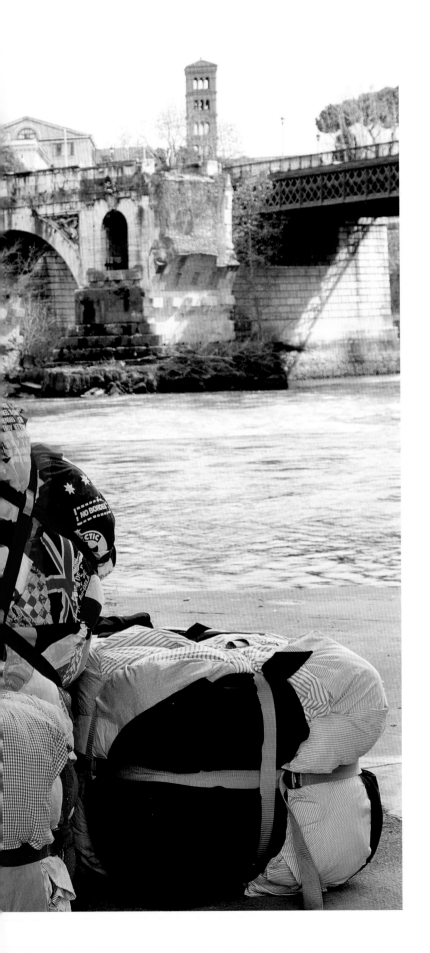

Still from *Spirits – Fabulae Romanae*, Lucy + Jorge Orta, filmed
video performance, 2012, commissioned by ZegnArt.

'Chanel Mobile Art'
exhibition pavilion

Touring Hong Kong, Tokyo and New York, the 'Chanel Mobile Art' exhibition, curated by Fabrice Bousteau, showcased the work of twenty international artists – including Soundwalk, Yoko Ono, Pierre & Gilles and Sylvie Fleury – who created pieces inspired by the elements and aesthetic of Coco Chanel's signature quilted bag. In 2008, Chanel's artistic director Karl Lagerfeld commissioned Iraqi-born British architect Zaha Hadid to create a futuristic exhibition pavilion to house the touring exhibition, bringing together two iconic brands – Chanel and Hadid. The external form of Hadid's pavilion was inspired by organic forms found in nature, resembling a mollusc with a white shell. Lagerfeld was enthusiastic about the collaboration and fluent in his public praise for Hadid's work: 'She is the first architect to find a way to part with the all-dominating, post-Bauhaus aesthetic. The value of her designs is similar to that of great poetry. The potential of her imagination is enormous.'[18] Following its tour, the exhibition was dismantled and shown in various iterations at department stores around the world. Chanel donated Hadid's mobile art pavilion to the Arab World Institute in Paris where, since 2011, it has been used to showcase contemporary art from Arab countries.

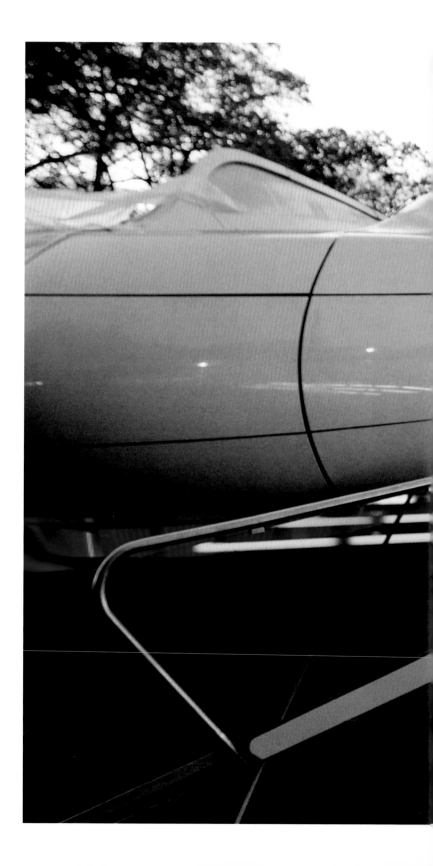

'Chanel Mobile Art' pavilion designed by Zaha Hadid, shown here at its opening in Central Park, New York, 2008.

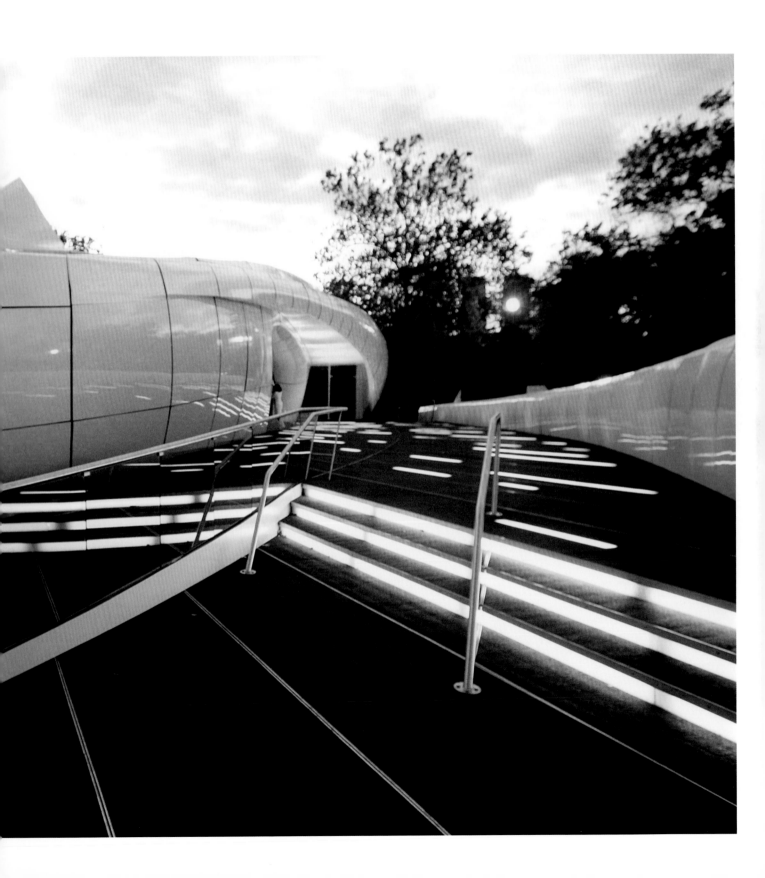

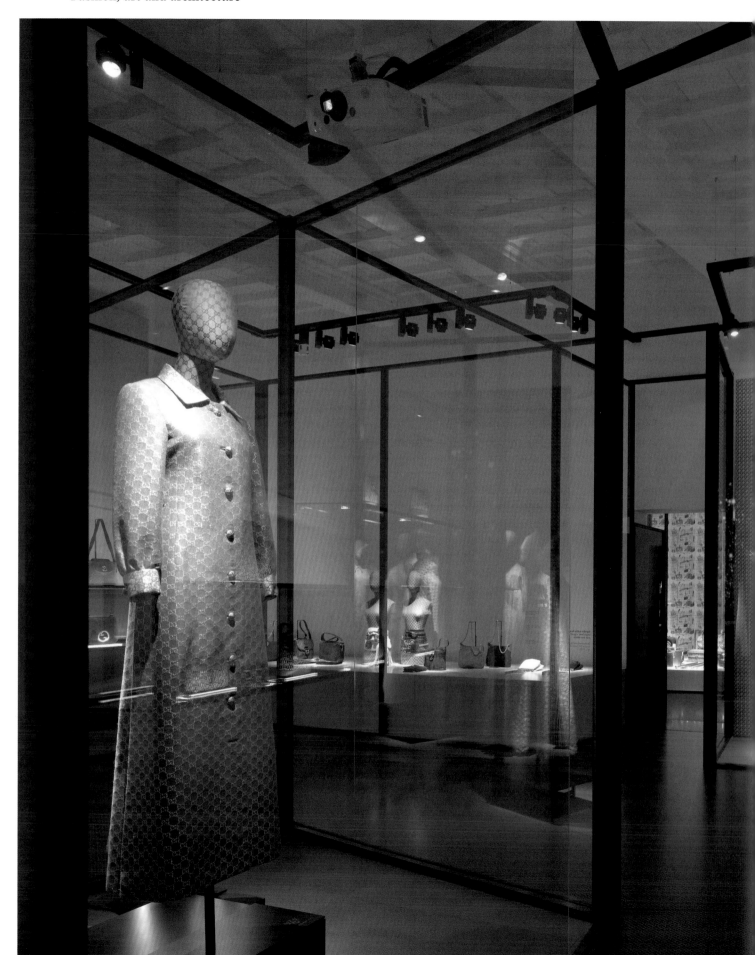

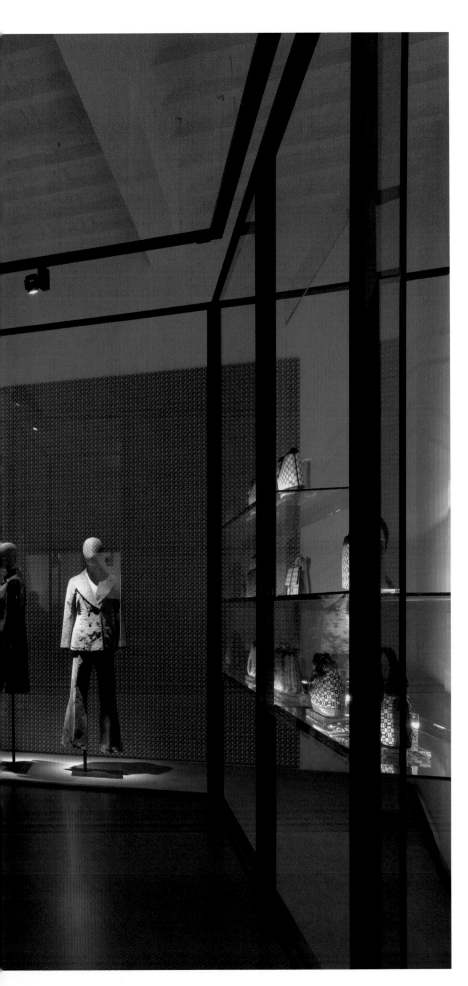

Gucci Museo

Gucci, founded in Florence in 1921, is the quintessential global luxury brand whose logo is synonymous with Italian design. Its Gucci Museo, which opened in 2011, spread across three floors of the historic Palazzo della Mercanzia near the Piazza della Signoria in Florence, showcases a permanent collection of garments and accessories from the company's archives alongside regular exhibitions of contemporary art sponsored by the foundation established by François Pinault, head of the French conglomerate Kering, which has owned Gucci since 2003. These exhibitions, which are presented in the museum's dedicated Contemporary Art Space, focus primarily on film and new media, reflecting Gucci's long association and sponsorship of the Film Foundation. The permanent collection is displayed in thematic galleries inspired by Gucci's iconic products and motifs, such as Flora World, which celebrates the famed floral scarf pattern, Logomania, which traces the evolution of the double-'G' logo, and Travel, which includes everything from a customized Cadillac to the luxury luggage that made Gucci a favourite brand of the wealthy jet set.

Gucci recognizes that its history is intimately tied to the development of 20th-century celebrity culture, and this is reflected in the presentation of the collection alongside numerous images of famous figures, such as Sophia Loren, wearing the label's designs. Head designer Frida Giannini developed the slogan 'Forever Now' that grounds the display, firmly locating the brand in both a historical and a contemporary context. Ultimately, however, the museum is a statement about Gucci's current status as a luxury titan. Rather than waiting for a conventional retrospective exhibition at an art museum, Gucci has founded its own gallery in which it can present its history as it wishes to be represented, while associating the brand with carefully curated contemporary art.

The Logomania thematic gallery at Gucci Museo, Florence.

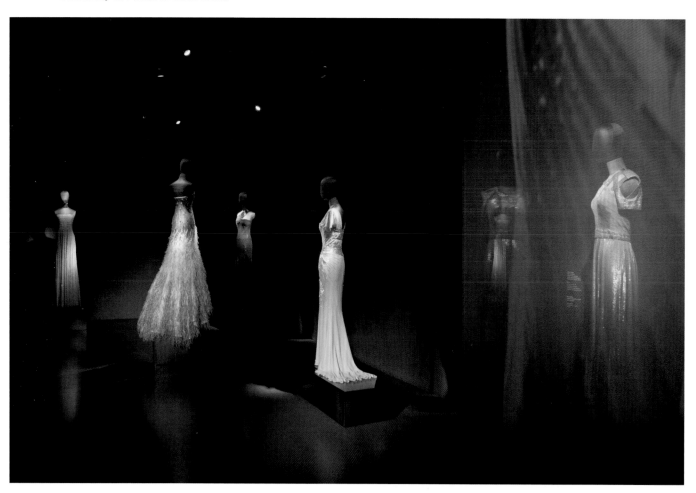

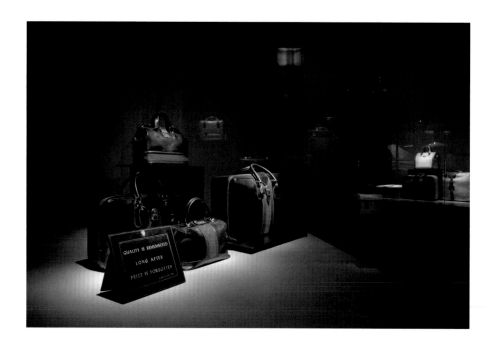

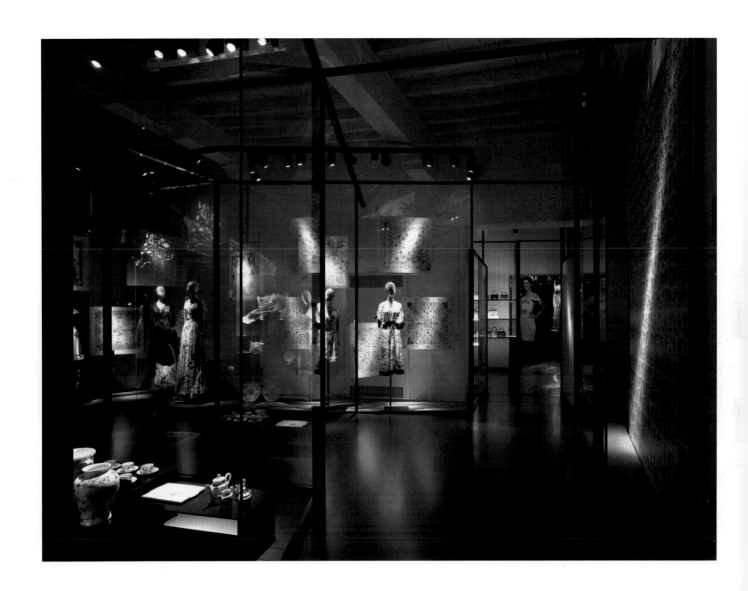

Above: The Flora World gallery at Gucci Museo
displays a wide variety of items imprinted with the
brand's signature floral motif.
Opposite above: The Evening gallery showcases the brand's
evening gowns, including pieces worn on the red carpet.
Opposite below: The Handbags gallery celebrates
Gucci's historic handbag models.

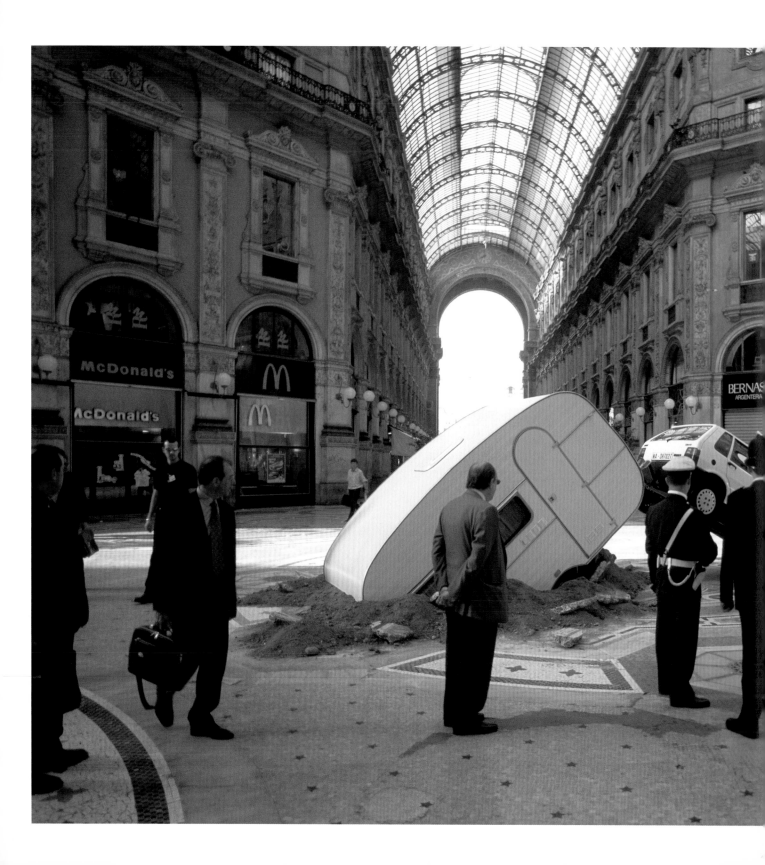

Fondazione Nicola Trussardi

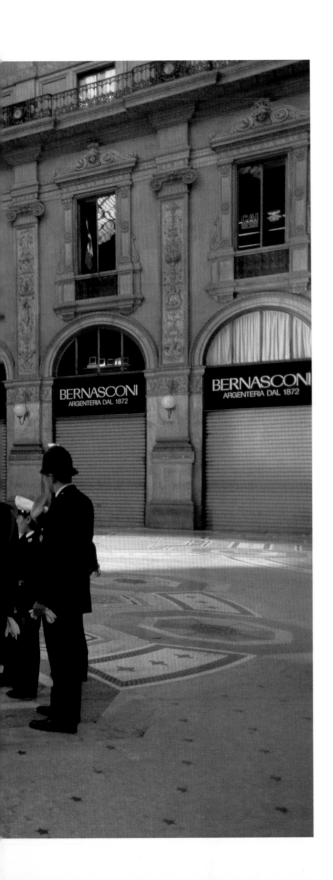

Italian label Trussardi established its namesake foundation in Milan in 1996. The Fondazione Nicola Trussardi initially invited artists to collaborate with its in-house artisans, but since 2003 it has focused on temporary installation projects realized on a grand scale in public spaces 'to demonstrate that art can give a new identity and international visibility to the city, entering our everyday, public existence to enrich it with unexpected languages and experiences'.[19] The foundation has worked with a wide range of prominent contemporary artists, including Maurizio Cattelan, whose installation *Untitled* (2004) depicting the bodies of three children hanging from an oak tree in Piazza XXIV Maggio, alluding to Italy's violent fascist past, caused considerable controversy. Other public installations sponsored by the foundation have included Polish artist Paweł Althamer's *Balloon* (2007), a giant inflatable nude scupture of the artist that was suspended outside the Renaissance Palazzina Appiani in Parco Sempione; and Swiss-born artist Urs Fischer's *Bread House* (2004), consisting of a small Alpine-style house constructed from sourdough bread, foam and wood, which was installed inside a church, where it was then devoured by fledgling parakeets over several days. In Elmgreen & Dragset's spectacular installation *Short Cut* (2003), located in the atrium of Galleria Vittorio Emanuele II, a white Fiat Uno towing a caravan appeared to burst through the floor of the famous arcade; another project, the film *Parts of a Film with Rat and Bear* (2008), saw Swiss artists Peter Fischli and David Weiss dress up as a giant rat and bear to roam the halls of the historic Palazzo Litta.

Fondazione Nicola Trussardi's collected projects were the subject of a major publication, *What Good is the Moon?: The Exhibitions of the Trussardi Foundation*, in 2012. In 2013 the foundation's director Massimiliano Gioni curated the Venice Biennale, demonstrating Fondazione Trussardi's ambitious artistic vision and the respect it has garnered since its inception.

Left: Elmgreen & Dragset, *Short Cut*, mixed media, Fiat Uno and camper trailer, 2003, installed in the Galleria Vittorio Emanuele II, Milan. The work was commissioned and produced by Fondazione Nicola Trussardi. Overleaf: Peter Fischli and David Weiss, *Rat and Bear Costumes*, costumes of the protagonists of the *Rat and Bear* films displayed in Perspex cases, 1981–2004, shown here at Palazzo Litta, Milan. The work was produced and organized by Fondazione Nicola Trussardi in collaboration with Tate Modern, London, and the Kunsthaus Zürich.

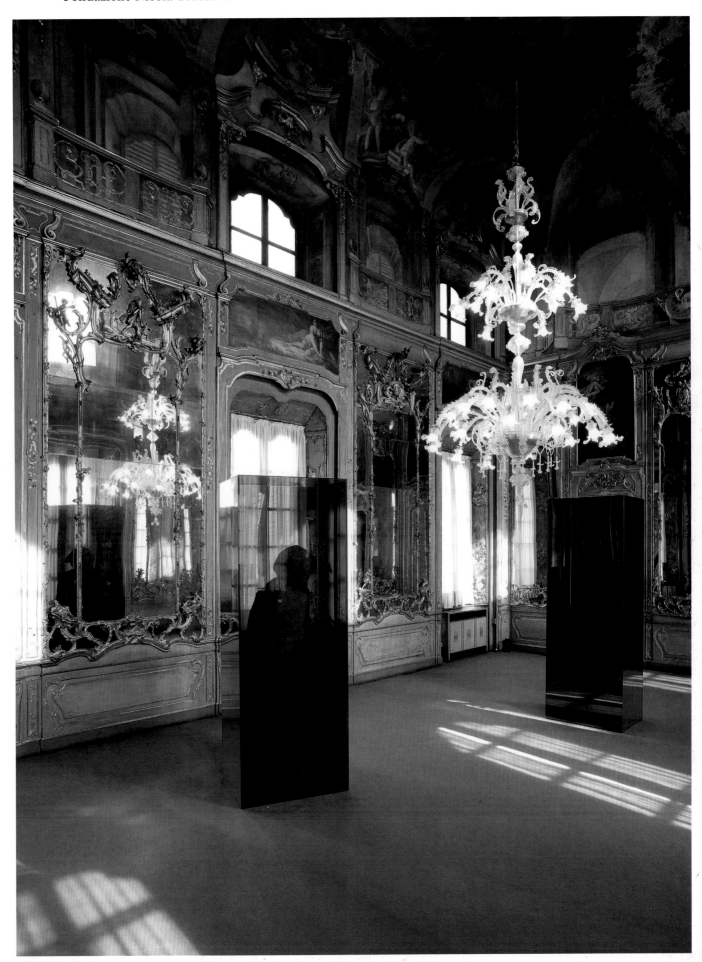

Notes

All references to *Vogue* imply the American edition unless otherwise indicated. Fashion seasons refer to the northern hemisphere.

Introduction: An artistic embrace
1. Andy Warhol, interviewed in *Mondo Uomo*, 1984, as quoted in the press materials for the exhibition 'The Fashion World of Jean Paul Gaultier: From Sidewalk to Catwalk', Montreal Museum of Fine Arts, 2011, available at <http://www.mbam.qc.ca/jpg/en/>, accessed 15 April 2013.
2. Walter Benjamin, 'The work of art in the age of mechanical reproduction' in *Art in Theory: 1900–1990: An Anthology of Changing Ideas*, ed. Charles Harrison and Paul Wood, 1992, pp. 512–20, at p. 513.
3. José Teunissen, 'Fashion and Art' in *Fashion and Imagination: About Clothes and Art*, ed. Jan Brand, José Teunissen and Catelijne de Muijnck, 2010, pp. 10–25, at p. 19.

Chapter 1 – More than clothes: Fashion as art
1. Diana Crane, 'Boundaries: Using Cultural Theory to Unravel the Complex Relationship between Fashion and Art', in *Fashion and Art*, ed. Adam Geczy and Vicki Karaminas, 2012, pp. 99–110, at p. 101.
2. Oscar Wilde, 'Phrases and philosophies for the use of the young', *Chameleon* 1 (December 1894), p. 1, repr. in Oscar Wilde, *Miscellanies*, ed. Robert Ross, 1908.
3. Karin Schacknat, 'Brilliant utopias and other realities', in *Fashion and Imagination: About Clothes and Art*, ed. Jan Brand, José Teunissen and Catelijne de Muijnck, 2010, pp. 314–29, at p. 315.
4. Valerie Steele, 'Fashion', in *Fashion and Art*, ed. Adam Geczy and Vicki Karaminas, 2012, pp. 13–27, at p. 20.
5. Schacknat, 'Brilliant utopias', p. 315.
6. Fiona Duncan, 'Martin Margiela's inside joke: Getting to the crux of MMM for H&M', *Bullett*, 14 November 2012, available at < http://bullettmedia.com/article/martin-margielas-inside-joke/>, accessed 15 April 2013.
7. Alexander McQueen interviewed for *The Fashion*, Spring/Summer 2001, and *Women's Wear Daily*, 28 September 2000, quoted from <http://blog.metmuseum.org/alexandermcqueen/tag/voss>, accessed 15 April 2013.
8. Linda Yablonsky, 'Close encounters: The art-and-fashion cachet' (review of *Rodarte, Catherine Opie, Alec Soth*, 2011), *artnet.com*, 19 September 2011, available at <http://www.artnet.com/magazineus/books/yablonsky/rodarte-catherine-opie-alec-soth-9-19-11.asp>, accessed 15 April 2013.
9. Deidre Crawford, 'Rodarte on art as inspiration for fashion', *California Apparel News.net*, 19 January 2012, available at <http://www.apparelnews.net/blog/2058_rodarte_on_art_as_inspiration_for_fashion.html>, accessed 15 April 2013.
10. All quotes in this section are from Emma Price in conversation with the authors, 14 January 2012.
11. All quotes in this section are from Jonathan Zawada in conversation with the authors, 17 August 2012.
12. All quotes in this section are from Susan Dimasi in conversation with the authors, 20 April 2012.
13. 'Viktor & Rolf: "There's very little regal glamour"', *The Talks*, 26 October 2011, available at <http://the-talks.com/interviews/viktor-rolf/>, accessed 15 April 2013.

Chapter 2 – Art meets fashion: Collaboration
1. Yves Carcelle quoted in Kate Betts, 'Art lessons', *Time*, 11 October 2007, available at <http://www.time.com/time/magazine/article/0,9171,1670494,00.html>, accessed 15 April 2013.

2. All quotes in this section are from press materials provided to the authors by the exhibition organizers.
3. All quotes in this section are from press materials provided to the authors by Christian Dior.
4. All quotes in this section are from Graeme Fidler and Michael Herz in conversation with the authors, 29 May 2012.
5. Olivier Saillard, *Louis Vuitton: Art, Fashion and Architecture*, 2009, p. 71.
6. Ibid.
7. Marc Jacobs, quoted in Christopher Bagley, 'Marc Jacobs', *W*, November 2007, available at <http://www.wmagazine.com/artdesign/2007/11/marc_jacobs>, accessed 15 April 2013.
8. Ibid.
9. Tim Roeloffs, quoted in 'Tim Roeloffs collaboration', *Wallpaper**, 26 February 2008, available at <http://www.wallpaper.com/fashion/tim-roeloffs-collaboration/2115>, accessed 15 April 2013.
10. Ibid.
11. All quotes in this section are from press materials provided to the authors by Pringle of Scotland.
12. All quotes in this section are from Natalie Wood in conversation with the authors, 18 July 2012.
13. All quotes in this section are from press materials provided to the authors by Coach.
14. Erwin Wurm in conversation with curator Mathias Schwartz-Clauss, Vitra Design Museum, available at <http://www.design-museum.de/en/information/texts-of-the-vdm/detailseiten/erwin-wurm.html>, accessed 15 April 2013.

Chapter 3 – Eye candy and ideas: Fashion as exhibition
1. James Laver, *Modesty in Fashion: An Inquiry Into the Fundamentals of Fashion*, 1969, p. 9.
2. Judith Clark, 'Looking at looking at dress', in *Fashion and Imagination: About Clothes and Art*, ed. Jan Brand, José Teunissen and Catelijne de Muijnck, 2010, pp. 184–90, at p. 185.
3. 'Prada: Nicholas Cullinan and Francesco Vezzoli in conversation', *Kaleidoscope*, Issue 13, 2012, available at <http://kaleidoscope-press.com/issue-contents/prada-nicholas-cullinan-and-francesco-vezzoli-in-conversation/>, accessed 15 April 2013.
4. Jonathan Jones in conversation with the authors, 11 March 2011.
5. Thierry-Maxime Loriot in conversation with the authors, 24 July 2012.
6. Ibid.
7. Ibid.

Chapter 4 – Beyond the photoshoot: New fashion media
1. Jens Grede and Erik Torstensson, opening manifesto of founding issue of *Industrie*, 2010, p. 12.
2. Jefferson Hack, *Another Fashion Book*, 2009, p. 3.
3. Ella Alexander, 'Snowdon Blue', *Vogue* (UK), 2 May 2012, available at <http://www.vogue.co.uk/news/2012/05/03/acne-and-lord-snowdon-launch-snowdon-blue-book-and-exhibition>, accessed 15 April 2013.
4. Jochen Siemens, *Inez van Lamsweerde & Vinoodh Matadin*, 2009, p. 6.
5. Steven Heyman, 'Photographers without Borders', *T Magazine, New York Times*, 28 December 2011, available at <http://tmagazine.blogs.nytimes.com/2011/12/28/photographers-without-borders/>, accessed 15 April 2013.
6. Ibid.
7. Cathy Horyn, 'When is a fashion ad not a fashion ad', *New York Times*, 10 April 2008, available at < http://www.nytimes.com/2008/04/10/fashion/10TELLER.html?pagewanted=all&_r=0>, accessed 15 April 2013.

8. All quotes in this section are from Liz Ham in conversation with the authors, 22 December 2011.

9. Tamara Abraham, 'Christian Dior slammed over "racist" images designed for Shanghai store launch', *Daily Mail Online*, 6 September 2006, available at <http://www.dailymail.co.uk/femail/article-1309512/Christian-Dior-slammed-racist-images-designed-Shanghai-store-launch.html>, accessed 15 April 2013.

10. All quotes in this section are from Deborah Turbeville in conversation with the authors, 26 June 2011.

Chapter 5 – From boutique to gallery: Fashion, art and architecture

1. Bradley Quinn, 'The Fashion of Architecture', in *Fashion and Imagination: About Clothes and Art*, ed. Jan Brand, José Teunissen and Catelijne de Muijnck, 201, pp. 260–75, at p. 261.

2. Taro Igarashi, *Louis Vuitton: Art, Fashion & Architecture*, 2009, p. 14.

3. James B. Twitchell, *Branded Nation: The Marketing of Megachurch, College Inc., and Museumworld*, 2004, p. 203.

4. Gilles Lipovetsky and Veronica Manlow, 'The "artialization" of luxury stores', in *Fashion and Imagination: About Clothes and Art*, ed. Jan Brand, José Teunissen and Catelijne de Muijnck, 2010, pp. 124–67, at p. 155.

5. Ibid.

6. Twitchell, *Branded Nation*, p. 226.

7. Ibid., pp. 225–26.

8. Andy Warhol quoted in Twitchell, *Branded Nation*, p. 227.

9. Desirée Heiss and Ines Kaag in conversation with Mitchell Oakley Smith, 27 March 2012.

10. 'BLESS Shop #03' on Bless company website, available at <http://www.bless-service.de/BLESS/BLESS_Shops/Eintrage/2000/7/5_BLESS_Shop_034th_Werkleitz_Biennale,_Werkleitz,_Germany.html>, accessed 15 April 2013.

13. Mohsen Mostafavi, *Louis Vuitton: Architecture & Interiors*, 2011, Foreword, p. 8.

14. Ibid.

15. All quotes in this section are from press materials provided to the authors by Louis Vuitton.

16. Germano Celant quoted in the monograph *Prada*, 2009, p. 455, no named author.

17. All quotes in this section are from press materials provided to the authors by Selfridges.

18. Fondation d'entreprise Hermès press release, available at <http://www.e-flux.com/announcements/h-box-a-nomadic-video-art-screening-room/>, accessed 15 April 2013.

19. All quotes in this section are from press materials provided to the authors by ZegnArt.

20. Karl Lagerfeld press conference quoted in 'Power couples: day 10', *Wallpaper**, 23 September 2006, available at <http://www.wallpaper.com/fashion/power-couples-day-10/1092>, accessed 15 April 2013.

21. All quotes in this section are from press materials provided to the authors by Fondazione Nicola Trussardi.

Further Reading

Essential texts on art and fashion:

Arts, Jos, et al., *Fashion and Imagination: About Clothes and Art*, ed. Jan Brand, José Teunissen and Catelijne de Muijnck (2010).

Barthes, Roland, *The Fashion System* (1992).

Benjamin, Walter, 'The work of art in the age of mechanical reproduction', in *Art in Theory: 1900–1990, An Anthology of Changing Ideas*, ed. Charles Harrison and Paul Wood (1992), pp. 512-520.

Blackman, Cally, *100 Years of Fashion* (2012).

Craik, Jennifer, *The Face of Fashion: Cultural Studies in Fashion* (1993).

English, Bonnie, *A Cultural History of Fashion in the 20th Century* (2007).

Geczy, Adam, and Vicki Karaminas, eds, *Fashion and Art* (2012).

Hack, Jefferson, *Another Fashion Book* (2010).

Laver, James, *Modesty in Fashion: An Inquiry Into the Fundamentals of Fashion* (1969).

Lutgens, Annelie, Richard Martin and Hans Nefkens, *Art and Fashion: Between Skin and Clothing* (2011).

Mackrell, Alice, *Art and Fashion: The Impact on Fashion and Fashion on Art* (2005).

Menkes, Suzy, and Valerie Steele, *Fashion Designers, A–Z* (2013).

Oakley Smith, Mitchell, *Fashion: Australian and New Zealand Designers* (2010).

Quinn, Bradley, *The Fashion of Architecture* (2003).

Steele, Valerie, *The Berg Companion to Fashion* (2010).

Stern, Radu, *Against Fashion: Clothing As Art, 1850–1930* (2005).

Twitchell, James B., 'Museumworld, Inc.', in *Branded Nation: The Marketing of Megachurch, College Inc., and Museumworld* (2004), pp. 223–27.

Monographs and exhibition catalogues:

Armstrong-Jones, Anthony (Lord Snowdon), Thomas Persson and Frances von Hofmannsthal, *Snowdon Blue* (2012).

Barnbrook, Jonathan, and Edward Booth-Clibborn, *Fashion and Art Collusion* (2012).

Bolton, Andrew, and Harold Koda, *Alexander McQueen: Savage Beauty* (2011).

Bolton, Andrew, and Andrew Koda, *Schiaparelli and Prada: Impossible Conversations* (2012).

Burton, Johanna, and Eva Respini, *Cindy Sherman* (2012).

Castets, Simon, et al., *Louis Vuitton: Art, Fashion and Architecture* (2009).

Chalayan, Hussein, *Hussein Chalayan* (2011).

Debo, Kaat, and Bob Verhelst, *Maison Martin Margiela: 20: The Exhibition* (2008).

Edelmann, Frederic, and Ian Luna, *Louis Vuitton: Architecture and Interiors* (2011).

Evans, Caroline, and Susannah Frankel, *The House of Viktor and Rolf* (2008).

Giannini, Frida, *Gucci – The Making Of* (2011).

Golbin, Pamela, *Louis Vuitton/Marc Jacobs* (2012).

Guinness, Daphne, and Valerie Steele, *Daphne Guinness* (2011).

Hasegawa, Yuko, *Hussein Chalayan: From Fashion and Back* (2010).

Heilman, Hannah, *Vibskov and Emenius: The Fringe Projects* (2009).

Loriot, Thierry-Maxime, *The Fashion World of Jean Paul Gaultier* (2011).

Miyake, Issey, *Pleats Please* (2012).

Mulleavy, Kate and Laura, Catherine Opie and Alec Soth, *Rodarte, Catherine Opie, Alec Soth* (2011).

Prada, Miuccia, and Patrizio Bertelli, *Prada* (2009).

Siemens, Jochen, *Inez van Lamsweerde & Vinoodh Matadin* (2009).

Teller, Juergen, *Marc Jacobs Advertising 1998–2009* (2009).

Turbeville, Deborah, *Deborah Turbeville: The Fashion Pictures* (2011).

Van Beirendonck, Walter, and Christian Lacroix, *Walter Van Beirendonck: Dream the World Awake* (2012).

Wilson, Mark, and Sue-an van der Zijpp, *Bernhard Willhelm and Jutta Kraus* (2010).

Photography Credits

Key to abbreviations: a=above; b=below; c=centre; l=left; r=right

2 Courtesy Studio Erwin Wurm; 4–5 Quentin Shih, *Hong Kong Moment* (no. 2, a project with Christian Dior), 2010, digital chromogenic print, 111.8 × 182.9 cm (44 × 72 in.), edition of 8; 9 Chad Buchanan/Getty Images; 10 Lord Snowdon, courtesy Acne Studios; 12a Quentin Shih, *Hong Kong Moment* (no. 8, a project with Christian Dior), 2010, digital chromogenic print, 111.8 × 182.9 cm (44 × 72 in.), edition of 8; 12b Copyright Azzedine Alaïa, photography Robert Kot/Groninger Museum; 13 Juergen Teller; 15 Courtesy Britain Creates, photo Matthew Hollow; 16 Peter Stigter; 17a Courtesy Studio Erwin Wurm; 17b Olaf Breuning; 19 Victor Boyko/Getty Images; 20 Courtesy Selfridges; 21a Geoff Ang; 21b Laurie Sermos, courtesy Prada; 23 Juergen Teller; 24 Lyn Balzer and Anthony Perkins; 26 Copyright Azzedine Alaïa, photo Robert Kot/Groninger Museum; 27a Lucas Dawson; 27b Alistair Wiper; 28 Amy Sussman/Getty Images; 31 François Guillot/AFP; 32–33 Karl Prouse/Catwalking; 34, 36–37, 38–39 Lucas Dawson; 41 Pierre Verdy/AFP; 42 Karl Prouse/Catwalking; 44, 45, 46–47 Marten de Leeuw/Groninger Museum; 49 Dominique Charriau/WireImage; 50–51 The Washington Post; 52, 53, 54, 55 Copyright Azzedine Alaïa, photo Robert Kot/Groninger Museum; 57 Heathcliff O'Malley/Catwalking; 58–59 Chris Moore/Catwalking; 60, 61, 62–63 Ronald Stoops; 64, 65, 66, 67 Jordan Graham; 69, 70–71 Elisabet Davids; 72–73 Uli Holz; 74 François Guillot/AFP; 77, 78, 79 Lyn Balzer and Anthony Perkins; 80a, b, 81 Adrian Mesko; 82 Alistair Wiper; 83 Shoji Fujii; 84–85 Alistair Wiper; 87, 88, 89 3Deep; 90, 92, 93 Peter Stigter; 94 Bec Parsons; 96 Courtesy Marni; 97 Olaf Breuning; 99 Courtesy Louis Vuitton; 100 Christophe Simon/AFP; 101a Courtesy Acne Studios; 101b Courtesy Christian Dior; 102–3 Courtesy Britain Creates, photo Gautier Deblonde; 105 Courtesy Britain Creates, photo Stephen White; 106–7 Steven Meisel, courtesy Prada; 108, 109, 110–11 Courtesy Acne Studios; 112, 113 Courtesy Christian Dior; 114–15 Olaf Breuning; 116, 117 Courtesy Bally; 118, 119 Courtesy Stella McCartney; 120 Copyright Tracey Emin, courtesy Longchamp; 122, 123 Stephane Muratet, courtesy Louis Vuitton; 124 Chris Moore/Catwalking; 126 Courtesy Louis Vuitton; 127 Angelo Pennetta; 128 Philippe Jumin; 131 Giuseppe Cacace/AFP; 132a, b, 134–35 Copyright Liam Gillick, courtesy Pringle of Scotland; 136, 137 Bec Parsons; 138a, b, 139 Six 6 Photography; 140–41 Copyright James Nares, courtesy Coach; 142, 143 Copyright Hugo Guinness, courtesy Coach; 144, 145, 146, 147 Courtesy Marni; 149, 150, 151 Courtesy Studio Erwin Wurm; 152 Sergio Pirrone, courtesy Prada; 154a Jerry Pigeon/Montreal Museum of Fine Arts; 154b Luc Boegly/Les Arts Décoratifs; 155 Copyright The Museum Metropolitan of Art, New York; 157 Marten de Leeuw/Groninger Museum; 158a Jerry Pigeon/Montreal Museum of Fine Arts; 158b Hyo Seok Kim; 159 Courtesy Calvin Klein Inc; 160–61, 162, 164–65 Copyright The Museum Metropolitan of Art; 166–67 Sergio Pirrone, courtesy Prada; 168, 169al, ar, b Luke Hayes/London Design Museum; 170–71, 172–73 Marten de Leeuw/Groninger Museum; 174, 176–77 Copyright The Museum at FIT; 179 Helen Oliver-Skuse; 180–81 Christian Markel; 182–83, 184 Courtesy Calvin Klein Inc; 185a, b Hyo Seok Kim; 186–87, 188–89, 190, 193, 194–95 Luc Boegly/Les Arts Décoratifs; 196 James Evans, courtesy Studio Elmgreen & Dragset; 198, 200, 201 Jerry Pigeon/Montreal Museum of Fine Arts; 202 Juergen Teller; 204 Cindy Sherman, *Untitled*, 2007/2008, colour photograph, frame 156.5 × 124.8 cm (61.625 × 49.125 in.), image 154.3 × 122.6 cm (60.75 × 48.25 in.), edition of 6, courtesy of the artist and Metro Pictures, New York; 205 Geoff Ang; 207 Quentin Shih, *A Chinese Woman with a Lady Dior Handbag* (a project with Christian Dior), 2011, digital chromogenic print, 111.8 × 111.8 cm (44 × 44 in.), edition of 8; 208, 209 Juergen Teller; 210–11 Bill Owens, courtesy *A Magazine Curated By Rodarte*; 214–15 Erik Madigan Heck, courtesy *A Magazine Curated By Giambattista Valli*; 216al, ar, c, b, 217 Original

photographs Lord Snowdon, published in *Snowdon Blue*, images courtesy Acne Studios; 219, 220–21 Daniel Askill, film stills from *Concrete Island*, 2010; 222–23 Inez van Lamsweerde and Vinoodh Matadin; 224, 226, 227 Juergen Teller; 228al, ar, b Liz Ham; 231 Cindy Sherman, *Untitled*, 2008, colour photograph, frame 198.8 × 150.2 cm (78.25 × 59.125 in.), image 196.5 × 148 cm (77.375 × 58.25 in.), edition of 6, courtesy of the artist and Metro Pictures, New York; 232–33 Cindy Sherman, *Untitled*, 2010/2012, colour photograph, image 203.2 × 356.2 cm (80 × 140 1/4 in.), frame 205.6 × 357.3 cm (80 15/16 × 140 11/16 in.), edition of 6, courtesy of the artist and Metro Pictures, New York; 234–35 Cindy Sherman, *Untitled*, 2010/2011, colour photograph, frame 206.2 × 351.3 cm (81 3/16 × 138 5/16 in.), image 202.6 × 347.7 cm (79 3/4 × 136 7/8 in.), edition of 6, courtesy of the artist and Metro Pictures, New York; 236a Quentin Shih, *Shanghai Dreamers* (no. 6; a project with Christian Dior), 2010, digital chromogenic print, 111.8 × 111.8 cm (44 × 44 in.), edition of 8 and 152.4 × 152.4 cm (60 × 60 in.), edition of 5; 236b Quentin Shih, *Shanghai Dreamers* (no. 7; a project with Christian Dior), 2010, digital chromogenic print, 111.8 × 111.8 cm (44 × 44 in.), edition of 8 and 152.4 × 152.4 cm (60 × 60 in.), edition of 5; 237 Quentin Shih, *Shanghai Dreamers* (no. 2; a project with Christian Dior), 2010, digital chromogenic print, (111.8 × 111.8 cm) 44 × 44 in., edition of 8 and 152.4 × 152.4 cm (60 × 60 in.), edition of 5; 238–39 Quentin Shih, *The Stranger in the Glass Box* (no. 17; a project with Christian Dior), 2008, digital chromogenic print, 111.8 × 190.5 cm (44 × 75 in.), edition of 8; 240–41 Quentin Shih, *Hong Kong Moment* (no. 1, a project with Christian Dior), 2010, digital chromogenic print, 111.8 × 182.9 cm (44 × 72 in.), edition of 8; 242, 243 David Armstrong, courtesy Scanlan & Theodore; 244–45 Deborah Turbeville; 246 Courtesy and copyright Ermenegildo Zegna and Lucy + Jorge Orta; 248a Courtesy Peter Fischli/David Weiss and Matthew Marks Gallery, New York, photo Roberto Marossi; 248b Courtesy Selfridges; 249 Courtesy Gucci; 250 Tom Sibley; 252 Courtesy Antonino Cardillo; 253a Alex Rodriguez, courtesy Prada; 253b Courtesy and copyright Ermenegildo Zegna and Lucy + Jorge Orta; 254–55, 256, 257 Courtesy Antonino Cardillo; 258 Peter Stigter; 259, 260–61 Ludger Paffrath; 263, 264–65 Stéphane Muratet; 266 Courtesy Louis Vuitton; 269 Gaye Gerard/Getty Images; 270 Universal Images Group; 271 Frederic Souloy/Getty Images; 272 Franco Rossi, courtesy Prada; 273 Floto & Warner, courtesy Prada; 274–75 Franco Rossi, courtesy Prada; 276al, ar, b Nacasa & Partners, courtesy Prada; 277al, ar, b OMA/AMO, courtesy Prada; 278–79 Courtesy Prada; 280, 281 Nacasa & Partners, courtesy Prada; 282, 283, 284, 285 Tom Sibley; 286, 287, 288–89, 290, 291 Courtesy Selfridges; 292–93 An exhibition of the Fondation d'entreprise Hermès presented at Third Floor, Singapore, image courtesy and copyright Shinji Ohmaki; 294, 295a, b, 296–97 Courtesy and copyright Ermenegildo Zegna and Lucy + Jorge Orta; 298–99 Andrew H. Walker/Getty Images; 300–1, 302a, b Courtesy Gucci; 303 Richard Bryant, courtesy Gucci; 304–305 Michael Elmgreen & Ingar Dragset, *Short Cut*, 2003, mixed media, Fiat Uno, camper trailer, 250 × 850 × 300 cm (98 7/16 × 334 10/16 × 118 1/8 in.), installation view at Ottagono, Galleria Vittorio Emanuele, Milano, commissioned and produced by Fondazione Nicola Trussardi, image courtesy Michael Elmgreen & Ingar Dragset and Galleria Massimo De Carlo, Milan, photo Ian Cumming; 306, 307 Peter Fischli/David Weiss, *Rat and Bear Costumes*, 1981–2004, costumes of the protagonists of the *Rat and Bear* films in Perspex cases, each 280 × 80 × 100 cm (110 1/4 × 31 1/2 × 39 3/8 in.), installation view at Palazzo Litta, Milano, produced and organized by Fondazione Nicola Trussardi in collaboration with Tate Modern, London, and Kunsthaus Zürich, image courtesy the artists and Matthew Marks Gallery, New York, photo Roberto Marossi.

Author Biographies
Acknowledgments

Author Biographies

Alison Kubler is a freelance curator and writer. She has a bachelors degree in Art History from the University of Queensland, Australia, and a masters in Post-war and Contemporary Art History from the University of Manchester, UK. She has worked for nearly twenty years as a curator in museums and galleries in Australia, and writes for leading art journals and magazines. She is currently associate curator of the University of Queensland Art Museum, where her projects have included the exhibitions 'Polly Borland: Everything I want to be when I grow up' (2012) 'The 2011 National Artists Self Portrait Prize', 'the more you ignore me, the closer I get' (2009) and 'Neo Goth: Back In Black' (2008). Other projects include 'Our Place in the Pacific: Recent Work by Adam Cullen', 'Moving Cities' at the Australian Embassy, Berlin, in 2000 and 'Quiet Collision: Current Practice/Australian Style' at Viafarini and CareOf contemporary art spaces in Milan. She also previously worked as arts adviser to Senator George Brandis, SC, the former Australian Federal Minister for the Arts and Sport. Alison is a co-director of mc/k art consulting, working on public art commissions, curatorial projects and publishing, and is a board director of the Museum of Brisbane. She is married to artist Michael Zavros, and together they have three children, Phoebe, Olympia and Leo.

Mitchell Oakley Smith is a freelance writer and editor. He is the author of *Fashion: Australian & New Zealand Designers* (2010) and *Interiors: Australia & New Zealand* (2011), both published by Thames & Hudson. He has held senior roles at Australian *GQ* and *GQ Style*, and has written for *Architectural Digest, Art Monthly, Belle, Harper's Bazaar, Monument, The Australian, Wish* and *Vogue Living*. He currently edits and publishes the quarterly men's fashion journal *Manuscript*. He appeared in the National Gallery of Victoria's 'ManStyle' exhibition (2011) and regularly judges the Australian Textile Institute National Student Design Awards.

Acknowledgments

The authors would like to thank the following people for their continued support and encouragement: Jolyon Mason, Nichole Walkling, Kate Venman, Michael Zavros, Lindsay Kubler, and Phoebe, Olympia and Leo Zavros.

Index

Art/Fashion in the 21st Century
© 2013 Thames & Hudson Ltd, London

Designed by Bianca Wendt Studio

First published in 2013 in hardcover in the United States
of America by Thames & Hudson Inc., 500 Fifth Avenue,
New York, New York 10110

thamesandhudsonusa.com

Library of Congress Catalog Card Number 2013932058

ISBN 978-0-500-23909-4

Printed and bound in China by C&C Offset Printing Co. Ltd

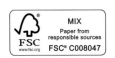